# Conflict and Catastrophe Medicine: A Practical Guide

Springer
London
Berlin
Heidelberg
New York
Barcelona
Hong Kong
Milan
Paris
Singapore
Tokyo

# Conflict and Catastrophe Medicine
## A Practical Guide

*Edited by*
James Ryan, Peter F. Mahoney, Ian Greaves and
Gavin Bowyer (Eds)

*Project Co-ordinator*
Cara Macnab

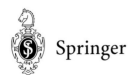 Springer

James Ryan, MB, BCh, BAO, MCh, FRCS, DMCC, FFAEM (Hon)
Leonard Cheshire Professor
Leonard Cheshire Centre of Conflict Recovery
Royal Free and University College Medical School
Academic Division of Surgical Specialties
4 Taviton Street, London WC1H 0BT

Peter F. Mahoney, TD, M Sc, FRCA, FFARCSI, FIMC, RCS (Edin), DMCC
Honorary Senior Lecturer
Leonard Cheshire Centre of Conflict Recovery
Royal Free and University College Medical School
Academic Division of Surgical Specialties
4 Taviton Street, London WC1H 0BT

Ian Greaves, MB, ChB, MRCP (UK), DMCC, DipIMCRCS (Ed)
Honorary Senior Lecturer
Leonard Cheshire Centre of Conflict Recovery
Royal Free and University College Medical School
Academic Division of Surgical Specialties
4 Taviton Street, London WC1H 0BT

Gavin Bowyer, MB, BCh, MChir, FRCS(Orth)
Consultant in Orthopaedic and Trauma Surgery
Trauma and Orthopaedic Directorate
Southampton General Hospital
Directorate of Orthopaedics
Trenoma Road, Southampton SO16 6YD

British Library Cataloguing in Publication Data
Conflict and catastrophe medicine: a practical guide
1. Disaster medicine
I. Ryan, James M., FRCS
616′.025
ISBN 1852333472

Library of Congress Cataloging-in-Publication Data
Conflict and catastrophe medicine: a practical guide
1. Disaster medicine
I. Ryan, James M., FRCS
616′.025
ISBN 1852333480

ISBN 1-85233-347-2 Springer-Verlag London Berlin Heidelberg
a member of BertelsmannSpringer Science+Business Media GmbH
http://www.springer.co.uk

Typeset by EXPO Holdings, Kuala Lumpur, Malaysia
Printed and bound at Kyodo Ptg (S'Pore) Pte Ltd, Singapore 628599
28/3830-54321 Printed on acid-free paper SPIN 10930021

*This work is dedicated to*
*Sir Patrick Walker KCB and*
*Commander David Childs RN (Rtd)*

# Foreword

The decision to produce this work sprang from the problems, some painful, experienced during projects by the staff and volunteers of the Leonard Cheshire Centre of Conflict Recovery in University College London. I shared with them the process of learning from their work in Azerbaijan, Kosovo, Bosnia and Namibia. We soon realised that a concise but comprehensive guide to the organisation of projects was needed.

The first important lesson we learnt was that a medical guide would not be enough; the book had to cover all aspects of operating in areas suffering the aftermath of natural and man-caused disasters. It therefore starts with a brief description of the disasters and conflicts which the world faces. Recent experience suggests that there is unlikely to be any improvement; there will always be disasters.

The first two sections are designed to assist individuals, especially junior health professionals, and organisations to decide whether to become involved in projects; to highlight the preparations needed before going to the area of a project; and to emphasise the approach required when working with people from very diverse social, political and cultural backgrounds. It then moves on to the medical factors and problems of working in post-disaster situations.

The immediate aim of post-disaster projects is to provide relief and help to the people suffering the effects of disasters. The longer-term aim must be to re-establish local medical and relief services. It is also important for an organisation taking on a project to plan how to withdraw in a way that will enable the local authorities to assume responsibility for the project and that will not adversely affect the standing of the organisation and its staff.

The editors of this book, under the lead of Jim Ryan, the Leonard Cheshire Centre Professor, who has been involved from the beginning, have been able to call on the great experience of the contributors. It is hoped that its concise style will enable it to be a valuable ready reference for all interested in becoming involved in the immensely worthwhile work of helping those suffering the after effects of disasters.

*Sir Patrick Walker, KCB*

# Preface

This work is intended as an *entry-level* text aimed at medical, nursing and paramedical staff undertaking work in a hostile environment.

It covers aid across a spectrum of hostile environments encompassing natural disasters, man-made disasters and conflict in all its forms, and extending to cover remote areas and austere industrial settings. The common thread in these situations is an increased risk of injury or death, which extends to both the local population and the expatriate workers.

Providing care in these environments needs an understanding of the situation, and how this constricts and limits what can be achieved. This understanding bridges the fields of medicine, politics, economics, history and international relations.

Many humanitarian and equivalent organisations have long recognised the difficulties which can be experienced, and run a wide variety of courses, workshops and exercises to broaden the skill and knowledge of the worker.

We hope this work will help in these endeavours, and provide a link to the more specialist texts and training available.

It should give the prospective volunteer a feel for the depth and breath of the subject, and make volunteers realise the importance of external factors which impact upon medical care. It should also heighten their respect and understanding of other professionals in the field, such as engineers and logisticians.

Finally, this work should educate and inform those who now, or in the future, volunteer to deploy into an environment of conflict or austerity.

*Jim Ryan*
*Peter F. Mahoney*
*Ian Greaves*
*Gavin Bowyer*

# Contents

## SECTION THREE
## Planning, Related Issues and Clinical Care

## SECTION FOUR
## Aftermath

## SECTION FIVE
## Resources

## SECTION SIX
## And Finally

---

*Cover Photos*

1. Difficulties of caring for some one in setting of the refugee camp: Azeri mother caring for a child who has undergone orthopaedic surgery
2. Poster from the conflict in Sarajevo
3. Child's drawing of everyday life during the Bosnian conflict
4. Ministry of Defense helicopter with a team off-loading a patient in training session

*Back Cover:* sign warning of mine danger in conflict zones

# Contributors

Mr Scott A Adams
Major RAMC
MDHU Derriford
Derriford Hospital
Plymouth, PL1 2LB
Devon
UK

D Rachel Aspögard
Freelance writer and journalist
Junohällsvägen 14A
S-11264 Storra Essingen
Stockholm
Sweden

Dr Peter J Baxter
Consultant Physician
Department of Public Health and Primary
  Care
Institute of Public Health
University of Cambridge
Forvie Site
Robinson Way
Cambridge, CB2 2SR
UK

Mr John P Beavis
Senior Lecturer
Consultant Orthopaedic and Trauma
  Surgeon
Leonard Cheshire Centre of Conflict
  Recovery
Royal Free and University College Medical
  School
Academic Division of Surgical Specialties
4 Taviton Street
London, WC1H 0BT
UK

Col C J Blunden
Commanding Officer
7 Medical Battalion Group
South African Military Health Service
Private Bag X1010
Lyttleton, 0140
South Africa

Dr Gavin Bowyer
Consultant in Orthopaedic Surgery
Trauma & Orthopaedic Directorate
Southampton General Hospital
Directorate of Orthopaedics
Trenoma Road
Southampton, SO16 6YD
UK

Mr Adam J Brooks
Specialist Registrar in General Surgery
Queens Medical Centre
University Hospital
Nottingham, NG7 2UH
UK

Mr Eddie J Chaloner
Senior Lecturer in Surgery
Leonard Cheshire Centre of Conflict Recovery
Royal Free and University College Medical
  School
Academic Division of Surgical Specialties
4 Taviton Street
London, WC1H 0BT
UK

Mr David J Childs
World Memorial Fund for Disaster Relief
Waterfall Cottage
Chicksgrove
Tisbury
Wiltshire, SP3 6NA
UK

**Dr A Christodoulides**
Senior Specialist in Accident and Emergency
Larnaca General Hospital
Cyprus

**Mr Charles Cox**
Consultant Obstetrician and Gynaecologist
Women's Hospital
New Cross Hospital
Wolverhampton, WV10 0QP
UK

**Dr Roger J Diggle**
Chief Medical Officer
King Edward VII Memorial Hospital
Stanley
Falkland Islands

**Mr Jonathan R A Duckett**
Consultant Gynaecologist
Medway Maritime Hospital
Windmill Road
Gillingham, ME7 5NY
UK

**Mr Peter V Dyer**
Consultant Maxillofacial Surgeon
Maxillofacial Unit
Royal Lancaster Infirmary
Ashton Road
Lancaster LA1 4RP
UK

**Mr Matthew Fleggson**
Coordinator
Overseas Programmes
Leonard Cheshire Centre of Conflict Recovery
Royal Free and University College Medical
School
Academic Division of Surgical Specialties
4 Taviton Street
London, WC1H 0BT
UK

**Mr M Gavalas**
Emergency Medicine Consultant
A & E Department
University College Hospital
Cecil Flemming Building
Grafton Way
London, NC1E 6AY
UK

**Mr Iain C Grant**
Consultant
British Antarctic Survey Medical Unit
Accident and Emergency Department
Derriford Hospital
Plymouth, PL6 8DH
Devon
UK

**Dr Ian Greaves**
Leonard Cheshire Centre of Conflict Recovery
Royal Free and University College Medical
School
Academic Division of Surgical Specialties
4 Taviton Street
London, WC1H 0BT
UK

**Mr Jeffrey Green**
Chairman
Asset Security Managers Ltd.
East India House
109-117 Middlesex Street
London, E1 7JF
UK

**Colonel Alan Hawley, OBE**
Chief of Staff
Army Medical Directorate
Keogh Barracks
Ash Vale
Aldershot
Hampshire, GU12 5RR
UK

**Major Peter F Hill**
Specialist Registrar
Trauma and Orthopaedics
Royal Defence Medical College
Fort Blockhouse
Gosport
Hampshire, PO12 2AB
UK

**Mrs N K Jyothi**
Consultant Obstetrician and
Gynaecologist
Warwick Hospital
Lakin Road
Warwick, CV34 5BW
UK

Mrs Caroline Kennedy
Journalist, author
31 North End House
Fitzjames Avenue
London, W14 0RT
UK

Dr Craig H. Llewellyn
Department of Military and Emergency
  Medicine
Uniformed University of the Health Sciences
Bethesda, Maryland
USA

Professor John Lumley
Department of Surgery
5th Floor, King George V. Block
St. Bartholomew's Hospital
West Smithfield
London, EC1A 7BE
UK

Dr Campbell MacFarlane
Head of Emergency Medical Services
  Training
Gauteng Provincial Government
Gauteng Department of Health
Emergency Medical Services
P.O. Box 8311
Halfway House
Johannesburg, 1685
South Africa

Ms Cara Macnab
Research Fellow
Leonard Cheshire Centre of Conflict Recovery
Royal Free and University College Medical
  School
Academic Division of Surgical Specialties
4 Taviton Street
London, WC1H 0BT
UK

Dr Peter Francis Mahoney
Honorary Senior Lecturer
Leonard Cheshire Centre of Conflict Recovery
Royal Free and University College Medical
  School
Academic Division of Surgical Specialties
4 Taviton Street
London, WC1H 0BT
UK

Mr Stephen J Mannion
Orthopaedic Consultant and Senior Lecturer
Lilongwe Central Hospital
and Malawi Against Physical Disability
PO Box 30333
Lilongwe 3
Malawi

Dr Bob Mark
Medical Advisor
Frontier Medical Services
Rank Xerox Business Park
Mitchledean
Gloucestershire GL17 0DD
UK

Miss A M McGuinness
Consultant in A & E Medicine
A & E Directorate
University College Hospital
Cecil Flemming Building
Grafton Way
London, WC1E 6AU
UK

Dr David J Morgan-Jones, MBE
Chief Instructor
Defence Medical Services
Training Centre
Keogh Barracks
Ash Vale
Aldershot, GU12 5RG
Hampshire
UK

Dr John F Navein
Consultant in Clinical Telemedicine
164 Banbury Road
Stratford upon Avon
Warwickshire, SV37 7HU
UK

Dr S Nazeer
GP Principal
Consultant in Primary Care in A & E
Clinical Assistant in Paediatrics
A & E
University College Hospital
Cecil Flemming Building
Grafton Way
London, WC1E 6AU
UK

Mr Simon J. O'Neill
Commercial Director
Unit 3
42 Worminghall Road
Ickford
Buckinghamshire, HP18 9JD
UK

Ian P Palmer, RAMC
Lt. Colonel
Tri-service Professor of Defence Psychiatry
Royal Defence Medical College
Fort Blockhouse
Gosport
Hampshire, PO12 2AB
UK

Professor A D Redmond
Emeritus Professor of Emergency Medicine
Keele University
UK

Professor James M Ryan
Leonard Cheshire Centre of Conflict Recovery
Royal Free and University College Medical School
Academic Division of Surgical Specialties
4 Taviton Street
London, WC1H 0BT
UK

Dr A J Thomas
Specialist Registrar in A & E Medicine
A & E Directorate
University College Hospital
Cecil Flemming Building
Grafton Way
London, WC1E 6AU
UK

Dr Claire S Walford
Consultant Primary Care / A&E
University College London Hospitals NHS
   Trust
A&E Department
Grafton Way
London, WC1E 6AU
UK

Sir Patrick Walker KCB
Lately Chairman Leonard Cheshire
   International and Chairman Leonard
   Cheshire Centre UCL
Leonard Cheshire
22 Millbank
London SW1P 4QD
UK

Dr Paul R Wood
Consultant Anaesthetist
University Hospital Birmingham
   NHS Trust
PO Box 881
Selly Oak Hospital
Raddlebarn Road
Birmingham, B29 6JD
UK

Dr Jane N Zuckerman
Senior Lecturer & Honorary Consultant
Academic Centre for Travel Medicine and
   Vaccines
Royal Free & University College Medical
   School
Rowland Hill Street
London, NW3 2PF
UK

# Medical Intervention and the World We Live In

# 1. The World in the New Millennium – Globalisation and Humanitarianism

Jim Ryan and John Lumley

**Objectives**

- To describe, in brief, the concept of humanitarianism.
- To introduce the concepts of globalisation and disintegration.
- To describe the failed state and its significance to the aid worker.
- To suggest means of staying safe in these new environments.

## Introduction

Confucius's phrase "May you live in interesting times" can be interpreted equally as a blessing or a curse. When directed at a prospective humanitarian aid volunteer, eager to embark on an overseas mission in the new millennium, the phrase leans more towards the latter. This may be an unexpected introduction to a manual directed at future volunteers, but this view is becoming widespread and bears dispassionate scrutiny.

We do live in interesting times, largely because of the radical restructuring of the world political scene that came about in the last quarter of the twentieth century. Humanitarian volunteers are already feeling the impact of these changes. To understand the current situation it is useful to look back at a number of historical watersheds.

In 1648, the Treaty of Westphalia was signed, which ended the Thirty Years War and the power of the Papacy. The *sovereign, independent state* as a discrete entity was born, and this ushered in a period of relative enlightenment, interspersed with wars. These new states embarked on a series of interactions, often resulting in *treaties* concerning such varied activities as trade, commerce and the conduct of war. This included the treatment of prisoners of war, wounded soldiers and non-combatant civilians. These attempts at reducing the appalling consequences of wars culminated in the next major watershed in affairs between states – the establishment of the International Committee of the Red Cross.

In June 1859, the battle of Solferino took place, which resulted in the usual mass slaughter on both sides and the abandonment of the wounded where they fell. The majority would die alone and untreated. A Swiss National, Henri Dunant, witnessed this battle and was so moved by the plight of the wounded that he organised care for them. In 1862, he published "*A memory of Solferino*", which recounted these events. Dunant then set in motion initiatives which resulted in the creation of the *International Committee for Relief to Wounded Soldiers*. As its flag, it adopted the distinctive Red Cross on a white background. The following year, members drawn from 16 states drew up the first Geneva Convention for *The Amelioration of the Condition of the Wounded in Armies in the Field*. In 1880, the name was changed to the International Committee of the Red Cross (*See also Ch. 7A*).

Thus was ushered in a period where the rights of wounded and captured soldiers, civilians and medical aid personnel were enshrined in a variety of treaties and memoranda of understanding. Humanitarian aid organisations, including international governmental organisations (IGOs) and non-governmental organisations (NGOs) concerned with caring for the victims of war and disasters, proliferated, particularly in the latter half of the twentieth century. In 1909 there were 37 IGOs and 176 NGOs. In 1997 these numbers had risen to 260 IGOs and a staggering 5,472 NGOs. Two reasons can be given for the increase in IGOs and NGOs – the ever-increasing demand for their services and their freedom to work in a climate of relative safety. The reasons for this climate of safety are worth noting. Within most nation states, even when at war, there was recognition of the institutions of law and order, and of the laws of war. In addition, there were codes of ethics and morality governing the activities of non-combatants and combatants alike. Although there were notable exceptions, these understandings pertained in most instances.

# Globalisation and Disintegration

As the new millennium begins the world political scene is changing – a change that began in the latter half of the last century. Far from looking to a future of certainty and an end to conflict, the world in the new millennium seems confused. Two distinctive processes can be identified – globalisation and disintegration – resulting in a troubling paradox.

## Globalisation

The nature of sovereign independent states is undergoing radical change. States are drawing together over a range of activities including trade, communications and defence. National economies are moving towards integration, and increasing political integration seems inevitable (witness the extent and speed of change within the European Union over the last 25 years). These moves have resulted in a global market which is changing for ever the way the world functions. This, in a word, is globalisation. In 1977, the General Secretary of the United Nations, Koffi Annan, stated that "Globalisation is a source of new challenges for humanity. Only a global organisation is capable of meeting global challengesWhen we act together, we are stronger and less vulnerable to individual calamity." It is not just the desire of individual states for closer integration that is driving the trend. New hierarchies, the IGOs, are wielding power and influence. World affairs are increasingly influenced, if not controlled, by IGOs such as the United Nations (UN), the World Trade Organisation (WTO) and the North Atlantic Treaty Organisation (NATO). Transnational regional organisations also exert influence – notably the European Union and the Organisation of African Unity. Although these organisations are composed of sovereign nation states, the power and influence of the individual states is often subsumed. These networks of international interdependence are concerned with a growing range of global issues. The more important are:

- defence and disarmament;
- trade and economic development;
- communication and information dissemination;
- humanitarian aid and development;
- human rights;
- health and education;
- the environment;
- refugees and internally displaced people (IDPs).

What is clear is that the power of states to act independently is being progressively eroded as the trend towards globalisation develops. While the benefits are enormous, problems lie in the resulting inequality between states and groups of states. Already a backlash is evident.

## Disintegration and Backlash

In opposition to moves by many major states towards integration and an acceptance of cultural diversity, other states and groups within states are resisting. The result is widespread instability with increasing threats to world and local peace. This backlash is occurring now and is gathering pace. Destructive and disintegrative trends are appearing in many parts of the globe. Globalisation and its dependence on commu-nication via the new information highway, the internet, favours the wealthier and more developed economies, leaving much of the less well-developed world, including Russia, trailing in its wake. There is an increasing view that territorial conquest by sovereign states is of less importance than economic dominance. This shift is occur-ring as the primary fault line in international affairs as conflict between communism and capitalism disappears. The change, often described as the end of the bi-polar distribution of power, has not resulted in stability or world peace. The rise of nation-alism, tribalism, transnational religious movements and racial/ethnic intolerance seems to defy the trend towards globalisation and a toleration of cultural diversity.

The backlash against globalisation is all the more worrying because of the prolif-eration of weapons, including weapons of mass destruction. The most powerful and lethal weapons are no longer controlled by great powers alone. With the collapse of the Warsaw Pact, vast quantities of small arms, explosives and a range of other weapons appeared on the international market at very low cost. Many of these weapons have fallen into the hands of terrorist, extreme nationalist and religious fundamentalist groups. Further, many smaller states have now developed nuclear weapons and the means to deliver them globally. Many of these states and groups are unstable and vehemently opposed to globalisation and integration.

Yet another factor must now be considered – the disintegration of states and the emergence of failed and failing states.

## The Failed State

The failure of Marxist–Leninist communism and the rise in nationalism has resulted in a convulsive and often violent disintegration of old alliances and power blocks. The collapse of the Soviet Union is the most obvious example, but there are others. Collapse, disintegration and armed conflict have occurred in the Balkans, the Caucasus, North and Central Africa and Asia. The result has been the emergence of dozens of new self-governing entities that have obtained, or are still seeking, recognition as sovereign independent states. United Nations membership statistics are illuminating. In 1991, the UN had 166 member states; in 1997, this number had increased to 185. Predictions for the future suggest a membership of up to 400; many of these will lack the means to survive independently without international assistance and will fail. The terms *failed state, failing state and defeated state* have now entered the literature of sociology, politics and journalism, although a consensus on their definitions has yet to be reached. They may be defined in terms of governmental mismanagement resulting in a loss of the loyalty of the population and leading to disintegration. Alternatively, they may be defined in terms of economic or political non-viability following the break-up of a larger state or union of states (parts of the former Yugoslavia are good examples). This definition fits many of the newly emerged states in Africa and Eastern Europe. The consequences of these entities for humanitarian volunteers are immense.

## Conflict in Failed States

Failed, failing and defeated states are characterised by conflict, which may be internal or external. Conflict from without may be the result of the new state breaking away from a larger entity. The larger entity may endeavour to ensure the new state's failure to survive by economic means or by direct military intervention. New or newly emerging states that have suffered in this way include Slovenia, Croatia, Bosnia, Kosovo, Chechnya and East Timor. Conflict from within may arise because of ethnic or religious divisions. Examples include Azerbaijan, Armenia and much of Central and West Africa. Some entities are affected by conflict from both without and within; Bosnia and Kosovo are examples.

These conflicts pose novel threats to the humanitarian volunteer. The climate of relative safety for humanitarian volunteers achieved in the late eighteenth century and much of the nineteenth is no longer to be taken for granted. The reasons for this are complex, and no single factor can be blamed. This is discussed in the closing section of this chapter.

## Natural Disasters

Thus far discussion has been confined to the impact of man-made conflicts and disasters. The next chapter discusses natural disasters in detail, but it is appropriate to consider them in relation to the foregoing discussion. Whereas the move towards globalisation has great attraction for the developed world, with state stability and growing economies, the move towards the disintegration of unstable and economically poor states, while undesirable, seems inevitable. These disintegrating states face a double jeopardy. In the last quarter of the twentieth century, natural disasters resulted in over three million deaths, and one billion people have been affected by their aftermath, with intolerable suffering and by the reversal of years of development. The World Bank, one of the key IGOs, estimates annual losses to be in the region of £23 billion, while the current annual mortality is in the region of 250,000 and is expected to rise. The escalating world population can only lead to a further deterioration in this situation, particularly as many of these people will be concentrated in zones which are prone to natural hazard. By the year 2100, 17 of the 23 cities estimated to have more than 10 million people will be in these areas. The double jeopardy arises from the fact that these are the very centres of population which face the greatest risk of disintegration and internal conflict.

## Humanitarian Volunteers at Risk

Deployment overseas on humanitarian missions has always been associated with risk, and workers have always known this – risk goes with the job. The humanitarian community have long accepted this fact and have coped with sporadic instances of death and serious injury. Historically these have been concerned with accidents or disease, and rarely has the humanitarian volunteer been deliberately targeted. There was a widespread belief that the flags and emblems of the humanitarian organisations provided shields for their volunteers. This is no longer the case.

The historical safety of the humanitarian volunteers and the non-combatant civilians was based on concepts developed within sovereign states, as already discussed. However, concepts such as neutrality, impartiality, human rights and the duties imposed by various Geneva Conventions assume a functioning state with its instruments of power (police and military forces, for example) intact and obeying the rules of national and international laws.

Within failed, failing or defeated states such institutions and codes of behaviour may cease to exist. This may also apply to states affected by natural disasters, at least for a time. Power or control may become vested in the hands of illegal bodies such as irregular militias, paramilitary groups or terrorists, often commanded by local warlords. Within failed states there may be a myriad of such groups engaged in conflict between themselves, but often forging short-lived alliances, making the climate even more dangerous and unpredictable for outside agencies. The particular tragedy of such conflicts is the deliberate targeting of civilians, including women, children and the elderly. In some cases, for example the aftermath of the fall of Vukovar in Croatia, this has extended to the slaughter of the ill and injured in hospitals. In past wars, the majority of the people killed or injured have been soldiers. The ratio has historically been 80% soldiers to 20% civilians. In modern wars and during conflicts in failed states this ratio has reversed as a matter of deliberate policy. It is salutary to note that between 1900 and 1987, about 130 million indigenous people were slaughtered by genocide within their own countries.

One of the features of conflicts within these states is an attempt to "purify" the regions ethnically by the enforced movement of populations perceived to be alien and posing a threat – this is the phenomenon of ethnic cleansing. On occasion this may extend to attempts at annihilation, the holocaust being an unsurpassed example. More recently, and on a smaller scale, the mass murder of refugees and IDPs has occurred in Rwanda, Bosnia, Kosovo and East Timor.

Humanitarian volunteers cannot remain immune. Non-state groups such as militias, or indeed state-sponsored organisations in the case of external conflict, increasingly find political advantage in targeting volunteers and their organisations. The aim has usually been to cause destabilisation. Aid organisations are also targeted because they may be seen to favour one faction over another. In Bosnia, Somalia, Sudan and Afghanistan this has led to the hijacking of food and medical aid convoys, and the kidnapping and beating of volunteers. At the time of writing, articles are appearing in international newspapers describing a climate of cold-blooded terrorism against aid volunteers. Volunteers working with the World Food Programme (WFP) are being targeted as they deliver food in refugee camps and many have been killed. WFP has the unenviable record of having lost more staff members to violence than any other UN agency. The statistics are grim – the UN has lost 184 civilians employees to violence between 1992 and 1999. In 1998, more civilian humanitarian aid workers died than armed and trained UN military peacekeepers. The risk extends to all humanitarian aid organisations. Volunteers working for the International Committee of the Red Cross, an organisation long considered immune, have been threatened and beaten in Africa and murdered in their beds in Chechnya.

## Staying Safe – the Way Ahead

With the close of the twentieth century, a paradox may be observed. On the one hand it was the most productive century in terms of social progress, education, health and wealth creation, while on the other hand it was the most destructive in the annals of human history. There were 250 wars and conflicts resulting in nearly 110 million deaths. These are grim statistics for humanitarian workers gazing into the crystal ball of the new millennium. One fact is clear – during this millennium, no aid worker should consider that donning a white uniform with an NGO emblem on the sleeve is a guarantee of safety. The opposite may be the case. What, then, are the implications for the humanitarian aid volunteer in the twenty-first century? To withdraw completely and ignore such conflicts is not an option – although many have suggested it. Highly motivated and skilled humanitarian volunteers have never been needed more urgently, and the numbers required will rise during the new millennium. Assuming that people will continue to volunteer, the question must be asked – how may they protect themselves and their colleagues? Should they be armed or work under the protection of armed groups? These are vexing questions and must be addressed. At last, the United Nations Security Council are debating these issues. Under discussion are initiatives to train future aid volunteers in techniques such as the anticipation of danger, recognition of mine fields, extraction from trouble at roadblocks, and ways to cope with kidnap, imprisonment and interrogation. Many of these difficult and contentious issues are debated in later chapters and sections of this manual. There are no easy or hard-and-fast answers, but preparation and training well in advance of deployment has never been more important. While other sections of this manual discuss personal preparation and training in detail, some of the more important aspects are emphasised here.

## Choosing an IGO or NGO

The proliferation of organisations engaged on humanitarian aid missions in areas of conflict and catastrophe has been noted. Many, if not the majority, of these organisations enjoy well-deserved reputations for their effectiveness. They take great care over the preparation of volunteers and look to their safety. However, there are numerous smaller organisations, which are often involved in single issues, that arise and then disappear. Volunteers should spend time checking the credentials of any IGO or NGO seeking their services. There are central clearing houses which hold extensive information on such organisations – notably the International Health Exchange. As a minimum, a volunteer should insist on the following information:

- Written details of the organisation, including annual reports and financial statements.
- Mission briefings, including clear aims and objectives.
- Political and security briefings.
- Details of local and international logistical support.
- The availability of health checks, including vaccination needs and disease prophylaxis.
- Medical insurance scheme, including repatriation.
- Mission-oriented training programmes and workshops.
- Provision of details concerning the mission end point and the return home.

In other words, volunteers should only work for organisations of good standing who prepare volunteers before deployment, transport them safely, house them adequately during deployment, give clear and achievable tasks, and then ensure their safe return.

## Personal Preparation

In a climate of increased danger, volunteers should examine their motivation and suitability. Physical and mental fitness are paramount. A history of cardiovascular, gastrointestinal or psychiatric illness should preclude deployment. This also applies to those on any form of long-term medication. If in doubt, seek expert advice (most reputable organisations demand rigorous heath checks); the exacerbation of a long-standing medical condition during deployment may have catastrophic consequences. A well-known aphorism states, "Do not become a casualty yourself and become a burden on already overburdened comrades". Personal preparation should extend to home and family. Consider "Will and bills". Check life assurance policies for their validity in conflict settings. Also consider the effects of deployments, particularly long and arduous ones, on family life. It is easy to forget that volunteers have to return home and pick up the threads of their personal and professional lives.

## Professional Preparation

Any volunteer must consider the professional task required during the mission and then question their ability to perform it. This extends beyond the individual's own ability and skills to include the means to carry out a task. It would be pointless to recruit and deploy a surgeon without an appropriate team and infrastructure in place, yet this has happened.

It is usually a requirement for volunteers to be multiskilled and adaptable in austere environments. At very least an individual should be capable of personal survival and should, for example, be able to prepare clean water and food, chose appropriate shelter, drive off-the-road vehicles and use a basic radio set. Many organisations would regard the above as a minimum set of skills over and above medical or related qualifications. Finally, if the volunteer is taking part in a basic or higher professional training programme, assurances must be sought that no time or professional penalty will be accrued because of the deployment.

# Conclusions

This is the uncertain future facing volunteers in 2001 and beyond. Yet taking part in a humanitarian aid deployment is an enriching experience and affords a unique opportunity to understand the plight of most of the world's population and to realise the good fortune of those living in stable and wealthy areas of the world. The prospect for future humanitarian volunteers is that they will *live in interesting times.* The authors of this chapter wish you all *bon voyage.*

# 2. The Spectrum of Conflict

Alan Hawley

<table>
<tr><td>**Objectives**</td><td>
<ul>
<li>To define conflict.</li>
<li>To describe the spectrum of conflict.</li>
<li>To indicate the changing nature of conflict.</li>
<li>To describe the impact of conflict on humanitarian assistance.</li>
</ul>
</td></tr>
</table>

## Introduction

From the beginning of recorded history, organised fighting between human groups has been a frequent occurrence. The genesis of this behaviour is a matter of debate; theories range from genetically driven to socially created. Regardless of this uncertainty, the fact of conflict is undeniable whilst its external manifestations vary. Patterns of conflict, purposes and end states have all varied through the thousands of years of human existence. There have been as many different organisations for conflict as there have been different human societies. Nor should this be a surprise, since the organisation of resources required to deliver violence is a social process which necessarily reflects the prevailing culture of the society from which it springs.

### The Changing Nature of Conflict

The nature of conflict has continuously evolved and changed, whilst reflecting some external factors and their interplay on each other. Hence, the available technology is a main driver. This has evolved from simple hand-held weapons (possibly derived from hunting tools) to stand-off precision munitions with satellite control systems. In the process, the actual physical component of conflict has altered. There has been an increasing depersonalisation of conflict as technology has allowed methods of killing at a distance to be utilised. Not that direct face-to-face violence has disappeared. There is a continuing tradition, and indeed a military requirement in certain circumstances, to close with the enemy and engage him in the most direct and intimate form of fighting.

However, for many armed forces this is not the preferred option since it gives free rein to the play of chance and fortune. Risk aversion has political attractions and requires the control, if not the elimination, of chance from the battlefield.

## The Essence of Conflict

Despite all the variations and evolutions witnessed throughout history, the essence of conflict remains the same; it is the defeat of one human group by another using the threat or actual delivery of organised and purposeful violence. By its nature, this involves injury and death. These are inevitable consequences of conflict. Indeed, they are more than this; they are the very currency of conflict. The rational intention of warring sides is to force the other to undertake a certain action. Violence is used to alter perceptions. Fundamentally, war is waged *in* men's minds *for* men's minds. It is this psychological basis which provides the key to understanding the utility and limits of conflict.

## The Nature of War

The essence of conflict is the actual or implied use of violence. This is also the fundamental nature of war, and so the relationship between the two becomes a matter of some significance. Is conflict the same as war? Are the words merely synonyms of each other? If not, what is the difference?

Conflict is the process of organised and purposeful violence of one human group against another. In the context of a consideration of war and conflict, violence is taken as actual physical action, although in different settings other forms of action, including verbal and emotional, may be appropriate. It can be seen that war can also be defined in the same terms as conflict. However, war has a forensic dimension with legal implications. Interestingly, there have been few declared wars since the Second World War. However, there have been hundreds of conflicts. Part of the solution to this conundrum is that *war implies an act by a sovereign nation state*, whilst many of the conflicts have been intra-state, or states have chosen not to engage in the formal process of a declaration of war. Clearly, there are contingent questions about legitimacy and authority in these deliberations. These can be complex and complicated and require a whole body of law to accommodate them. Nevertheless, there may be ramifications for all parties involved in a conflict or in immediately post-conflict operations. As a simple rule, war contains conflict and conflicts; the reverse does not apply.

## Massacre, Genocide and Criminal Behaviour

Recent experience has seen the continued play and existence of massacre and genocide on various violent stages throughout the world. Not only are these distinct from each other, they are also different from conflict and war. Whilst there is a linkage between them (it is difficult to conceive of genocide occurring without conflict), they are patently not the same concepts. All forms of criminal behaviour may become prevalent, especially crimes against the person. Rape has become a distressingly common feature of wars with an ethnic edge to them. Similarly, assault and murder are also more common in these circumstances. Massacre can be thought of as wanton or indiscriminate killing in large numbers. It may occur in conflict as the result of a temporary loss of control in the heat of battle or as a result of moral and disciplinary laxity. Sadly, there are many examples of this type of behaviour and they can be found in the annals of all armies. It seems that the rasp of war may sometimes fray the leash of civilisation a little too vigorously. Recognising this fact, additional moral limits have been applied by outlawing such conduct.

Genocide is a rather different matter. This is the deliberate use of violence to kill and eventually eliminate an entire racial, cultural or ethnic population. It is a perennial fact of human life that such campaigns have been frequent visitations on the species. They have clearly varied in effectiveness, but have not disappeared with the growth of literacy and assumed knowledge. Whilst the experience of the holocaust brought the issue of genocide to an appalled and shocked Europe, recent similar episodes in the Balkans, Rwanda and Cambodia serve as sad reminders of the tendency to genocide within the human condition. It is a tendency to be guarded against, and to this end, the developing structure of international and human rights legislation is welcome. For the purposes of this chapter, the concepts of conflict, war, massacre and genocide need to be borne in mind since they reflect recent practitioner experience. An insight into how the extent of philosophies of conflict and war has evolved is both a useful and necessary adjunct to understanding conditions in a post-conflict context. Without such comprehension, avoidable mistakes and errors will ensue, and in humanitarian operations such failings may cause distress and death.

## Traditions of War and Conflict

Attempts have been made throughout the history of conflict to make sense of it and to define its purpose. Given the significance and consequences of conflict, it is hardly surprising that effort has been invested in considerations of organised inter-group fighting. The risks are generally high and the results are unpredictable. In addition, there are real moral questions of the legitimacy of killing which require examination and analysis. In general, there are two such generic approaches to these ethical considerations: the absolutist and the pragmatic.

## The Absolutist Views of Warfare

There are two differing absolutist views of warfare, which can be viewed as polar opposites. The pacifist contention would suggest that no killing and violence can be justified and so it is wrong. Policies which incorporate the acceptance of conflict are ethically unacceptable. Such a view is clear and unambiguous. Conversely, the tradition of a Holy War also bases itself on absolute moral principles and legitimacy, but comes to a different conclusion. In this approach, the sanction, or even the command, of a deity is taken as the driving force behind the conflict. Further, the omnipotent nature of the deity is such that the norms of human intercourse can be overridden. In such a view, all manner of atrocities can be visited upon an opponent because of the support of the Supreme Being. Such support places the action beyond human sanction or consideration. Hence, morally absolute ethical positions, whilst having the advantages of clarity and simplicity, do not sit comfortably with the realities of compromise and negotiation which are the tools and instruments of international politics. Apart from noting that these two traditions exist and that they are mutually exclusive (pacifism defines an absolute moral duty not to fight), no further consideration of them will be made. Instead, the more general approach of pragmatism and politics will now be addressed.

## Moral Basis of Conflict

Difficult decisions about the moral basis of conflict have existed throughout history. A justification for shedding blood has been a necessary concomitant to declarations of war as well as other forms of fighting. Such concerns clearly spring from a need in many people to have a clear basis and purpose before committing themselves to the demanding process of fighting. Supplying that justification has been a main preoccupation of leaders before conflict is openly commenced. Throughout history, there have been a myriad such reasons, ranging from trade, hegemony, security and principle to sheer covetousness. What such a list also suggests is that conflict can be seen as a not unusual form of human intercourse with both ethical and political dimensions. The emergence of this tradition within the Western world began with the acceptance of Christianity by the Roman Empire. The early Christian movement was a pacifist organization, but the welcome accommodation with the temporal power of the Empire required some re-thinking of this issue. The eruption of barbarian threats and invasions gave added point to this development. Accordingly, Saint Augustine and others laid the foundations of the theory of a "Just War".

## Just War Theory

This approach attempts to set the context in which conflict and war are acceptable. Inevitably, such a philosophy requires there to be an acceptance of certain limitations. These limitations are applied in two separate but linked areas.

The first approach sets down criteria for the war itself. This is the "jus ad bellum", and lays down a set of conditions to be followed if a war is to be accorded the description of just.

1. There must be a just cause.
2. There must be a right intention; the stated reason for war is the crucial determinant, and ulterior motives are unacceptable.
3. The decision to go to war must be made by a legitimate authority.

4.  There must be a formal declaration of war.
5.  There must be a reasonable prospect of success; the evils of war must not be lightly entered upon.
6.  War must be used only as a last resort.
7.  The principle of proportionality must apply. This means that the good coming from the war must be of such significance as to outweigh the evils of the war itself.

Once war has been entered upon a different set of conditions apply; "jus in bello". These are used to codify and define the conduct of the conflict. These are essentially simple and linked concepts.

1.  Non-combatant immunity must be respected. Fighting must be directed against other combatants.
2.  Proportionality of means must also be used (as well as that of ends). The means adopted must not be such that the evils and harm inflicted outweigh any possible good to be achieved.

This corpus of philosophy has become ingrained in the norms of state conduct and personal ethos. It has provided the underpinning for much of the current body of international law in this area. It is now uncontentious and widely accepted. However, there are other strands in the philosophical foundations for war, and some of these substantially pre-date the Christian church. Many of them spring from China.

## Sun Tzu and the Art of War

The most well known of the oriental military philosophers is Sun Tzu. He was a Chinese warlord who lived about 600 BC. His life was spent in the hard pragmatic school of field soldiering. He accrued experience and expertise in warfare during a series of campaigns within China itself. Much of this knowledge was then recorded in a book, *The Art of War* [1], that has survived in part to contemporary times. In this book, a series of aphorisms and advice has been recorded. Whilst many of these are of limited relevance to the actual physical conditions of modern conflict, the underlying philosophical approach still has relevance. Indeed, much of it has provided the intellectual foundations for the manoeuvrist approach that has become enshrined in much contemporary Western military thinking. An important element of this philosophy is the requirement to match one's strength against an enemy's weakness. Sun Tzu enjoins his readers to avoid unnecessary bloodshed by avoiding matching strength against strength; it is the exploitation of weakness which is central to this doctrine. It also implicitly recognises the central significance of psychology in this process. The creation and exploitation of uncertainty in the mind of an enemy is the essence of Sun Tzu's doctrine. This is a lesson in applied psychology.

## Von Clausewitz on War

Whilst it is invidious to select just a few examples from 3,000 years of military experience, any such collection would always include the musings of Carl Von Clausewitz.

He was a Prussian officer who fought throughout the French Revolutionary and Napoleonic wars. His personal experience started at the age of 12 and extended to his death from cholera in 1832 aged 51. He never quite achieved the distinction as an operational commander which he craved. However, this frustration was sublimated into a deep consideration of war and its nature. This analysis formed the basis of his great seminal work *On War* [2], which has been studied and discussed endlessly since its posthumous publication. In this book, the actual form, purpose and character of war and conflict were examined and analysed. Von Clausewitz used the examples of conflicts that he had witnessed, and illustrated points by reference to recent historical events. He surmised that the purpose of war lay in seeking political advantage over an opponent. Indeed, he postulated that war was itself part of the process of political intercourse. As such, he recognised and gave voice to the realist position in politics and strategy; war was a process of cost –benefit analysis in the endless struggle between states. However, his own experience in battle and campaigns against the French convinced him that conflict has a dynamic of its own. It possesses a tendency to escalate from a limited form into the absolute. Nor should this be a surprise, since the actual physicality of combat means that chance and uncertainty have a major effect on the events of that conflict, and the process of bloodshed serves to harden and change perceptions. Such alterations in commitment and engagement require a dispassionate analysis of the political purpose and goals of the conflict to be continued. Von Clausewitz believed that this ultimate rationality should remain the duty of the government. Further, he felt that the state consisted of three elements: the government, the military and the people. There was a necessary interplay between them in order that the political benefits of the conflict could be achieved, and each component had its own specific part to play. A successful outcome could only be achieved if all elements did their duty within this relationship. Fundamentally, as an experienced practitioner of warfare, Von Clausewitz understood the psychology of conflict. He knew how to use the methods of applied psychology in the realm of uncertainty which was the battlefield. Highlighting this truth by an analogy with a wrestling match in which each opponent seeks to gain an advantage and eventually to secure victory by throwing the other, he explained the central essence of conflict. The exercise of maximum effort, chance and free will helps to guarantee a probability rather than a certainty. Nothing can be taken for granted, since there is a universal potential for disruption. This he described as friction due to the interplay on the battlefield of chance, fatigue and fear. Together, this combination ensured that human failure and frailty continued to affect the outcomes of conflict. Furthermore, Von Clausewitz memorably described the requirement for character in a commander by asserting that in strategy all things are simple, but not on that account necessarily easy. It is an admirable description of the reality facing a commander and his troops on the battlefield. Clarity and fortitude are basic requirements to meet the challenges of combat.

## Marx, Lenin and Political Conflict

For Prussia and Von Clausewitz, the security problem faced by the state was one of survival against stronger neighbours and no natural defensive positions or features.

In such a situation, the central organisation of the state so that all of its resources could be most efficiently deployed was of paramount importance. This set of geo-strategic realities led to a communitarian orientation of society, with the *rights of the individual being subordinated to the security of the whole*. It also coincided with the political instincts of revolutionary movements, especially those of Marx and Lenin [3].

The political nature and dimension of conflict dovetailed with their perception of revolutionary struggle. Accordingly, Von Clausewitz was embraced by the new schools of revolutionary thinking and enshrined in their philosophy of action. In particular, his understanding of applied psychology, the political nature of conflict and the relationships between the components of society were adopted. Implicitly accepted in this analysis was the communitarian view of society. This was the antithesis of the libertarian view, which placed the individual at the heart of society, and then placed rights and obligations around him in order to maximise personal liberties. Such a view was the predominant philosophy in the Atlantic maritime states with a global trading viewpoint and the geo-strategic security which that geographical position gave.

## Mao, Giap and Revolutionary Warfare

The revolutionary warfare concepts developed by Mao [4] and Giap [5] bore clear evidence of their genesis from Sun Tzu and Von Clausewitz. The essential political nature of conflict was derived from the latter, whilst attacking the enemy's weaknesses and subsequent exploitation of that vulnerability came from the Sun Tzu camp. Both Mao and Giap pioneered the struggle by a movement against a stronger government establishment. The importance of politics and the need to win men's minds were central to successful revolutionary warfare. The pursuit of these ends was to be ruthlessly maintained. Since the eventual result was to be a revolution, conventional means and methods were not necessarily to be used. Thus, the creed of *the end justifies the means* became enshrined in this revolutionary doctrine. Reprisals and violent acts against those identified as enemies of the revolution were to be routinely employed. Terror and intimidation were used alongside conciliation and reward. Such a heady mixture of outrage and selflessness bore fruit in a number of different campaigns. The retreat from empire in the post-war period saw many examples of this approach. It also witnessed some successful campaigns against revolutionary war, notably in Malaya and Dhofar. Such examples owed their effectiveness to the early recognition of the political process enshrined in revolutionary action, and the appropriate coordinated politico-military response. However, such successes were not easily won, since they required an investment in time and in military, financial and political resources. The conflict itself was often highly destructive and had many of the unpleasant features of civil war. Frequently, populations were the targets of direct military action, with the recognised effects of migration, disenfranchisement and poverty, as well as trauma in all its guises. Humanitarian aspects became increasingly significant.

Terrorism has been spawned from the ideas of revolutionary warfare and is the antithesis of humanity in conflict. Sadly, it is a commonplace problem in the contemporary world and is always a possible option open to opponents. It can be waged either nationally or internationally, with varying degrees of discrimination and violence. However, it is based on Mao's advice, "Kill one, frighten 1000". Once more, it can be seen that violence is being used to change and manage perceptions. The moral context may differ from that of conventional conflict, but the underlying purpose does not.

## Modern Military Philosophy

Modern military thinking is inevitably derived from historical, philosophical, cultural and technological imperatives. Essentially, its basis is the realist view of international relations in which the pursuit and promotion of the national interest in a competitive world is underpinned by the exercise of power. This approach implicitly depends upon an understanding of and commitment to the rationality of force; military power is cast in the Von Clausewitzian role of political action. For most developed nations, the likelihood of conflict is seen in terms of fighting against either comparable powers or less well-developed opponents. This division is usually referred to as *symmetric* and *asymmetric* warfare.

## Symmetric Warfare

Symmetric conflict occurs between two opponents who have similar capabilities. Furthermore, these capabilities are matched by similar commitments to targeting policies, limits of action and acceptability of risk. In many ways, symmetric conflict can be viewed as traditional warfare between approximately equal nation states. It is a quintessentially Von Clausewizian perspective. There is some degree of commonality in ends, ways and means between the competing sides. Thus, in modern times the Falklands Campaign and the repeated Indo-Pakistan conflicts are representative of this genre. There is an understood and usually implicit commitment to the common standards of acceptability. Within this overall commitment, both sides will seek to gain maximum advantage in order to prosecute their case most effectively. As Von Clausewitz emphasised, bloodless battle is a chimera; fighting means the expenditure of money, resources, sweat and blood. Nevertheless, symmetric warfare presupposes equivalence in capability and commitment.

## Asymmetric Warfare

On the other hand, asymmetric conflict reflects the divergence in ends, ways and means between two antagonists. Such a conflict highlights the fundamental asymmetry between both warring parties. Differences in targeting policies are frequently key areas of asymmetry. Thus, one side may adopt a more terrorist-like targeting approach, aiming to hit selected individuals by assassination or frighten whole populations by arbitrary acts of indiscriminate violence. Meanwhile, a whole raft of considerations (political, ethical and military) may restrain the other side to a more traditional engagement of opposing military forces only. Equally, substantial differences in available military power may be reflected in these opposing approaches.

Indeed, classic revolutionary warfare enjoins the insurgents not to match strength against strength. For the weaker force, attempting to match an adversary's strength with one's own is a recipe for military defeat. Instead, using one's strength against his weakness, along the lines of Sun Tzu, is a more profitable line of operation. A corollary of this is the concept of protracted struggle.

## Protracted Struggle

In order to circumvent the greater military strength of an opponent, the weaker party needs to avoid quick solutions and adopt a strategy to prolong the struggle. Such a philosophy would tie up increasing proportions of the enemy's resources and render it increasingly expensive in all dimensions, including casualties. For this strategy to become effective, time is required for the commitment to grow in terms of resources engaged, while the commitment in terms of political will declines in the face of burgeoning bills for finance, materials and manpower. This strategy was perfected by Mao and was termed a "protracted struggle". The strategy recognised the disparities in ways, means and ends in asymmetric warfare, and outlined the approach by which the militarily weaker party might eventually prevail. Time was the critical component. As an example of the successful waging of asymmetric warfare by a weaker side, the Vietnam War is a classic. In this conflict, the most powerful nation on the earth failed to subdue an insurgency from a small peasant-based economy. At heart was Giap's belief that the Vietnamese could maintain being killed for longer than the Americans could maintain killing them. The disproportion in casualties between the two sides underlines this contention (55,000 US troops, 1.3 million Vietnamese) [6]. In the end, the strength of political commitment to the cause was greater on the Communist side.

## Manoeuvrist Approach

The complexities of symmetric and asymmetric warfare may differ from each other in both kind and degree. However, they both share an understanding that it is the human mind that is the real battlespace. Conflict is the process by which perceptions may be changed; it is at heart a political process. The contexts may vary, but this essential truth is recognised by both streams of warfare. Equally, both approaches recognise an underlying doctrinal view known as the *manoeuvrist* approach. Basically, this approach is derived from an amalgam of historical and philosophical antecedents which have produced a military doctrine enshrining the importance of the psychological elements within it. In this philosophy, uncertainty is recognised as being unavoidably intermingled with conflict and the battlespace. The recognition of this central fact then allows the military to exploit it by seeking to reduce their own uncertainty, whilst accepting that an irreducible minimum exists, and simultaneously increase that of the enemy. Uncertainty can be most debilitating, especially to organisations that require detailed planning and coordination to deliver their capability as military forces.

Hence, the central significance of uncertainty to the applied psychology of the battlespace is enshrined in a series of training, organisational and equipment issues for most armed forces.

## Technocentric War

Military development is an iterative process of an intensely pragmatic nature tempered by intellectual rigour. Consequently, the future direction of military development in a climate of increasing resource constraint and increasing unit costs for personnel and equipment is a matter of much debate and consideration. This process has been loosely called a revolution in military affairs, and is an attempt to resolve the competing issues of the utility of the military, the contexts in which development and deployment might occur and the structure of future military organisations. Many of these questions are complex and opaque in nature. However, in accordance with Von Clausewitz's direction to use recent history for illumination, the significance of the Gulf War of 1991 has been central to this debate.

One school of thought which might accurately be described as technocentric suggests that the Gulf War is the first of the modern wars. In this view, conflict will be characterised by a reluctance to engage the enemy closely. Instead, stand-off weaponry will be used to reduce casualties. In addition, modern technology will allow an increasing precision of effect, so that the need to risk a close engagement, with all the uncertainties of casualty generation and loss of materials, will be avoided. Instead, the relatively risk-free, clean option of conflict at arm's length will be attainable. In order to achieve this, the importance of the air dimension is emphasised. Indeed, the only way in which this option can be maximally developed is by switching resources into the creation of capabilities delivered from air/space. Target acquisition, reconnaissance, surveillance and weapons deliveries are all to be effected from the air and aerial platforms. The importance of traditional military structures in armies and navies is then greatly reduced. Instead, the air element is emphasised. Such a view is profoundly challenging to many military orthodoxies.

## Van Creveld: An Alternative View

Equally challenging is the approach of Van Creveld, the eminent Israeli strategist and military writer. Whilst agreeing that the Gulf War has a central significance, his view is markedly different from the technocentric perspective. Far from being the first of the modern wars, Van Creveld argues that the Gulf War was the last of the old-style conflicts. At heart, his argument rests on the nature of political organisations in the future. The Gulf War model implicitly accepted the existence and relevance of the nation state with the interplay of the traditional three players: the government, the armed forces and the people. This is the trilogy as described by Von Clausewitz. However, political and economic realities are increasingly undermining the existence of the nation state, with many of them foregoing sovereignty for reasons of economic or security interests. In addition, the nature of conflict is becoming less inter-state and increasingly intra-state in nature. Thus, the usual pattern is for a state to suffer separatist tensions that evolve into political and military campaigns with potential overlays from terrorism, organised crime and interested outsiders, some of whom may be commercial organisations. This is a complicated welter of influences and ideologies to which the technocentric view of warfare has at best only limited applicability. Instead, the military requirement is for close engagement almost in a policing role with the ability to escalate up to full military action for particular objectives. Whilst the advantages of better surveillance and target acquisition capability which are central to the technocentric view would be useful in Van Creveld's picture of future conflict, technocentrism is irrelevant to the core question of the political problem. On the contrary, the importance and relevance of the traditional military organisations and structures are confirmed. Thus, these two views of future conflict set the parameters for the debate on the revolution in military affairs. Within these poles there is a range of views and beliefs which are part of a continuing and complex debate.

## Aspects of Conflict

The contemporary world is composed of a mixture of states in varying degrees of economic, political and military development. The passing of the Warsaw Pact and the decline of superpower rivalry have resulted in a patchwork of national tensions and rivalries across all the continents of the world. In many ways, the loss of the certainties associated with the superpower ideological struggle has made the globe a more dangerous place. Instead of the control exercised by the two superpowers over their respective satellite states, there is now no effective, extant, overarching control mechanism for international conflicts other than the United Nations (UN). Recent experiences in the Balkans, sub-Saharan Africa and Asia illustrate the problems that the UN faces in preventing and then engaging in these sorts of conflicts. As a consequence, a series of bloody conflicts has arisen and these have resulted in thousands of deaths, many of which have been in civilian populations. The spectacle of migrant populations and poorly targeted, if not indiscriminate, military action had become all too familiar a sight on the television screens of the world. Conflict has re-established itself as one of the prime drivers of population movement. Frequently, humanitarian disaster follows forced migration.

## The Changing Pattern of Conflict

The pattern of conflict has altered over the last 200 years. During this period, warfare has moved from being predominantly an inter-nation state affair (largely European and north American in extent), through three major world wars (the Napoleonic, and the First and Second World Wars), to the age of wars of national liberation (the retreat from empire by colonial powers). This process has seen a decreasing likelihood of developed nations waging war against each other. Instead, a pattern has emerged of war being waged between developed and developing nations or between two developing nations. Many of these are legacies of colonial political or economic affairs. In these conditions, symmetry and asymmetry apply to both sets of circumstances. In contrast, processes of negotiation, trade sanctions and compromise resolve disagreements between developed nations. Nevertheless, all nations remain vigilant about their own security and are reluctant to forego the means of guaranteeing it, and so the military option remains available.

## Failed States

Not infrequently, circumstances may change so that the actual viability, or even the existence, of a state is called into question. Prolonged civil strife, war or economic failure that is severe enough to threaten the fabric of a society may cause such conditions. In such a situation, the delicate balance between the needs of the individual and the requirements of the community is completely disrupted, causing the failure of normal social and economic relationships.

Hardship and destitution follow, with the young, the women and the elderly frequently being the most vulnerable. In such a society there may be reversion to gun law and a complete failure of social norms. Sadly, such examples abound in Africa (notably Rwanda, Somalia and Angola at various times). Regrettably, the problem of the failed state is likely to be a continuing challenge in the future. It presents a particular challenge for humanitarian involvement because of the complex of security, political, logistic, legal and ethical dilemmas that may ensue.

Conflict will almost always be a further complicating factor in the mixture, and its nature may vary from the symmetry of deployed military groups with the concomitant pattern of fighting to the vagaries of gun law and arbitrary violence.

## The Spectrum of Conflict

Attempts have been made to codify and simplify the pattern and nature of conflict. One of the best known is the spectrum of conflict depicted in Fig. 2.1. In this model there exists a gradual gradation of the level of conflict from assistance to the civil power up to full high-intensity warfare. Usually, this top end of the spectrum refers to the type of conflict seen during the 1991 Gulf War, using the full range of conventional weaponry in an integrated strategy within the battlespace. This type of warfare would ideally be waged at high tempo and continuously until the objectives had been attained. Such conflict demands the full synchronisation of air, land and maritime elements throughout all weathers and regardless of night or day.

Figure 2.1 also usefully illustrates the possibilities of escalation and de-escalation within a particular conflict. Indeed, there might simultaneously occur a range of conflicts within the same theatre of operations. Thus, high-intensity operations could be prosecuted in one sector whilst low-intensity conflict is being waged, all this being coterminous with humanitarian relief. It is a potentially complicated mixture that the model illustrates with some clarity.

An alternative model of conflict portrays the process as a continuous cycle varying between pre-conflict, conflict and post-conflict stages, as shown in Fig. 2.2

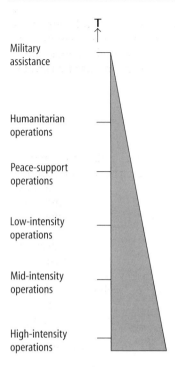

**Fig. 2.1.**  Spectrum of conflict.

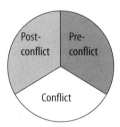

**Fig. 2.2.**  Cycle of conflict.

This view allows for the different stages of the conflict process to occur simultaneously, and demonstrates how they may meld from one to another. It is a useful construct since it gives some idea of the dynamism which conflict generates. It also indicates the element of confusion that always exists with conflict. The confusion is an aspect of Von Clausewitz's friction as well as being inseparable from the complexities of simultaneous operations. The concept of a cycle with ease of passage between the different stages of the continuum is extremely useful in conveying the operational and philosophical reality.

# Conclusions

Conflict has existed throughout recorded history. It has evolved to accommodate cultural, economic, political and technological aspects. As a result it is a multifaceted process with distinctive differences between peoples and countries. Whether it is the cause of instability or the product of it is a difficult question that would require a detailed case-by-case analysis. Probably, the truth lies somewhere between the extremes, with an acceptance that conflict may *exacerbate* instability but is more usually the *manifestation* of it. At any rate, it has become a perennial factor in the process of human relations.

## Humanitarian Law and the United Nations

There has been a slow change in both the acceptability and utility of conflict in the world. With the emergence of a body of humanitarian law ᴀnd the establishment of the UN, a vehicle for the analysis and expression of the rationale for conflict has been provided. Whilst in many quarters there is a deep cynicism about the value of the UN in conflict prevention and resolution, there is an undeniable requirement for states to justify a resort to arms in settlement of a dispute.

Even the most powerful states feel compelled to invest effort in public defence of their actions and if possible to seek UN support for such action. A significant example of exactly this process was the detailed negotiations and dealing that preceded the arrival of the British Task Force in the Falklands in 1982. Both the British and the Argentineans mobilised their supporters and the UN in support of their particular cause and actions. Similarly, the American-led coalition against Saddam Hussein in 1991 expended considerable effort to ensure UN support. These examples may be interpreted as an acceptance by states that there are legal, political and moral considerations in the choice of conflict to resolve differences between them.

## The Role of Law

The increased significance of the role of the law on the international stage is a recent development. The gradual evolution of a coherent body of humanitarian law is a major element in this success. However, compliance with the law is still patchy at best. Recent captures and successful prosecutions of war criminals by the War Crimes Tribunals are notable developments. Nevertheless, the process is still in its infancy and has a long way to go. Similarly, the attempts to outlaw war itself seem to be premature given the state of the world political stage and the lack of an enforcing mechanism. The trend is easily identifiable, but a successful imposition of a single international criminal code regulating inter-state relationships seems a far distant prospect.

In the interim, it is likely that conflict will continue to afflict mankind. This means that all the uncertainties, brutalities and vicissitudes of the battlespace will continue to be visited upon combatant and non-combatant alike. An understanding of why a particular conflict is being waged and its nature will remain invaluable to a successful humanitarian operation. Only if the essence of conflict is comprehended can maximally effective humanitarian assistance be applied. Shortcomings in this crucial comprehension can only worsen the prospects for humanitarian actions as well as the security of all involved. Knowledge is power in all fields of human endeavour. On the other hand, in the situation of conflict, ignorance may represent failure and even death rather than bliss.

# References

1. Gray CS Modern strategy. Oxford: Oxford University Press, 1999; 124–7.
2. Howard M, Paret P Carl Von Clausewitz – on war. Princeton: Princeton University Press, 1976; 3–58.
3. Neumann S, von Hagen M Engles and Marx on revolution, war and the army in society. In: Paret P, editor. Makers of modern strategy. Oxford: Oxford University Press, 1986; 262–80.
4. Mao Tse Tung. On guerrilla warfare. (Translated by Griffiths S) New York: Doubleday, 2000; 61–101.
5. Giap VN People's war people's army. Delhi: Natraj, 1974; 41–74.
6. Lomperis TJ From people's war to people's rule. Chapel Hill: University of North Carolina Press, 1996; 108–10.

# 3. Catastrophes – Natural and Man-Made Disasters

Peter J. Baxter

<table>
<tr><td>**Objectives**</td><td>• To define natural and man-made disasters.<br>• To introduce the concept of vulnerability.<br>• To indicate the scope and extent of the problem.<br>• To discuss the medical implications.</td></tr>
</table>

## Introduction

Natural disasters are a growing public health problem in the increasing number of events and the numbers of people affected. This chapter focuses on some of the background health issues behind this global trend as they apply to aid workers. Technological disasters differ in many important respects from natural disasters in their causes and health impacts, and their frequency is much lower as they are inherently preventable by engineers and government regulation. Avoiding technological disasters is more straightforward than mitigating natural hazards, but disaster workers should include both types of disaster in an all-hazards approach to planning and preparedness. Thus an earthquake may trigger the failure of a hazardous installation such as a nuclear reactor, or floodwaters may become contaminated with toxic materials. Man-made humanitarian emergencies from conflicts or political repression (*complex disasters*) may also be complicated by natural hazards, or responses to events such as floods in war zones can be inhibited by the threat of landmines.

## Natural Disasters

There is no completely satisfying definition of a disaster, but the following is probably the most useful for health-care providers [1].

> A *disaster is the result of a vast ecological breakdown in the relation between humans and their environment, a serious and sudden event (or slow, as in drought) on such a scale that the stricken community needs extraordinary efforts to cope with it, often with outside help or international aid.*

The important element in a disaster is a breakdown in society, which prevents the mounting of a planned response; i.e. the disorganisation of normal functioning to a point of chaos. In Britain we plan our response to major incidents, since disasters according to the above definition are very rare (we could say that the last disaster was the east coast flood in 1953, see below). Therefore, the response by the emergency services is essentially planned to be on a larger scale than, but not qualitatively different from, the most typical adverse events.

Deaths from natural disasters do not number amongst the world's top thirty causes of mortality, but they present a rising global trend that runs counter to falling premature mortality from most other causes. In the last half of the twentieth century about 250 great natural disasters hit the planet, killing at least 1.4 million people and disrupting the lives of many millions more. Ninety per cent of natural disasters and 96% of the deaths they cause occur in the developing world. The number of people affected by disasters every year is at least 130 million, and the number is rapidly climbing. Most of the losses have been from earthquakes, windstorms and floods (Fig. 3.1). Between 500 and 700 natural catastrophes are recorded every year, with the late 1980s and 1990s being marked by individual events with extremely large economic losses. Natural hazards are not discernibly becoming more frequent, but human populations, both in numbers and distribution, are spreading into more highly exposed regions and into larger urban settlements. In the last decade the human population grew by nearly another billion, mostly in the developing world, where millions of people who are desperate for work have moved into cities and crowded into substandard buildings in once-marginal land. About one billion people now live in unplanned shantytowns. These and other global trends, such as deforestation for maximising farmland or logging profits and other forms of environmental degradation, are thought by many to be increasing the vulnerability of human settlements to natural disasters.

Sudden-onset disasters (Tables 3.1 and 3.2) can be classified as being due to extreme weather events such as severe winds (hurricanes or tropical cyclones, tornadoes and temperate windstorms), geological events (earthquakes, volcanic erup-

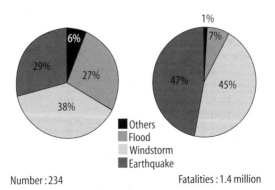

**Fig. 3.1.** Great natural catastrophes 1950–1999 (Source: Munich RE Group)

**Table 3.1.**  Environmental disasters

| Geophysical |
| --- |
| Earthquakes |
| Volcanoes |
| Weather-related |
| Hurricanes |
| Tornadoes |
| Floods |
| Drought |
| Technological |
| Air pollution |
| Chemical releases |
| Fires |
| Nuclear reactor incidents |

tions), geomorphic events (landslides, debris flows) or hydrological events (river and coastal floods, tsunamis). These categories can overlap, so a volcanic eruption may trigger a landslide which then crashes into the sea to produce a tsunami that floods the opposite shoreline and causes massive loss of life. Heavy rainfall from a tropical cyclone can lead to floods and landslides, the death tolls from which may far exceed those from the devastation caused by the high winds. Disaster from extraterrestrial impacts such as asteroids is not too remote: in 1908 a rocky asteroid exploded in Siberia, felling the forest over an area larger than Greater London. In contrast, famines, drought and desertification are subject to long-term processes, and may lead to migrations of populations with all the problems of dealing with large numbers of refugees. These disasters are seen today as not simply meteorological, or another instance of extreme weather, since their development also follows an array of social, economic and political responses to environmental perturbation. An extreme example of this was the largest famine in human history, which took place in China during 1959–1961, when some 30 million Chinese people starved to death. The deeper causes of this extraordinary catastrophe lay in Communist Party ideology that led to the abandonment of private food production and were only partly to do with drought [2].

The natural background rate of extreme weather events – heatwaves, droughts, floods, storms – and their severity can be disturbed by climatic perturbations. Most scientists now agree that the effect of anthropogenic influences on global temperature is becoming discernible, but there is less agreement on the future effects of this change over the next century on extreme weather events and where these are likely to occur. The Intergovernmental Panel on Climate Change – a multidisciplinary scientific body established by the United Nations – forecasts an increase in the average world temperature of 1.0–3.5°C over the next one hundred years. Global sea levels are likely to rise by 50 cm on average over the next century, but in some places the rises may be greater. Undoubtedly, a sea level rise would increase the frequency and severity of coastal flooding events, but other influences on severe windstorms and rainfall (floods and drought) in the future are less clear. Thus it has

**Table 3.2.**    Selected sudden-onset natural catastrophes in the twenty-first century (Source: Munich RE Group)

| Date | Event | Location | Approximate death toll |
|---|---|---|---|
| 8 Sep. 1900 | Hurricane | Galveston, USA | 6,000 |
| 18 Apr. 1906 | Earthquake | San Francisco, USA | 3,000 |
| 28 Dec. 1908 | Earthquake | Messina, Italy | 85,926 |
| 12 Jan. 1915 | Earthquake | Avezzano, Italy | 32,610 |
| 16 Dec. 1920 | Earthquake | Gansu, China | 235,000 |
| 1 Sep. 1923 | Earthquake | Yokohama, Japan | 142,800 |
| Jul.–Aug. 1931 | Flood | Yangtze Kiang, China | 140,000 |
| 30 May 1935 | Earthquake | Quetta, Pakistan | 35,000 |
| 10–22 Sep. 1938 | Hurricane | New England, USA | 600 |
| 25 Jan. 1939 | Earthquake | Concepción, Chile | 28,000 |
| 26 Dec. 1939 | Earthquake | Erzincan, Turkey | 32,740 |
| 16 Oct. 1942 | Cyclone | Bangladesh | 61,000 |
| 1 Feb. 1953 | Storm surge | The Netherlands; UK | 1,932 |
| Aug. 1954 | Flood | Dongting, China | 40,000 |
| 26–27 Sep. 1959 | Typhoon | Honsh, Japan | 5,100 |
| 29 Feb. 1960 | Earthquake | Agadir, Morocco | 12,000 |
| 7–12 Sep. 1965 | Hurricane Betsy | Florida, USA | 75 |
| 12 Jan. 1970 | Cyclone | Bangladesh | 300,000 |
| 31 May 1970 | Earthquake | Chimbote, Peru | 67,000 |
| 4 Feb. 1976 | Earthquake | Guatamala City, Guatamala | 22,084 |
| 27–28 Jul. 1976 | Earthquake | Tangshan, China | 290,000 |
| 19 Sep. 1985 | Earthquake | Mexico City, Mexico | 10,000 |
| 13–14 Nov. 1985 | Volcanic eruption | Armero, Columbia | 24,740 |
| 9–17 Sep. 1988 | Hurricane Gilbert | USA, Caribbean, Central America | 355 |
| 7 Dec. 1988 | Earthquake | Spitak, Armenia | 25,000 |
| 17 Oct. 1989 | Earthquake | USA (Loma Prikea) | 68 |
| 25 Jan.–1 Mar. 1990 | Winter storms | Western Europe | 230 |
| 29–30 Apr. 1991 | Storm surge, cyclone Gorky | Bangladesh | 139,000 |
| 26–28 Sep. 1991 | Typhoon Mireille | Kyushu, Japan | 62 |
| 23–27 Aug. 1992 | Hurricane Andrew | Florida, USA | 62 |
| 30 Sep. 1993 | Earthquake | Maharashtra, India | 9,475 |
| 17 Jan. 1994 | Earthquake | Northridge, CA, USA | 61 |
| 17 Jan. 1995 | Earthquake | Kobe, Japan | 6,348 |
| May–Sep. 1998 | Flood | Yangtse Kiang, China | 3,650 |
| 25 Oct.–8 Nov. 1998 | Hurricane Mitch | Honduras, Nicaragua | 9,200 |
| 17 Aug. 1999 | Earthquake | Izmit, Turkey | 17,000 |
| 20 Sep. 1999 | Earthquake | Taichung, Taiwan | 2,400 |
| 26 Nov. 1999 | Hurricane, storm surge | Orissa, India | 10,000 |

been suggested that a warming of the oceans would create the potential for more intense hurricanes, and widen the area of the world at risk. Impacts on agriculture and droughts could lead to famines that trigger large population movements and ensuing complex emergencies [3].

Climate cycles affecting the tropical Pacific Ocean and associated with El Nino and La Nina are now well-recognised phenomena. More recently, evidence has grown for their association with world-wide impacts on regional weather patterns and "cycles of disaster" that leave a trail of worldwide epidemics of disease, droughts, forest fires and floods in their wake [4]. Twenty-three El Ninos have affected the earth since the beginning of the century, and the four strongest have occurred since 1980; the last one waned by the end of 1998. On 24 September 1998, for the first time this century, four Atlantic hurricanes were active at once, which was consistent with the developing La Nina conditions. One of the four was Hurricane Mitch, which was one of the most destructive storms in the Western hemisphere for 200 years, killing at least 10,000 people in landslides and floods in Central America. Advances in forecasting El Nino events with adequate lead times may assist countries in disaster preparedness. How a warmer world as a result of climate change might influence these cycles is unknown.

## Vulnerability

Sudden-onset natural disasters strike with little, if any, warning and leave their impact over a short period of time. Survivors are left to pick up the pieces of their homes and communities and rebuild their lives. The return periods of disastrous events are most often many years, or even several generations, in any one place, even in disaster-prone countries, and human memory being short the circumstances leading to the catastrophe are highly likely to recur. Poverty is an important factor in this cycle of disaster, combined with a fatalism that little can be done to offset such unpredictable events. For a given type of event, the loss of life will typically be much greater in developing countries, but the economic losses may be much greater in richer countries when the damage to buildings and infrastructure and the disruption of business are considered. Even for an earthquake of the same magnitude striking two cities, the damage and loss of life may vary enormously depending upon the country in which such an event occurs. Thus, in 1993, an earthquake of magnitude 6.5 struck Maharashtra (India) killing 10,000 people, but a year later an earthquake of almost the same size hit North Ridge, California, and fewer than 60 people died, the difference being a reflection of the different building standards in the two countries.

What makes the difference is termed the *vulnerability* of the area, which is almost invariably higher in the developing world. This is founded on a cluster of political and socio-economic factors not at all dissimilar to those determinants which are responsible for public health inequalities in general and which provide similar scope for prevention. These include such measures (and examples) of social deprivation as poor housing (a key factor in earthquake risk), lack of education (awareness of risk and an understanding of science), being socially marginalised (unable to influence decision-makers), and unemployment (leading to a more fatalistic approach to risk in order to earn a living). Promoting health and protecting security are inseparable from these social, economic and political factors, and are inextricably linked with promoting and protecting human rights.

Many people see vulnerability as springing from a web of human actions, decisions and choices at different levels in society [5]. Disasters are not unpredictable, chance visitations by cruel nature or divine retribution raining on the just, the unjust and the innocent, but are essentially man-made. Vulnerability is the result of ignorance, a failure to educate, a lack of intervention or regulation by governments, or a global economic system that forces people to become marginalised. Living in ignorance in defective dwellings and in exposed areas, and destined by poverty to have limited choices, the vulnerable bear the brunt of natural disasters. Any solutions will attack the political and social causes of such vulnerability. However, there are examples of natural disasters where such evidence is not apparent. It is important to separate vulnerability in terms of determining what lessons can be learned to prevent loss in the future from the more futile exercise of apportioning blame (whether it is to the builders of defective buildings, scientists, the government or God).

## Vulnerability and Risk

In this age of low-cost international air travel, tourists or business travellers rarely worry about the risk of natural disasters when making their plans, although occasionally they can be caught out when their honeymoon in the Caribbean is wrecked by a hurricane, or they are unlucky enough to be in a resort during an earthquake. The chances of an inhabitant of even a high-risk area being killed in a natural disaster is very low compared with other life risks such as road traffic accidents and the general mortality from infectious and chronic diseases. You are indeed more likely to be struck down by a bus. However, the risk of a catastrophe occurring *somewhere* is increasing, both on a national and on a global scale. It is therefore in the interest of governments and *international government organisations* to do something about it, even though individuals may not see the situation in the same light. Unfortunately, in many developing countries government intervention to devise mitigation measures may be viewed with suspicion by populations hardened to natural risks, or more accustomed to political corruption.

Risk is a function of vulnerability: the probability of the occurrence of a hazardous natural event and the number or proportion of those exposed. Previously, when the role of vulnerability was not understood, it was supposed that risk was a combination of an event's characteristics and incidence in places where people were at risk. Accordingly, an accurate prediction of an extreme event coupled with a technological or engineering solution would be all that was needed to protect people and property successfully. This approach is the philosophy behind preventing technological disasters such as accidental nuclear and chemical releases. If it were that simple, losses would be falling as our technical capacity increased, but the reverse has happened. Only in recent years has it be shown that the scientific ability to forecast natural hazards and protect against them are far from being as straightforward as human hubris would lead us to believe.

Climatological, historical and geological records can put a limit on risk estimates by providing evidence of the *return periods* (recurrence rates) of earthquakes, hurricanes, floods, volcanic eruptions and other natural hazards. Thus the number of Atlantic hurricanes in a forthcoming season might be based on a historical average figure, but the drawback is that in any one year there may be wide variations depending on the many causal factors that apply. As we learn more and more about these influences, numerical weather forecasting models will become more sophisticated and predictions of the hurricane count should become more accurate; however, there is also a fundamental randomness or *uncertainty* that cannot be eliminated with any amount of improvements in knowledge of how hurricanes work. Statistical estimates of return periods for natural hazards should be viewed with an estimate of their uncertainty, and for various reasons should be applied with caution when advising decision makers on the interventions they should seek to make to protect populations. Of course, the statement that the Thames Barrier was built to protect London from flooding events so large that they occur only once in every thousand years refers to a constant probability, so although it appears remote, the event could occur in any one specific year (with probability of 0.001%) – perhaps the next one! Understanding and being able to interpret probabilities is not easy, and ultimately we cannot measure risk in the same way that we can take a temperature or record someone's weight.

Another aspect of risk is *lead-time*, or the time period between the first signs of a natural hazard developing and when it strikes. This may be days for a hurricane, hours for floods and minutes after a premonitory event for a volcanic eruption. In earthquakes there may be little time for warning at all. Clearly one of the goals of scientists is to continue to find ways to identify early signs of trouble so that adequate warning time can be given to the population to evacuate from, or protect themselves in, the area exposed to risk. Unfortunately, it is a fact of life that as the sensitivity of a method to detect a premonitory change increases, the potential for false-positive warning signals usually increases as well. The dilemma faced by authorities of when to heed a warning and advise a population can be the most difficult decision in disaster management, especially when major evacuations of large populations may be needed or the alternative is large loss of life.

## Limitations of Emergency Medical Aid

The world responds to disasters by sending relief teams and supplies to the stricken area, but for at least 25 years it has been recognised that the only way to reduce human losses significantly is by taking preventive measures *before* the disaster occurs. Medical teams invariably arrive too late to make much impact, since most deaths occur when the disaster strikes. Emergency surgical treatment for major trauma has to be performed within a "golden" hour or two if it is going to be effective, but in the chaos of a major event casualties cannot even be rescued in that time let alone be sent to a hospital which is functioning. Training a community in "frontline" measures such as first-aid as part of long-term community preparedness, so that survivors of an earthquake can extricate the injured and apply basic life-support measures, may save many more lives than any other form of post-disaster response. Thus Safar, who studied the 1980 earthquake in Italy, concluded that 25–50% of victims who were injured and died slowly could have been saved if life-saving first-aid had been administered immediately [6]. Relief teams of engineers and others who restore roads and bridges, and bring potable water, solid-waste management, food protection, vector control and sanitation to the disaster area play a vital part in preventing further loss of life (*See also Ch. 17*).

Nowadays, harrowing images of stricken people are flashed onto TV screens across the world soon after a disaster strikes, with commentators highlighting delays by national or international relief teams. What is not pointed out is that aid will almost always be too late to save most lives in sudden natural disasters.

Finding the evidence to support the value of mitigation will never be easy when it is difficult to show that an event has not occurred as a result of an intervention, and when the disaster situation is not conducive to well-controlled investigation. However, we do have the technology to radically reduce the impacts of disasters and it needs to be shown to be cost-effective – despite much hand-ringing over the economic losses in disasters these are not calculated consistently and loss estimates can vary widely [7]. Until a generally acceptable framework for loss estimation in disasters is used, the cost-effectiveness of hazard mitigation measures will always be difficult to demonstrate to a sceptical world, which is much more easily persuaded by TV pictures of relief teams picking out survivors from the rubble. It is also difficult, or even impossible, to fully measure the human losses in disasters in terms of short- and long-term morbidity and mortality, especially when the mental and social effects can last for many years.

## The Search for Solutions

### Applying Science and Technology

The case for technological warning systems, where they can be applied, is overwhelmingly and regularly demonstrated on the world's media. Every year in the Atlantic tropical cyclone season, meteorologists use a combination of radar, satellite and reconnaissance aircraft and screen images to predict the path of hurricanes heading towards the US coastline, thereby enabling people in their thousands to evacuate from the shorelines in time. New satellite-based technology is also emerging which allows the total rainfall to be estimated as well as the water flow in rivers, and thus forecasting floods will become more accurate. Hurricanes demonstrate the importance of *forecasts and warnings, together with evacuation measures*, and earthquakes show the need for *engineering measures*, to mitigate and/or prevent loss of life. Other key measures are *land-use planning* to prevent people living in exposed areas in the first place, and *community preparedness and planning*. The reality is that the world recognises the effectiveness of these mitigation measures but fails miserably to put them in place, so that disaster cycles recur. Even after a major earthquake, new buildings which are not seismic-resistant will be put up in the same area. This may be through ignorance, or because they are cheaper or because no one enforces the building codes. Settlements will be rebuilt in flood plains or on the flanks of destructive volcanoes, and the affluent will flock back to new houses on hurricane-prone shores. For individuals, this behaviour is not entirely irrational, as they perceive that over years, or decades or even longer the benefits outweigh the potential for loss, although it is sure to come eventually. This is especially true in a rich country like the United States, where insurance companies or government will provide compensation. However, in view of growing economic losses and bankrupt insurance companies that are the direct result of these behavioural strategies, support for future victims may be less forthcoming.

In 1999, a super cyclone struck the coast of eastern India, the worst the country had experienced in a century. At least 10,000 inhabitants of the state of Orissa were drowned by the surge that swept in from the coast, and over a million were made homeless. Although meteorologists watched the hurricane approach, inadequate warnings were given to the population by the authorities, who in any event were not sufficiently prepared to know what to do. This is another example of the failure to apply existing technology, and to incorporate it into community preparedness.

Forecasts and warnings are clearly applications of science that can make a huge difference, but despite much costly work, scientists are no nearer predicting when and where an earthquake can strike in a seismic fault zone. The next big earthquake on the San Andreas Fault in California, or in Tokyo, will be as sudden and without warning as in disasters in the past. Scientists will always be wary of using words such as *prediction* because, since its publication in the 1960s, chaos theory has opened up a natural world in which a situation can be both deterministic *and* unpredictable. Although numerical simulation models and statistics are still the main tools for assessing natural hazard risk, the closer we try to predict the natural world the less predictable it becomes. Unfortunately, misunderstanding these limitations of science can lead to the blame for a disaster being placed at the door of scientists. The public, if they understand science at all, may have illusions that mankind has some mythical mastery over life and death as well as control over the environment.

### The 1990s: The International Decade for Natural Disaster Reduction

When we start to study and analyse natural disasters we find that there are at least four distinct phases:

- the pre-impact phase, or the time for alarm and warning;
- the impact phase when the disaster strikes;
- the relief phase when assistance from outside starts to reach the disaster area;
- the rehabilitation phase, which should lead to the restoration of pre-disaster conditions.

The phases of a comprehensive hazard management plan for disasters are:

- pre-disaster planning and preparedness;
- emergency response;
- recovery and reconstruction.

The recognition that a huge scientific and technical input is needed to inform and assist in these phases, the most important being the planning and preparedness of communities rather than relying on ad hoc relief responses in the aftermath of a disaster, has been long overdue. In the 1980s, scientists (the US Academy of Sciences) led the call to reduce the impact of natural disasters by advancing and applying scientific and technical know-how. In the 1990s, the UN declared a decade of international effort to increase awareness of natural disasters, and called for governments, scientists, disaster professionals and communities to work towards the common goal of disaster reduction [8]. The International Decade for Natural Disaster Reduction (IDNDR) was not an unqualified success. Halfway through, it became evident that insufficient emphasis had been given to the socio-economic and political causes of vulnerability, and that technological disasters had been left out. Raised hopes of greater funding for scientists were not borne out. Many governments in developed countries took the attitude that disasters were a problem of the developing world, whereas many examples existed of inadequate preparedness for disaster risk in their own countries. As with preventive measures in general, it was hard to show the benefits that planning and preparedness may bring, and most non-government organizations continued basing their strategies upon providing disaster relief. The insurance industry showed interest, but mainly remained aloof. By the end of the decade the UK government was spending only 1% of its overseas disaster budget on preparedness, the same as when the decade began, with the rest mostly going on relief. As for the health professions, the workers in the specialities most closely linked to disaster medicine and who were engrossed in providing ever more technologically driven treatment barely gave disaster mitigation a glance. When the decade passed, the challenges for the new millennium looked greater than ever. Fortunately, initiatives are likely to continue in many countries in the twenty-first century, and also in the UN under the new International Strategy for Disaster Reduction.

However, the International Decade for Natural Disaster Reduction had one important and unrecognized achievement in that it had brought together a large number of people working in quite disparate fields and showed them how the whole area of disaster mitigation could become more than just the sum of their own individual parts. The decade had begun with a Scientific and Technical Committee laying out a long list of aims achievable by scientists if funding could only be found. Amongst these was one that would involve medical scientists, working with engineers and seismologists, who could determine more exactly the types of injury that would be produced in earthquakes. This was in order to optimize building technologies and corresponding building codes in disaster-prone areas. However, the decade ended before this laudable aim was fulfilled. Earthquakes are one of the most common and devastating causes of disaster, and they present outstanding problems to the most affluent of countries, such as the United States and Japan, as well as the poorest. Perhaps more scientific work has gone into studying these than any other natural disasters. Long before the decade started, investigators were developing models to predict building damage in earthquakes of different seismic intensities. These were for the benefit of insurance companies who were underwriting future losses, and seismic engineers who were designing earthquake-resistant buildings. From this work, it was a short step to using the models to estimate the potential number of casualties in an earthquake of a given magnitude, as the majority of deaths and injuries in earthquakes are due to trauma from buildings or parts of buildings collapsing onto the occupants. But what is possible for earthquakes is possible for other types of natural disaster. Predicting the numbers and types of casualties, or answering questions about *how* people are injured, is a fundamental prerequisite if we are serious about devising the most appropriate mitigation measures and emergency response plans for high-risk areas. With the advent of increasingly powerful computers, not only can hurricanes and floods be predicted with greater accuracy, but simulations of the natural hazards themselves become possible, and these can be used to predict their behaviour in exposed areas. These tools are being developed, and offer a whole new approach to understanding how impacts and human trauma may occur.

## Post-disaster Assessment

Post-disaster assessment of needs is now accepted by international agencies in order to counter the indiscriminate sending of relief supplies and teams as a humanitarian knee-jerk response by external governments. The sending of uninvited medical teams is now frowned upon, as they can become part of the problem themselves, adding to the confusion. It is now accepted that a rapid needs assessment must be done before aid is sent. This should focus on the survivors' needs, tomorrow's needs and reasonable unmet requirements. Disaster management is essentially an exercise in information management, but obtaining an accurate and culturally attuned view in an emergency may be extremely difficult, with separate agencies relying on their own observers instead of a on a single coordinated team. Statistics of dead and injured can be notoriously unreliable, sometimes with many thousands of people unaccounted for. Mortality and morbidity in the recovery phase, which may take years, is rarely, if ever, included. Social and mental health problems will appear when the acute crisis has subsided and the victims feel (and often are) abandoned to their own devices. A feature of all disasters continues to be the sending of out-of-date medicines and inappropriate foodstuffs, clothing and shelter by governments and agencies of prosperous countries. To overcome these problems, the Pan-American Health Organization (PAHO) established the Humanitarian Supply Management System (SUMA) for the integral management of food and other relief supplies. Some myths surrounding post-disaster relief include [1]:

- any kind of international assistance is needed;
- the affected population is too shocked and helpless to take responsibility for their own survival;
- natural disasters trigger secondary disasters through outbreaks of communicable diseases;
- life gets back to normal after a few weeks.

Most of the post-disaster need is in the restoration of normal primary care services, water systems, housing and income-producing work.

## Role of Epidemiology

Investigating deaths and injuries and identifying risk factors is the stuff of modern epidemiology. In disaster epidemiology, for risk factors read vulnerability and we find we have a powerful tool for analysing risk and hence developing risk-reduction measures. In the 1976 Guatemala earthquake, which left 23,000 dead, an epidemiological study showed that the risk of being killed was far greater inside an adobe building than in any other type of collapsed building [9]. For many years it has been known that masonry buildings are weaker in quakes than reinforced concrete or frame and timber types, for example. There could be no clearer demonstration of structural vulnerability and the need to incorporate classes of building structure and their specific strengths and weaknesses against natural impacts into any risk classification of disaster. In extreme weather, few people remain outside, and the protection provided by the building becomes crucial in a hurricane or flood. "The house that stands up" to natural disasters is the difference between life and death in many types of event. The results of epidemiological studies can be passed on to engineers who can devise the necessary protective measures, and so the method lends itself easily to interdisciplinary work. The down side is that accurate data collection is not easy in the chaotic aftermath of a disaster, the time when the collection of perishable data is most critical. Relief teams rarely include epidemiologists, and a very committed research project would need to be mounted to include them. However, teams of structural engineers from universities or insurance sectors do visit the scene of earthquakes to study the effects of the shocks on buildings, and incorporating epidemiologists in these teams is more feasible. Many fewer useful epidemiological studies have been undertaken than might be expected, leaving many large gaps in our understanding of the acute and long-term impacts on health of disastrous events. Without doubt there is ample scope for scientific observational studies in the acute and long-term phases of disasters, especially to improve the evidence base for interventions, and they remain an important goal in the new century.

Epidemiological surveillance, however, is a key tool in monitoring and helping to assess the health needs of displaced groups and communities affected by disaster, e.g. nutritional status and communicable diseases in refugee camps [1].

## Deaths and Injuries in Natural Disasters

### Earthquakes

The greatest recorded loss of life in an earthquake this century was in China in 1973, when at least a quarter of a million people (over a quarter of the population of the city) were killed in the Tangshan earthquake. In August and September 1999, three destructive earthquakes struck one after the other in Turkey (Izmit), Greece (Athens) and Taiwan (Taichung), leading to substantial loss of life and alarm within the affected countries. The magnitudes of these eruptions were 7.4, 5.9 and 7.6, respectively, on the Richter scale. In Izmit, the earthquake occurred on the North Anatolian fault, where ten previous major shocks have occurred since 1939 [10]. Over 15,000 bodies were recovered, about 40,000 persons were missing, and the number of injured exceeded 43,000. In the aftermath, investigators blamed the poor construction of buildings and the lack of inspection in a known earthquake-prone area. In Athens, over 100 people were killed and 1,600 received severe injuries in a part of the city previously considered to be at little risk. The quake in Taiwan also took the community by surprise, leaving over 2,000 dead and another 9,000 seriously injured. These figures show the scale and range of the loss of life and the size of the response needed by medical services to deal with the injured.

The number of people killed will depend on the total number of collapsed structures and the level of their damage, the population per building (average family size in residential building stock), the time of day that the quake occurred, the proportion of occupants trapped by the collapse (based on the extent of the collapse), the proportion killed outright, and the additional mortality of trapped victims after the collapse [11]. The last is the "fade away" time for people with different injuries, and is a function of the capability of the rescue and medical services together with the survival time of those trapped in the rubble. Other factors influencing the "fade away" time include the climatic conditions, aftershocks, fire outbreaks and rainfall. Factors that determine the effectiveness of search and rescue efforts include, amongst others, manpower, equipment and skills. Unfortunately, little is known about the survival times of those trapped inside rubble. There is some evidence that different types of buildings (timber, masonry, reinforced concrete) inflict injuries in different ways and with different degrees of severity when they collapse. In masonry buildings, it is suspected that the primary cause of death is often suffocation from the weight and powder of the wall or roof material which buries the victim. In reinforced concrete structures as well, very large amounts of dust are generated by the collapse, which would also suggest that many deaths would be rapid and due to asphyxia, regardless of the injuries incurred. Lethal injuries caused by building collapse are crush injuries to the head and chest, external or internal haemorrhage, and chest compression. Delayed death occurs within days, and can be due to dehydration, hypothermia, hyperthermia, crush syndrome or post-operative sepsis. The majority of those requiring medical assistance suffer minor injuries such as lacerations and contusions. Infected wounds and gangrene were major problems following the 1988 Armenian earthquake.

Most authorities agree that more people would be saved if they were extricated sooner. Victims who are not removed within 12 h have a very low probability of survival. In Izmit, the first of the 112 Turkish teams arrived about 6 h after the shock, and the first from other countries about 16 h later. These teams were too late to undertake immediate life-saving interventions [10]. The greatest demand for emergency medical services is within the first 24 h, with injured people requiring emergency treatment only during the first 3–5 days. After this time the hospital case-mix patterns may return to normal. At Iznit, the conditions presenting to the medical services by 7 days after the big shock were minor injuries, psychological trauma, respiratory infections, diarrhoea, scabies and chronic diseases that had been aggravated by the breakdown in routine treatment. Thus, restoration of a primary care service becomes a major priority within a few days after a disaster.

Few investigations of the response of the emergency services under these conditions have ever been undertaken, so the findings at the Great Hanshin earthquake that struck Kobe City in Japan at 15.46 on 17 January 1995 are of special interest [12]. This disaster exposed serious flaws in the Japanese emergency services, as well as showing the need for comprehensive planning for medical care and welfare in earthquake-prone countries. The earthquake had a recorded magnitude of 7.2 on the Richter scale, and the scale of the disaster was beyond all expectations. The immediate victims included 5,520 dead (10% killed in fires) and 41,527 wounded. Four days later, 342,000 people (10% of the total population of the region) were staying in shelters at a time of sub-zero temperatures because their houses were totally or partially damaged. The plight of elderly people was not appreciated at first, with many of their carers in ordinary life either dead or surviving as victims themselves. It was difficult to secure medical staff to provide emergency care for disaster injuries. About 80% of the hospitals in the area were damaged, and 7% were completely destroyed. Undamaged hospitals were found to lack the structural means to adapt rapidly to deal with overwhelming numbers of casualties requiring emergency care, and the breakdown of supplies of water, electricity and gas and the failure in communications badly hampered other still-functioning hospitals. The transfer of pharmaceuticals and medical equipment also took longer than expected. Many lessons were learnt by the Japanese authorities about future earthquake preparedness. The economic losses exceeded 100 billion US dollars, making it the costliest natural disaster in the world to date.

## Hurricanes and Windstorms

A hurricane is one of a broad class of extreme weather phenomena that include winter storms (snow, sleet, freezing rain and freezes), thunderstorms (e.g. tornadoes, heavy rains, lightning, wind and hail), extreme precipitation (e.g. floods and flash floods) and windstorms. Hurricanes (or typhoons as they are called in the western Pacific) are tropical cyclones that form over warm oceans from pre-existing regions of relatively low surface pressures with an associated cluster of thunderstorms [13]. Their intensity is well correlated with ocean surface temperature (over 26°C), with wind gusts attaining speeds of 70 m/s (250 km/h or 155 m.p.h.). Once over land, they soon run out of energy and rapidly abate, but can still cause flooding from heavy rains. Very high wind speeds in a hurricane are restricted to a relatively narrow track, perhaps 150 km wide, within which localized gusts may even achieve tornado speeds and be exceedingly destructive. Contrary to expectations, most deaths and injuries in hurricanes are not from the effect of wind on people (who stay inside) or from building damage (buildings blown down on to their occupants taking refuge or people being struck by flying debris). Deaths and injuries are very commonly associated with flooding (extremely severe concurrent rainfall is typical over a larger area and extending further inland than wind speed), consequential landslides and the sea surge. These devastating impacts are more common in slow-moving hurricanes.

The parts of the world which experience hurricanes are the western Pacific, the north Indian Ocean and the Bay of Bengal, and the North Atlantic Ocean. On average, six hurricanes a year develop in the Atlantic, usually in the months of August, September and October. The coastlines most at risk are those of Central America, the Caribbean, the Gulf of Mexico and the eastern seaboard of the United States from Florida to the Carolinas. Every hurricane lifts the sea below it, and the sea surge typically rises 3-4 m on top of existing tides, with the wind generating waves on top of that. Flooding of coastlines where the hurricane makes landfall can easily be envisaged. The most destructive natural disaster in the history of the United States was Hurricane Andrew in August 1992, the third most intense storm to strike the United States in the twentieth century, although mitigation measures held the death toll at 43. Andrew developed sustained wind speeds in excess of 250 km/h and even greater localised gusts. It was expected to strike Miami head-on, but in the event its narrow path of destructiveness passed 24 km to the south, completely flattening some small towns. It subsequently moved across the Gulf of Mexico where it renewed its energy and struck the Louisiana coastline with a large storm surge that flooded a swathe of the coastline. About 700,000 of the one million who were advised to leave the path of the hurricane left their homes and drove out of the area or moved into hurricane shelters in the hours before it struck. That 300,000 ignored this advice is a striking testimony to how disaster mitigation measures can fail in even the most economically advanced countries with all the advantages of the latest communications and advanced-warning technology. For those who stayed and survived, perhaps even more harrowing than the hurricane passing was the shooting and looting that followed. Andrew is reported to have generated about 5 million tons of debris: an immense waste management and disposal problem.

During a 2-week period in October/November 1998, Central America was battered by Hurricane Mitch, one of the most severe storms in the history of the region. It formed off the coast of South America and gained strength moving northwards with gusts of more than 250 km/h. It then unexpectedly slowed to a tropical storm and turned a right angle to crawl across Honduras dumping a year's rainfall on Central America in a few hours as it went. The rains then shifted to Nicaragua, precipitating mudslides on the Casitas volcano, and further flooding in El Salvador, Guatemala and Belize. Central America's rampant deforestation added to the flooding and landslide risk. The result was about 13,000 slope failures, which added to the destruction of the flooding. Over 20,000 people were known to have died or were missing, 13,000 were injured and over 2 million were left homeless. Health services, water and sanitation networks, roads and communications were all disrupted in large parts of the region. Subsequently, the incidence of cholera and other water-borne diseases, leptospirosis, dengue and malaria increased, particularly in the urban areas and among the more impoverished and marginal groups [14].

The cause of 90% of the fatalities in hurricanes is drowning associated with storm surges or floods. Other causes of death include burial beneath houses collapsed by wind, penetrating trauma from broken glass or wood, blunt trauma from floating objects or debris, or entrapment in mudslides. As in floods, the number of severe trauma patients among survivors is usually small; the greatest need in the post-impact phase is the provision of adequate shelter, water, food, clothing and sanitation. Most patients who seek care after hurricanes can be treated as outpatients. Most suffer from lacerations caused by flying glass or other debris, or minor trauma such as closed fractures and puncture wounds. The wounds may be heavily contaminated, and primary wound closure may need to be avoided. Most of the presenting conditions can be dealt with through primary care facilities by physicians and nurses skilled in minor surgical emergencies.

## Floods

Countries at most risk from coastal flooding include those at the mercy of hurricanes and their sea surges. Most other floods result from moderate-to-large events (rainfall, snowmelt, high tides) occurring within the expected range of streamflow or tidal conditions. Although floods are more or less natural phenomena, the flood hazard is largely of human origin, where human encroachment onto river flood-plains and coastal lowlands has occurred and is increasing. In most countries, migration towards river and coastal flood-zone areas has been a feature of economic development in the last century. For this reason alone, the human and economic losses from floods will continue to mount. Almost three billion people live in coastal areas where the population is continuing to rise with in–migration at twice the global average [15].

In Britain, as in many countries with low-lying coastal land, the hazard of coastal flooding from sea surges and high tides is more serious than that of river flooding. Extraordinarily high casualty tolls have been reported from floods in China, a country whose flood history is inseparable from its destiny, and where 40 million inhabitants are estimated to be affected by flood each year. Flooding of the Hung Ho in 1887 and 1931 claimed 900,000 and 3.7 million lives, respectively. Historically, engineers have sought to fight floods with bigger and better coastal defences, improvements to river channels to increase their conveyance capacity, or the construction of flood-relief channels or flood embankments to protect vulnerable areas. However, a growing awareness of the weaknesses of this approach in technical as well as vulnerability terms has led to more flexible and adaptive measures directed towards living with floods, and acknowledging that complete protection from flooding is impossible. Thus, in the 1993 Mississippi flood brought on by months of heavy rain in the Mid-West USA and compounded by snow and melt, hundreds of levees (embankments) failed. Some of these were subsequently left unreconstructed to allow future floodwaters to spread more naturally and reduce the scope for severe flooding in narrower channels flowing through towns and cities.

Thus, as with hurricanes, there is an inevitability about future flood disasters as human populations continue to expand in coastal and other low-lying areas of risk. Extreme weather events will recur sooner or later, with overtopping or breaching of sea/river defences in various states of repair. Even in the UK, local planning departments give consent to about a third of the applications for developments in at-risk coastal areas against the advice of the government's Environment Agency. Flood warning and forecasting, combined with effective land management, community preparedness and evacuation planning, are therefore as essential as engineering work to build river and coastal defences.

The flood on the east coast of England in 1953 was the most devastating flood affecting the UK in recent times. On top of a moderate spring tide, a large surge was whipped up by gale-force winds and was amplified as it progressed southwards along the east coast. Sea levels rose more than 2 m higher than tidal predictions. The wind drove waves as high as 5 m against the sea walls and dunes until they were battered and breached. The damage extended over 1,000 miles of coastline, and involved breaches in the defences at some 1,200 sites, 307 people died and over 32,000 were evacuated from their homes. No warning system had been established for the population, so many people drowned in their beds as torrents of water suddenly poured into their homes. In The Netherlands, 1,795 people drowned as the surge swept further south. The probability of such an extreme combination of severe wind and high tide is put at once every 500 years, but this could be reduced by an order of magnitude (to once every 50 years) by a rise in sea level due to global warming over the next 50–100 years. This is an indication of the threat of severe flooding presented by climate change in the UK, but in addition, the population along the coastal areas and in large areas at risk inland has increased substantially since 1953. Given the aged state of the defences that were built following the 1953 event, the management of future flood risk is becoming an increasingly greater priority for government agencies.

The primary cause of death from floods is, of course, drowning, but trauma from impacts with floating debris and hypothermia due to cold exposure are also important. The proportion of survivors requiring emergency medical care is small, since most injuries are minor things such as lacerations. This absence of victims with severe or multiple trauma may reflect the long delay in reaching the badly injured in such disasters, so they die from their wounds or from exposure before being rescued. In the year following a major flood, non-specific morbidity and mortality appear to increase amongst those who were flooded.

In July 1997, heavy rains caused severe flooding in Central Europe, with over 100 people killed and tens of thousands made homeless. The region had been left vulnerable by decades of neglect of flood control under the old Communist regime. Substantial mental ill-health due to the flooding was recognised, and studies in Poland found that most victims suffered from some degree of post-traumatic stress disorder. Alcohol abuse and suicides were also encountered.

## Volcanoes

Earthquakes, hurricanes and floods can be extremely devastating or deadly, as well as disrupting the lives of many thousands or even millions of people, but survivors do often rebuild their lives and homes once the event has passed. Major volcanic eruptions differ from these events in that their threats are more drawn out over time and their impacts can change the landscape, giving visible weight to the saying that "life will never be the same again" for those who live in the volcano's shadow. A few volcanoes, e.g. Kilauea on Hawaii, mainly have lava eruptions whose flows do not normally travel fast enough to kill people, but they leave a deep, rough rock-hard layer that may take decades, or even centuries, to break down into a fertile and habitable surface. Most hazardous volcanoes are mainly explosive in character and are capable of producing pyroclastic flows and surges (hot clouds of ash and gas) that threaten to destroy areas up to many kilometres from the crater. A volcanic crisis can last years, resulting in economic disruption and/or evacuation.

As with other natural disasters, the growth of dense urban settlements in exposed areas has greatly increased the risk of volcanic disaster. At the time of writing, tens of thousands of people are threatened by on-going eruptive crises from Popocatepetl (near Mexico City) and Colima (near several towns, including Colima) volcanoes in Mexico, and Guagua Pichincha (Quito) and Tungarua (Baños) volcanoes in Ecuador. Vulcanologists are anxiously watching these volcanoes for signs of any build-up of activity. This would lead to the evacuation of thousands of people who would be at risk. The potential for disaster is huge. In the worst case, over a million people could be killed by pyroclastic flows if Popocatepetl suddenly repeated one of its huge eruptions. Even wider areas are affected by heavy ash falls from the eruption columns of explosive volcanoes: at the eruption of Mount Pinatubo, in the Philippines, in 1991, over 300 deaths were caused by the roofs of houses collapsing due to the weight of the ash, which had been augmented by rain from a passing typhoon. This was despite tens of thousands of people having been evacuated away from the paths of pyroclastic flows around the volcano itself. As well as causing floods, heavy rain (triggered by eruptions) can mobilise large volumes of ash and other debris deposited on the slopes of the volcano to produce lahars, or wet debris flows, capable of travelling under the force of gravity for tens of kilometres and sweeping away or burying everything in their path. The eruption of Ruiz del Nevado volcano in Colombia in 1984 triggered a lahar by rapid melting of the glacier at the summit. The melt waters rushed down the valleys and mixed with debris as they went. The muddy mass swamped the town of Armero, taking the inhabitants by surprise; altogether around 24,000 people died. The town itself had been built on a lahar from a previous eruption over a hundred years previously. Living memory may indeed be short – 15 years after the worst volcanic disaster of the twentieth century, new buildings were mushrooming on top of the buried town.

Most deaths and injuries in eruptions are caused by people being engulfed in pyroclastic flows and surges, and lahars. Injured survivors may suffer from severe burns and inhalation injuries in the former, and multiple trauma and infected lacerations in the latter. The number of survivors in major eruptions may be quite small. However, care of large numbers of evacuees is often required. Years after the Pinatubo eruption, thousands of people remain displaced because of the threat of lahars in every wet season, even though the eruption is long over. In the small Caribbean island of Montserrat, thousands of people had to be evacuated from their homes in 1996 because of the threat from the Soufriere Hills volcano. By 1997, the growing threat of pyroclastic flows meant that thousands had to leave the island all together to make new lives in the UK and elsewhere. A new cycle of activity began in 1999, making it unlikely that the southern half of the island will be reoccupied for many years to come.

About 500–600 volcanoes are known to be capable of eruptive activity and several major eruptions occur every year. So far major cities have been spared in modern times, but this reassuring picture will not last. The worst foreseeable disaster facing Europe in the years ahead is an eruption of Vesuvius, Italy, one of the world's most dangerous volcanoes. Land-use planning has been ignored, making the slopes of the volcano one of the most densely populated areas in Europe. At least 600,000 people will need to be evacuated out of the potential paths of pyroclastic flows, floods and lahars. The successful management of such a crisis will depend upon effective monitoring and warning by vulcanologists so that a planned evacuation of this large mass of people can be achieved in time.

## Mental Health in Natural Disasters

Whilst it is agreed that it is essential to include the psycho-social aspects of health in national disaster plans and in the provision of care during disasters, the instruments to make appropriate assessments and the personnel to use them are usually lacking in the post-impact phase. Nevertheless, it has been shown in all types of disaster that a proportion of survivors will suffer psychological problems including post-traumatic stress disorder, depression, alcohol abuse, anxiety and somatization. There is a large and growing literature which should leave sceptics in no doubt about these effects. Although a psychiatric history and exposure to previous traumatic events may increase a person's susceptibility, there is no way of predicting who will be affected. Emergency and disaster workers are also now known to develop post-traumatic stress disorder. Less clear is the effectiveness of interventions for victims or emergency workers such as stress debriefing following exposure to traumatic events. Organisations sending relief workers to conflict or disaster areas should have appropriate stress management programmes [16].

## Natural Disasters – What We Have Learnt

Human and economic losses in natural disasters are increasing in a seemingly inevitable way as human settlements grow in exposed areas. However, certain effective mitigation measures can be identified. Thus losses in earthquakes can be massively reduced by the adoption of appropriate anti-seismic construction methods and the application of buildings codes: no warning of earthquakes seems possible at present. In contrast, meteorologists can track the path of hurricanes and at least reduce the human losses by giving warning so at-risk groups can evacuate, but community preparedness is essential if such warnings are not to be ignored by thousands of people. In floods, a combination of engineered flood defences, meteorological warnings and community preparedness, together with land-use planning, is required. As floods can be caused by hurricanes, the same broad mitigation issues apply to both. With volcanoes, the example of Vesuvius shows that the only reliable measure to save lives is timely evacuation, but predicting the timing and size of an eruption is an impossible task for scientists [17]. Developing controls over land use is no longer an option for most areas of active volcanism, where populations have already moved in, as around Vesuvius. There are no complete answers to the dilemmas posed by natural disasters, and people must not be led to believe that scientists and officials have the means of eliminating the threat of natural hazards. Ultimately, the mitigation of natural disasters in the twenty-first century will depend upon the world learning to live with risk and understanding human limits in the face of Nature.

## Technological Disasters

Disasters resulting from modern technology are also most commonly acute-onset events which threaten many lives and are shocking to those involved. Major air-pollution events in the past were associated with the combustion of fossil fuels combined with adverse meteorological conditions leading to a build-up of pollutants in cities, the most serious incident occurring in London in 1952. The smog led to at least 4,000 excess deaths over 4 days. Today the inexorable growth of traffic threatens to lead to acute incidents from the build-up of exhaust emissions, but in developed countries controls over smoke and traffic emissions have nevertheless made severe smogs a problem of the past. A disturbance of weather patterns as a result of El Nino resulted in unusually dry conditions in Indonesia, and slash and burn practices led to uncontrollable fires for weeks, with the smoke extending over a wide area of south-east Asia. The health impact of these fires is unknown.

Accidental releases of toxic gases and flammable vapours from storage sites and during transport are now well-recognised hazards of the modern petrochemical industry. Worldwide initiatives and legislation have been put in place over recent decades to reduce plant failures. The world's worst chemical disaster occurred in Bhopal, India, in 1984, when a cloud of methyl isocyanate gas, a potent respiratory irritant, escaped from a pesticide plant and flowed over the city at night. About 4,000 people died that night from pulmonary oedema and related lung damage, or from sequelae in the following weeks. Tens of thousand were left with chronic respiratory problems. In the same year in Mexico City, over 500 people died when a liquid petroleum gas plant exploded. Chemical releases and fires can present additional problems of contamination requiring the evacuation of communities – the most notorious was in Seveso, Italy, in 1976, when a chemical plant accidentally discharged a chemical cloud containing dioxin, a persistent human carcinogen. Then 28,000 residents had to be evacuated rapidly when the hazard became known.

The threat of accidents and releases of radioactive materials from nuclear power or reprocessing plants has for many years fuelled public fears of technology and industrial pollution, with the horrors of Hiroshima and Nagasaki not far from the world's consciousness. The nuclear industry was successful in playing down these fears until the reactor fire at Chernobyl in 1986, when the most feared type of event nearly happened – an uncontrollable meltdown of the atomic pile. The radioactive emissions (iodine-131, caesium, strontium and plutonium) from the graphite fire, which burnt out of control for several days, spread over a wide swathe of northern Europe. In the Ukraine region around the reactor, several tens of cases of thyroid cancer attributable to this release have appeared in children since 1992. The absence of a strong safety culture contributed to this incident, as well as to those at Three Mile Island, USA, in 1979 and Tokaimura, Japan, in 1999.

Technological disasters are "man-made" because they arise from human activities, but there is also the sense, as in natural disasters, that they are intrinsically preventable by the application of knowledge and organizational measures. Some authors favour the view that modern societies and complex technologies lend themselves to accidents, but the role of human error and ignorance, and cultural and political factors is not far below the surface of most of these events, as in many natural disasters. Nonetheless, efforts to prevent technological disasters have mainly been directed towards improving engineering controls and safety cultures inside organizations, with little emphasis on the vulnerability of populations living around plants. Recent experience shows that this approach is successful judging by the limited number of major incidents reported, but the potential for disaster is not far away. There is always the possibility that progress will lead to new processes and products the environmental effects of which will be unknown until it is too late. This fear of modern technology cannot be dispelled, and is indeed rational, but the use of the word "accident", which means a harmful event that is entirely unforeseeable, is overused in our society today.

The distinction between "natural" and "technological" disasters is less clear when natural sudden-onset events may have the potential to trigger releases of chemical or nuclear materials. Fortunately, major secondary disasters of this type ("Na-Techs") have not occurred to date, but the potential again shows the importance of adopting an "all hazards" approach to risk mitigation.

# Conclusions

Growing human populations in areas exposed to natural hazards are the most important reason why the public health impact of disasters will continue to rise inexorably. Nevertheless, the impacts of natural disasters are capable of being reduced by the application of our current scientific technical knowledge. That a wide gap exists between our technical capabilities and their application is evident on our TV screens, and is shown by the inexorable rise in human and economic losses in global natural disasters. The reasons for this delay in applying mitigation measures are complex and are rooted in socio-political and cultural factors, as well as poverty. Most natural disasters are in this sense partly "man-made", with mitigation having emerged in the last decade as the major strategy for reducing future losses. Risk perception is an important limiting factor in taking preventive action, since there is no agreed measure of risk, and scientific forecasting of the timing and size of natural disasters is limited. Climate change could have a major impact on the number of severe weather and flood disasters in the twenty-first century, but much scientific uncertainty remains over this issue.

The fact remains that most deaths occur at the time a disaster strikes, and to prevent these deaths requires long-term attention to preparedness in disaster-prone areas. Emergency medical teams arrive too late to make any real difference. Re-establishing public health priorities, such as food, water and sanitation, and primary care are the most important relief measures. In technological disasters, engineering control measures, organisational safety cultures, and health and safety legislation play essential preventive roles. One consequence of globalization is the growing realisation that disasters are an important issue in sustainable development: for example, linking emergency aid with long-term development, and partnerships with the private sector in the interests of the commercial sustainability of multinational business. Linking aid and investment with sustainability, which includes disaster mitigation measures, involves recognition of the complex factors that make human populations vulnerable to disaster.

# References

1. Nojij EK, editor. The public health consequences of disasters. New York: Oxford University Press, 1997.
2. Smil V China's great famine: 40 years later. BMJ 1999;319:1619–22.
3. Epstein PR. Climate and health. Science 1999;285:347–8.
4. Bouma MJ, Kovats RS, Goubet SA, Cox JStH, Haines A. Global assessment of El Nino's disaster burden. Lancet 1997;350:1435–8.
5. Blaikie P, Cannon T, Davis I, Wisner B. At risk: natural hazards, people's vulnerability, and disasters. London: Routledge, 1994.
6. Safar P. Resuscitation potentials in mass disasters. Prehosp Disaster Med 1986;2:34–47.

7. National Research Council. The impacts of natural disasters: a framework for loss estimation. Washington, DC: National Academy Press, 1999.
8. Board on Natural Disasters. Mitigation emerges as major strategy for reducing losses caused by natural disasters. Science 1999;284:1943-7.
9. Glass RE, Urrutia JJ, Sibornis S, Smith H. Earthquake injuries related to housing in a Guatemalan village. Science 1979;197:638-43.
10. Guhar-Sapir D, Carballo M. Medical relief in earthquakes. J R Soc Med 2000;93:59-61.
11. Coburn A, Spence R Earthquake protection. Chichester: Wiley, 1992.
12. Baba S, Tanaguchi H, Nambi S, Tsuboi S, Ishihara K, Osato S. The Great Hanshin earthquake. Lancet 1996;347:307-9.
13. Pielke RA Jr, Pielke RA Sr. Hurricanes: their nature and impacts on society. Chichester: Wiley, 1997.
14. International Federation of Red Cross and Red Crescent Societies. World Disasters Report. Geneva, 1999.
15. Smith K, Ward R. Floods: physical processes and human impacts. Chichester: Wiley, 1998.
16. McCall M, Salama P. Selection, training and support of relief workers: an occupational health issue. BMJ 1999;318:113-6.
17. Scarpa R, Tilling RI. Monitoring and mitigation of volcanic hazards. Berlin: Springer, 1996.

# 4. Refugees and Internally Displaced People

Jim Ryan and David Childs

**Objectives**

- To understand the distinction between refugees and IDPs.
- To understand the principles of planning a care programme.
- To understand the importance of multidisciplinary and multi-agency team work.
- To recognise the immediate and urgent needs of a refugee/IDP community.
- To recognise the need for on-going surveillance, impact measurement and transition from acute care to long-term development.
- To recognise and respect refugees and their community.

## Introduction

The terms "refugee" and "internally displaced person" (IDP) are widely used in the literature of humanitarian assistance and require definition and distinction. Refugees are migrants who must have crossed an international frontier because of a well-founded fear of persecution. IDPs are people who have involuntarily been uprooted and displaced but still remain in their own countries. The distinction is important, as the United Nation's High Commissioner for Refugee (UNHCR) is legally bound by international law to protect and assist refugees. While care of IDPs is undertaken by UNHCR – witness the conflict in the Balkans – the arrangement is not legally binding. Although there are distinctions under international law, humanitarian assistance organisations make little or no distinction, and attempt to access and assist all displaced people.

The world's refugee problem is growing steadily. In 1960, numbers reached 2 million, by 1995 the figure had risen to almost 28 million. There are perhaps another 20–30 million living in their own countries as IDPs. War and conflict, leading to persecution and ethnic cleansing, is the common thread running through this picture of human misery.

Refugees and IDPs are faced with unique problems that go beyond medical care. Most victims have suffered human rights abuses, and experienced brutality resulting in death and injury to loved ones, forced migration, exposure to famine and communicable disease, and not least the break-up of family and community. The provision of care is multifaceted, demanding a multidisciplinary approach. Therefore, no attempt is made here to provide comprehensive instruction on the care of refugees and IDPs. That is done elsewhere, and there are a number of admirable texts which are exhaustive on the subject. They are listed in the resources section of this handbook. Here, the attempt is to summarise the central issues and problems and is directed at the humanitarian volunteer, irrespective of speciality or grade, with little or no prior experience of working with refugees or IDPs.

What, then, are the duties and responsibilities of the humanitarian volunteer? The humanitarian volunteer's first task is "not to become a casualty yourself". The first task is to remain dispassionate and objective. It is all too easy for the inexperienced to be overwhelmed when first confronted by mass gatherings of refugees (and IDPs). Spokespersons for the refugees/IDPs will invariably describe the sufferings of their people in graphic detail, including tales of murder, rape and torture. These tales may or may not be factual, and it is not for the volunteer to decide on veracity or make judgments. Listening and an impartial expression of sorrow are both reasonable and expected.

Volunteers will vary widely in their abilities and will need to work within teams. A wealth of skill and expertise is demanded when caring for refugees and IDPs; this normally requires not merely teamwork by individuals, but also collaboration among international aid agencies. Particular areas demanding special expertise include:

- provision of food and water;
- provision of sanitation;
- provision of shelter and energy;
- provision of immunisation programmes;
- public health surveillance;
- control of communicable disease;
- mother and child health.

The above list is far from exhaustive. Experience over the past quarter century has shown the overriding importance of the first three areas listed – food and water, sanitation and shelter. The lack of these basic facilities is the greatest determinant of death (and not, as might be imagined, the absence of acute medical care). In short, medical care is just one element in an overall integrated care plan.

The question most often asked is "who should carry out these functions?" Primary responsibility for refugees lies with the UNHCR. The UNHCR coordinates refugee aid programmes in collaboration with host government, international governmental organisations (IGOs) and non-governmental organisations (NGOs). In the main, the IGOs are other United Nations (UN) agencies, including the World Food Programme (WFP) who transport food aid by air, sea or land to reach the refugees, where it is then distributed by the UNHCR. NGOs, who are often specialised, usually work within the camps covering the provision of clean water, disposal of waste, health assessments and, where necessary, preventative or therapeutic programmes. Most readers of this manual will be destined for work with the NGOs operating on the ground rather than the larger, permanently staffed IGOs (although IGOs often employ humanitarian aid volunteers on short contracts).

Before turning to the practicalities of participating in a refugee/IDP aid programme, it is important to clarify some important issues around refugees as people, their displacement, their part in helping themselves, and resolution of their problems.

## Refugees/IDPS as a Community

Although some refugees/IDPs may become dispersed within settled population groups, they are most often concentrated in camps or similar discrete locations. Like any community, they are a collection of individuals with their own backgrounds, culture, religion and experiences. Often, the whole strata of society is mirrored in camps. Well-educated academics and wealthy businessmen are found alongside the less privileged. Teachers rub shoulders with shopkeepers and skilled craftsmen. The previous ruling elite may be present, including mayors and local politicians (*see also Ch. 6*). Also included may be religious and ethnic leaders. Attempts to impose an aid programme without consulting and seeking assistance from the community itself will result in the neglect of traditional beliefs, gender issues, culture and religion. The result may be friction, hostility and mission failure.

Refugees and their communities must be involved in the planning and implementation of aid programmes. In fact, without such involvement, most aid programmes will fail, or at least will be unsustainable.

The earliest planning will require detailed demographic and other data – in particular for vulnerable groups such as the elderly, children and women. Much of this may well be known by the refugee community and will be forthcoming if asked for. The principle from the outset should be to get the community to help itself and build long-term self-reliance. The community should, as far as possible, be allowed to govern itself through its familiar power structures.

### Anticipating and Dealing with Conflict

Much conflict can be avoided by adherence to the advice given above. However, there may be circumstances where conflict is present and unavoidable. Armed gangs such as militia or paramilitary groups may control refugee camps. These may or may not be hostile to the refugees/IDPs. Aid agencies may be accused of failing to be impartial. The may even advertently assist armed gangs by the provision of food and other aid. There is no single answer to this problem except to reiterate the need for scrupulous and transparent impartiality, which may be difficult when faced with the persecution of refugees by armed gangs as was evident in refugee camps in West Timor in 1999.

## Planning and Implementation

The aphorism "first do no harm" is as apt for refugee/IDP care as it is for any form of medical management. The most powerful weapon in preventing further harm is *knowledge* – the obverse, *ignorance*, will result in harm. Therefore, in formulating planning, knowledge of the problem is required.

## Planning – Pre-deployment

Before agreeing to a deployment, the following accurate information (knowledge) in the following areas is vital and should be requested by a volunteer.

- Where (which country or region) is the problem?
- What is most the urgent and/or immediate problem?
- Who is in charge? Who is the lead agency?
- The political and, if applicable, military background.
- Is there a plan?
- Is the plan feasible?
- Is there an end point for withdrawal?
- Do volunteers require vaccinations/malaria prophylaxis?

Further information is needed if the decision is made to deploy. Some typical examples are listed below.

- Has an initial assessment defined the immediate health problems?
- If so, what are they?
- Ethnic, religious, national or any other divisions.
- Language and traditions.
- Diet and taboos.

In the emergency phase of refugee/IDP care, the aim must be to limit excess mortality and to control morbidity.

## Planning – Arrival at Destination

When working with refugees it is very unlikely that a volunteer will arrive alone. Care of refugees/IDPs is a team-based activity. Ideally the volunteer should arrive in country as part of a specialised NGO invited to participate by the UNHCR or a similar agency. The following principles are recommended:

- if you arrive alone, find your team/agency and report;
- listen to instructions and briefings carefully;
- clarify what is expected of you;
- clarify the chain of command and reporting system;
- identify pre-agreed working practises (if they exist).

## Scope and Extent

You should be briefed on the scope and extent of the problem. Ask the following questions:

- How many refugees are there?
- Where are they located?
- What is the crude mortality rate (number of deaths per 1,000 per day)?
- Are more expected?
- What is the case mix, e.g. families, individuals or entire communities?
- Are there particularly vulnerable groups, e.g.
     women and female-headed households,
     elderly and the disabled,
     children,
     minority groups – religious, ethnic, political?

Other useful information on the extent of the problem should include:

- whether the group is urban, rural, sedentary or nomadic;
- their skills and languages;
- their customs and habits.

Most of the long-established NGOs have their own planning template for each phase of a refugee crisis from the emergency phase, through the post-emergency phase, and on to consolidation and long-term development. There is increasing agreement among NGOs and IGOs on priorities. For example, Médecins Sans Frontières (MSF) have listed the following top ten priorities for the emergency phase of a refugee crisis.

1.  Initial assessment.
2.  Measles immunisation.
3.  Water and sanitation.
4.  Food and nutrition.
5.  Shelter and site planning.
6.  Health care in the emergency phase.
7.  Control of communicable disease and epidemics.
8.  Public health surveillance.
9.  Human resources and training.
10. Coordination.

MSF have produced a comprehensive text on refugee health and this is listed in the resource section. Volunteers with a particular interest in refugee health are recommended to study this work in detail.

# Conclusions

This brief chapter serves as an introduction to refugees and internally displaced people. Problems relating to disease prevention and health care will be covered in detail in later chapters. Further discussion on refugees can be found in chapter 6, pages 92–96.

# 5. Medicine and Medical Aid in Remote Settings

Robert C. Mark, Roger Diggle and Iain C. Grant

**EDITORS' NOTE** – Much of this chapter is written in the first person as it is a very personal account from a highly accomplished trio of doctors with a vast experience of working in remote and hostile settings. Readers will note that most of the pearls of wisdom written here are echoed in many of the sections and chapters of this work.

## Part A – Medical Aspects of Oil and Gas Exploration
Robert C. Mark

### Acknowledgements

The author gratefully acknowledges the invaluable advice and assistance of Mr. Mark Tomlins, Operations Director, Exploration Logistics plc, and Mr. Leo Aalund, Technical Editor of the Oil and Gas Journal.

| **Objectives** | • To briefly describe exploration and production.<br>• To describe the working environment.<br>• To define health risks.<br>• To outline preventive measures against disease and injury.<br>• To describe a medical care plan. |
|---|---|

## Introduction

The term "remote" is used here to describe situations which are isolated in terms of distance or time, and where any immediately accessible medical facilities fail to meet acceptable standards. The business of searching for oil and gas and extracting them is often conducted in such areas, which are also subject to more than their fair share of conflict and catastrophe. The following review will give an insight into the industry and guidance on how to set up its medical provision, thereby emphasising principles common to all medical operations conducted in austere environments. Particular attention will be paid to the prevention of illness and injury, and involvement with the local community and its health workers. Examples of how these industrial projects have been directly involved in both conflict and catastrophe will be described.

## Oil Exploration and Production

The process of utilising oil or gas deposits begins when competing oil companies bid for an exploration and drilling licence issued by the host country. To ensure a close working relationship, the division of the potential revenues and other contractual obligations are agreed at the outset by company and state.

The initial phase of exploration is conducted by seismic survey. Pressure waves are set off in a grid pattern over the search area. The echo is then analysed and provides a picture of the underlying geological structures. The company may also conduct other geological and aeromagnetic surveys. If any of these appear to show potential oil-bearing formations they are subjected to exploratory, or "wild cat", drilling. Production facilities and pipelines must be constructed once oil is discovered that is both recoverable and marketable. These various steps are often conducted discontinuously depending on factors such as seasonal climatic changes, contractual issues or funding.

The driving force behind the whole process is, of course, financial success for both the oil company and the host country. Success depends on the ability to sell the product of this immensely complex and expensive enterprise. The economic limiting factor is the projected price of a barrel of oil on the international market, bearing in mind the readily available "bath tubs" in the Middle East.

The oil exploration company will nearly always bear the initial costs, which can be between £10 million and £50 million or more, before oil is even found. They will therefore have the controlling decision on whether to abort the project at any of the various milestones.

## Local Health Risks: Identification and Control

### Reconnaissance and Planning

The military adage "time spent on reconnaissance is never wasted" is readily applicable to the medical preparations for these projects. The wise medical operator will research both the area and the proposed activities before leaving home. Talk to colleagues who have recently returned from the area, and use the available telecommunications to converse with helpful sources in-country. The best use can then be made of the time available for inspection on the ground. Time and effort spent in this way will always be repaid.

Diligent enquiry will reveal such hazards to health as extremes of climate, standards of accommodation, hazardous plants and animals, local diseases, food safety standards, the potential for dangerous lifestyle habits (e.g. abuse of drugs and alcohol) etc. If you are dependent on reacting to problems, rather than being able to plan for them, the project and its staff will pay a price in morbidity and mortality, lost working time, medical evacuations and economic stress.

The risks to be identified and controlled will now be examined in greater detail using the format outlined in the Exploration and Production Forum's Health Management Guidelines for Remote Land-Based Geophysical Operations.

# Camp Standards

## Food and Drink

Food handlers should be screened for infectious diseases and trained in the safe preparation of food. Set standards for food supplies together with those for storage, preparation and cooking. Safe drinking water must be provided. This may require the importation of bottled water or the chemical sterilisation or filtration of local supplies, together with boiling.

## Camp Hygiene

Set standards for living quarters, toilet and washing facilities, lighting, ventilation and temperature control, and the safe disposal of sewage, laundry effluent, water and rubbish, including kitchen leftovers. Arrange for the safe disposal of clinical waste, including "sharps".

## Mosquito Control and Bite Avoidance

In malarial areas the prevention of this disease will be a crucial task. Site the camp at a distance from, and upwind of, open water. Breeding grounds should be eradicated as far as possible. Windows should have intact mosquito screens. Insect repellents should be used and fogging with insecticide carried out. Dress must be appropriate (e.g. long trousers and long-sleeved shirts). Permethrin-impregnated bed nets should fitted in particularly high-risk areas, especially in tented camps. Closing windows and staying indoors at dusk can further avoid bites.

## Other Hazardous Animal and Plants

Reduce the risk of animal bites through education, suitable clothing (especially calf-length boots in areas where snakes are found) and by siting the camp judiciously. Stinging and spiky plants will call for the wearing of robust clothing that covers the arms and legs.

## Local Diseases

Determine the prevalence of infectious diseases. Minimise their impact by strategies including immunisation courses, which must be commenced before leaving the home country. Resist the temptation to swim, wash or paddle in open water in areas with water-borne diseases such as schistosomiasis.

In malarial areas, give advice on the options for chemoprophylaxis depending on the risk of exposure, the existence of drug resistance, the efficacy of recommended drugs and their side effects. The final choice of regime must be determined by the patient and their physician, taking into account individual patient factors. Emphasise bite-avoidance methods.

Non-medical personnel must be educated in the recognition of the early symptoms of these diseases, and medical personnel must be trained in their diagnosis and treatment.

Consideration must be given to providing the diagnostic aids that will be required, such as bedside immunochromatographic testing kits for malaria together with the drugs needed for treatment.

Once in-country, disease surveillance will highlight the efficacy of preventative measures.

## Life Style Habits

The abuse of drugs, and especially alcohol, can be a problem for workers who are under stress, away from home and with little else to occupy their leisure hours. In some cultures, the social pressures to drink one's self into oblivion can be extreme. Strategies must be developed, implemented and monitored to prevent drug and alcohol abuse.

## Fitness for Work

In 1923, Macklin, a medical officer with Shackelton's 1914–1915 Trans-Antarctic Expedition, wrote:

> *"The chief work of the surgeon of a polar expedition is done before the ship leaves England, and if it has been properly carried out, there should be little to do during the actual journey".*

This sentiment still holds true for operations in remote areas, particularly in ensuring that personnel are fit for the job. The oil industry requires that its workers in remote areas are medically examined before deployment and at intervals thereafter to ensure that they meet agreed medical standards. Failure to do this will lead to unnecessary illness, injury or death amongst the workforce, with the attendant problems of lost working time, the search for a replacement worker and the cost of repatriation. Occasionally the company will employ a worker who does not meet the usual standards if his particular skills are commercially necessary. Both parties must take this decision on the basis of informed consent. Medical screening on returning home is advisable, and is covered elsewhere.

The need for dental fitness must not be forgotten. Severe toothache will prevent the toughest worker from performing his duties, not to mention sleeping. Dental care before departure can prevent personal misery, an extraction in the field, and unnecessary and embarrassing repatriation.

## Sexually Transmitted and Blood-borne Diseases

There will often be high local rates of infection with these diseases. Control measures will include education, restraint in personal relations, the availability of good-quality condoms, appropriate clinical working practices and the use of universal precautions.

# Work and Work Environment

## Stress, Fatigue and Work Cycles

The project planners must consider equipment standards, ergonomics, conditions of work, physical fitness, time for adaptation to the workload, recreation and sleeping conditions.

## Heat, Sun, Cold and Altitude

The debilitating effects of these phenomena can be ameliorated through education, appropriate clothing, acclimatisation and realistic working patterns.

## Chemical and Physical Hazards

These must be identified and the relevant technical and procedural control measures put in place. Appropriate personal protective equipment must be provided, together with education and training.

## Transportation and Driving Accidents

Road traffic accidents are the commonest cause of major trauma in remote areas. Vehicles must be maintained and inspected regularly. Pay particular attention to tyres, tyre pressures and brakes. Learn how to conduct the necessary daily checks yourself. Do not use vehicles which do not conform to required standards. Speed limits for the project must be set and rigorously enforced. Defensive driving will be called for at all times and risks must never be taken. Vehicles must carry written instructions for emergencies, safety equipment and survival kits. The skills required for both defensive and off-road driving should never be underestimated or assumed. Training programmes are often required for both local and expatriate drivers.

Initiate a journey management system. This is a simple scheme whereby all departing vehicles log out from a central control point recording the persons travelling, their route and expected time of arrival. Drivers report in at their destination and any available checkpoints en route. Using radio or telephone, the control point should confirm their safe arrival. Failure to arrive will trigger a search.

## Personal Hygiene

The facilities required to maintain high standards of personal hygiene must be provided, particularly in hot environments. Anyone whose standards start to slip should be tactfully encouraged to address the problem.

## Health Management System

A health management system is used to ensure that policy and objectives are agreed and achieved. An organisational structure will be needed. Responsibilities must be agreed and resources acquired. Standards and procedures should be developed and plans implemented. Performance monitoring will lead onto the improvement of processes, thus completing the cycle of audit.

## Medical Support: Local, Imported and International

To ascertain the acceptability of local medical facilities they must be audited using recognised standards. Comparing the level of medical care available locally with the environmental and occupational health risks will enable you to decide whether to contribute to the upgrading of local medical facilities, to import medical care or to combine both approaches. Requirements will change as the project develops. Whichever system is used, international medical support will also be required.

Arrange an itinerary in advance when visiting local facilities and personnel. Appointments should be sought with the most senior staff available. Provide a candid explanation of the purpose of the visit and the nature of the project. Find out what the local view is on what improvements are needed. Emphasise that mutual cooperation is sought for the good of all parties. However, remember that your agenda and that of the local community are unlikely to be the same.

## Local Medical Support

### Training

It is sometimes possible to upgrade the standards of the existing medical infrastructure by providing training for the local health carers. This must be done diplomatically. It is crucial to remember that they are professionals in their own right and will have their own unique experience and expertise. It is all too easy to give offence by adopting a high-handed approach: relations must be nurtured over time. Remember that the locals will have much to teach the incoming staff.

## Facilities

The buildings used for health care may need improving. Alternatively, new buildings might be constructed. Hygiene practices may need attention.

## Drugs and Equipment

It may be necessary to contribute equipment and supplies, but this approach must be carefully controlled. It has been known for drugs and equipment to be donated through the front door and then to go straight out of the back door as a source of extra income. Ensure that the use of these drugs and other supplies is clinically appropriate.

## Administration

Agree procedures for in-patient and out-patient treatment in local facilities before the event. This may include a method of payment.

## Communications and Transport

Do not take these aspects of the infrastructure for granted. Reassurances that everything required is in place should not be taken at face value. It is far better to see the system in action.

# Imported Medical Support

The need to import medical care will increase with the number of personnel on the project and its hazardousness and isolation, together with the paucity of local medical support.

## First Aiders and First Responders

All staff must be qualified in first aid or as emergency first responders (see bibliography). Arrangements must be made to ensure that they maintain their qualifications. An accredited first aid trainer can do this in the field. This is both cost-effective and occupies time when workers are off-shift. Small, low-risk projects may rely solely on first aiders, some of whom may require advanced training.

## Remote Area Medics

As the requirement for dedicated medical support increases, medical professionals will be required. The commonest requirement is for a nurse or "paramedic". The latter will not usually have the same skills profile as, for instance, a UK National Health Service paramedic. A better title might be "remote area medic".

The person filling this role will have a wide range of duties. These can include the supervision of environmental health, catering hygiene and other aspects of illness prevention, routine general medical care, emergency medical care, aero-medical evacuation, disaster planning, first aid training, and storage, supply and re-supply of medical equipment and drugs. They may also be called upon to act as a social worker during episodes of personal stress. The medic will work closely with the staff who are responsible for safety. If other duties allow, this person may also fulfil other roles such as in-camp administration.

The ideal candidate for this job is a mature and sociable character who is accustomed to working on his own in the middle of nowhere. Medically trained former military non-commissioned officers are often right for the job.

In the UK, the Offshore Medic's Certificate course is designed for medics operating on the North Sea. This qualification is issued under licence from the Health and Safety Executive. It is also the most frequently recognised qualification for remote land-based projects. In this environment, medical and traumatic emergencies are rare but particularly demanding. Therefore frequent refresher training in emergency medical care is necessary. Trauma courses such as Pre-Hospital Trauma Life Support or Basic Trauma Life Support should be considered. The Pre-Hospital Emergency Care Certificate and the Diploma in Immediate Medical Care are ideal pre-hospital emergency qualifications.

## Doctors

Doctors may sometimes be found in the field. This may be because the project is large, isolated or hazardous, or a combination of these factors. Occasionally a doctor may be employed from the host or another Third World country in preference to an expatriate Western medic solely on the basis of cost. Doctors may be employed when particularly extensive projects employ other subordinate medical or paramedical staff.

## The Camp Clinic

This should be housed in a clearly identifiable, prefabricated or other temporary building, sited close to the camp's administration and communication centre. There should be good vehicular access, and if possible aircraft should be able to land nearby. The entrance should allow access and egress for a stretcher. Air conditioning and/or heating should be installed and functioning. A telephone with a hands-off function and a radio with the same channels as used by the project and any relevant aircraft are invaluable assets.

In addition to equipment for routine medical care, the clinic should be equipped to a high standard for the management of medical and traumatic emergencies. Remember that seriously ill or injured patients may have to be treated for some hours before evacuation. Supplies of oxygen and intravenous fluids must be extensive if patients are to be treated along advanced trauma life support/battlefield advanced trauma life support (ATLS®/BATLS) guidelines.

## Medical Transport

A four-by-four ambulance, purpose-built or converted, is an expensive but often necessary provision. It must be fitted with communications equipment, a suitable stretcher and medical equipment, including oxygen. It must have air-conditioning or heating equipment appropriate to the climate. Extreme environments may require mechanical adaptations.

For some projects, local evacuation may be by fixed-wing aircraft or helicopter. Most of these will be multipurpose "work horses" rather than dedicated air ambulances.

## Emergency Planning

Draw up plans for medical emergencies, and then test, develop, publish and practise them on a continuing basis. These plans should concentrate on defining responsibilities, alerting procedures, communications and getting the medic to the casualty's location or vice versa. The medicine is often more straightforward than the logistics.

The project will have plans for major incidents, including fire, security threats and technical problems such as blowouts. It is important that you develop plans for multiple casualty incidents: command and control and much of the casualty care will be delegated to others who are not medically trained.

## Substandard Medical Provision

Regrettably, medical planning does not always take place. A project in a remote area will then rely solely on the existing local medical support, whatever its standard.

# International Medical Support

Although it might sometimes feel like it, you should not be operating in splendid isolation.

## Repatriation

Expatriate workers must be insured for medical repatriation and carry their membership card with them. You should keep a register of these and the relevant procedures. Plan how to get your patient to the nearest airport which the evacuation agency can use, and how to care for them there whilst awaiting the arrival of the repatriation team. The head office of the company in its country of origin should be involved, and the services of a locally retained physician can be of great assistance. It is essential that you maintain control of your patient until they are handed over to the personnel responsible for the aero-medical evacuation. Do not allow the patient to be side-tracked into an unsuitable local hospital.

*Topside Support*

Access to specialist medical advice by telecommunication is invaluable in assisting the remote professional to come to the right medical management decision in difficult cases. It will also make you less anxious. Confirm voice conversations and instructions in writing by fax or e-mail. Reliable international communications and the availability of the right senior colleague are essential if the arrangement is to function. Telemedicine is covered in detail elsewhere.

## The Oil Camp

In contrast to its surroundings, the oil camp may appear luxurious. The more permanent installation will have air-conditioned, semi-permanent offices and accommodation with a modern kitchen, dining rooms and opportunities for recreation. The communications room will contain an array of various radios, satellite phones and fax machines.

The staff will include expatriates from the developed world who will often be on a 4- or 6-week on/off rota. There will also be personnel who have been hired in-country. They may live locally or be accommodated in the camp. There may also be workers from elsewhere in the Third World who work on site for months at a time. Access to the camp may be controlled by security staff. There is great scope for social interaction and both formal and informal professional cooperation between the oil workers and those providing medical care for the local population. Take the time to visit each other and talk.

## The Local Community

In areas of unemployment, underemployment and poverty, the arrival of the oil industry is a major event. Hiring of locals can give a boost to the local economy. To be usefully employed can be a source of personal satisfaction and dignity.

However, community relations can be fragile and must be developed sensitively. Issues of land rights, rights of way and environmental protection must be addressed.

The project's medical staff must reach agreement with all parties regarding the treatment of local people. A common arrangement is that the company will take responsibility for the treatment of locally hired personnel and their families. The local definition of "family" may be broader than that with which you are familiar. Remember to take into account the sensibilities of the local medical workers.

It will be necessary to perform some medical screening of local workers. For example, check the eyesight of drivers (using an illiterate E chart), and ensure food handlers are free from tuberculosis, gastrointestinal infection and parasites.

However, the opportunities provided by the industry can be divisive. Competition for jobs may exacerbate religious or tribal hostilities. The influx of petro-dollars may inflate the prices of a range of goods and services to the disadvantage of local consumers and businesses alike. Purchase or rental of land may lead to resentment amongst those landowners who have not profited by providing property for the project.

Above all, it is essential to avoid encouraging long-term dependency on company support. The project will eventually close through failure to progress at one of the stages of development, when the deposit runs dry or if overwhelming contractual, economic, environmental or security problems ensue.

## Security

The industry can be subject to security risks for a number of reasons other than conventional war itself.

State control tends to be weaker in remote areas. Foreign investment can engender political and xenophobic hostilities against these high-profile projects. Terrorists can attempt to disrupt the industry's activities as an economic weapon. Both criminals and rebel groups use extortion by threats of violence.

Criminals and terrorists may kidnap personnel, including expatriates. A ransom demand may be for money, medical supplies, improvements in public services, arms, the cessation of company activity or the release of members of the group held prisoner by the government.

Theft, from the opportunistic to the organised, will take its toll. Extreme violence may result if you try and stop a thief whom you have disturbed: life is very cheap in some parts of the world.

Oil installations are sometimes vandalised in order to cause environmental damage. The perpetrators will then seek compensation for the damage done to their crops and other property.

The police and judicial system may not be wholly supportive. They can sometimes be part of the problem.

Security risks will make exploration and production more expensive, sometimes prohibitively.

# Examples of the Industry in Conflict and Catastrophe

## Kuwait Oil Fires February 1991

At the end of the Gulf War in Kuwait, Saddam Hussein's troops detonated explosive charges on more than 900 oil wells. Some of the wells burnt, producing huge clouds of smoke, whilst others failed to ignite and produced massive oil lakes. The operations to cap these wells were probably the largest and most expensive peacetime logistical exercise in history. On 5 November the same year, the Emir of Kuwait ceremonially extinguished the last fire.

Kuwait's oil fields do not contain significant levels of hydrogen sulphide, which is a highly toxic contaminant. If wells were to be blown up on a large scale in other fields which have a high concentrations of this "sour gas", the immediate threat to life could be huge.

## AIDS Amplification in Africa

An oil pipeline is to be built in Chad and Cameroon. Experience has shown that linear construction projects of this nature are associated with migration of the transient working population up and down the line. This leads to a thriving local sex industry and increased HIV infection rates amongst the oil workers, the sex workers and the community at large. Companies involved in this project are required to put in place approved measures to prevent the potential AIDs amplification.

## Pipeline Fires

### Ufa, Siberia, June 1988

Whilst the world's attention was focused on events in Tian An Men Square, Beijing, a large gas pipeline near the town of Ufa in the Former Soviet Union was leaking gas into a railway cutting. As two passenger trains crossed in the cutting, the gas ignited. An explosion followed which felled trees 2 miles away and shattered windows at a distance of 7 miles. Of the 1,200 passengers on the trains, hundreds died immediately and hundreds were injured as result of the explosion and fireball. The final toll of dead and injured has never been publicised. Casualties were treated as far away as Moscow. Plastic surgeons assisted from countries around the world.

### Warri, Nigeria, December 1998

A crude oil pipeline near this village developed a leak. Sabotage, theft or accidental damage have all been alleged. The villagers turned out in their hundreds to collect the free fuel. This ignited, perhaps as the result of a motorbike back-firing. The resulting fire caused more than a thousand casualties, with hundreds of deaths.

## Summary

Oil and gas exploration and production may take place in areas affected by conflict or catastrophe. Medical operations in remote areas, for whatever purpose, need to be carefully planned, equipped with suitable supplies, staffed by the right people and provided with international support. Good relationships must be established with the local community in general, and its health workers in particular.

## Further Reading

British National Formulary 36, September 1998, p. 284.

Macklin AH. Medical appendix V. In: Wild F, editor. Shackleton's last voyage: the story of the "Quest". London: Cassell, 1923; 352.

Mark B. None but ourselves: medical management of major incidents in the oil and gas industry in remote areas. SPE 46746. Society of Petroleum Engineers International Conference on Health, Safety and Environment in Oil and Gas Exploration and Production, Caracas, Venezuela, 7–10 June 1998.

Wasserstrom R, Reider S. Petroleum companies crossing new thresholds in community relations. Oil Gas J 1998; 14 December.

# Part B – The Falkland Islands, Expedition Medicine and Ship's Doctor

Roger Diggle

| **Objectives** | • To give a personal insight into working in a remote and austere environment.<br>• To describe the breadth of responsibility when working alone or in small teams.<br>• To point to some solutions. |
|---|---|

## What Is Remote?

A teaching hospital consultant in a capital city would no doubt regard his colleague in a district general hospital as being remote, and would certainly regard a rural general practitioner as being extremely so.

I am writing this chapter in the Falkland Islands, just off the tip of South America, and our logistic base and tertiary referral centres are in the United Kingdom some 8,000 miles away. By anyone's definition we are certainly remote. Within the Falklands, the medical services are centred in the capital, Stanley, with flying doctor services to the outlying farms and settlements. The hospital in Stanley is effectively the referral centre for a large part of the South Atlantic, with patients being sent from Antarctica, South Georgia, Tristan da Cuhna and many fishing vessels and cruise liners.

The British Antarctic bases are very remote, and expeditions from them are remoter still. It is clear that the definition of remote is a relative term and depends on ones own perspective. I will define remote as being far away from large centres of population, resulting in the need to deal with factors relating to isolation beyond the norm that most doctors will have experienced during their training and career within mainstream medicine.

## Standards

Does being remote mean lower standards? No, not necessarily. A lot of isolated islands and communities are indeed Third World in economic and social terms, since these communities cannot afford sophisticated medical care and have to accept very basic facilities. On the other hand, islands such as the Falklands are relatively wealthy and can afford good standards of care. Large employers such as the Ministry of Defence, the British Antarctic Survey, oil companies and other multinationals expect First-World care for their employees even when they are deployed to very remote, hostile environments.

Even if the location is aspiring to First-World standards, the way that this is achieved may be radically different from "back home".

## Expectations

When working in a new medical environment, it is essential to understand the basic political philosophy of the location and the local expectations for health care. Awareness of these factors is crucial, since one could be providing a level of care that is wholly inadequate, or one could be raising false hopes which are not sustainable. The level of care that is to be provided in any country is essentially a political decision rather than a medical one. What priority does the country put on medical care in relation to defence, education, roads, and the provision of water and sewerage?

Moving from the First World to the developing world, one may come across many paradoxes. We can all think of developing nations where the proportion spent on defence is extraordinarily high, and others where the infrastructure is well developed but the medical services are very basic indeed. There are others where there are superb hospital facilities but no safe water to drink, or children are dying of easily preventable diseases.

In the Falkland Islands, the politicians have put the highest priority on education and medical services. (We already have drinkable water and a reasonable sewage disposal system.) There are modern telecommunications and air links both within the islands and to the outside world. Yet until very recently there were no roads outside of the capital, Stanley. Even now there are only gravel tracks over many of the islands. Most of you will be aware that in 1982 the Argentines invaded the Falklands and a British task force liberated them. Prior to 1982, I think it is fair to describe the medical services as being of Third World standard. With the task force came military medicine, and for the first time the Islands had consultant standard British-style medical services available. Thus overnight, and really without any planning or forethought, the medical services changed dramatically and permanently. In 1984, the existing hospital was totally destroyed by a fire and rapid decisions were required regarding a replacement. A modern, First World complex was constructed within 2 years.

This highlights the crucial point that once standards and public expectations have been raised it is very difficult to revert to previous lower standards. Often these decisions are thrust upon a community by some major catastrophe, and are made very rapidly without careful analysis of the subsequent situation. This is a problem that is particularly relevant to medicine, as these are often the first services to arrive in a country after a catastrophe. Careful thought needs to be given by the aid agencies to avoid raising expectations to levels which are not sustainable.

Expectations of First World medicine in remote areas can create significant dilemmas for clinicians: for example, in the Falkland Islands we are considering whether to set up facilities for cataract surgery rather than send everyone to the UK. Should we consider Third-World type cataract extractions and accept a significant failure rate, or should we insist on First World standards, with some modifications, and accept the increased costs that this would incur? When we have a patient with a complex or difficult medical condition, do we manage the case ourselves or refer the patient to a specialist in the UK knowing that each referral costs the Government significant sums?

## Logistics

There are particular problems in providing a high level of provision 8,000 miles from a logistic base. The supply chain is so long that stock control and the ordering of supplies becomes even more vital than elsewhere. Small numbers of patients cause significant variation in demand; we may have only one patient taking a particular medication when another patient is started on the same treatment, which represents a 100% increase in usage and means that stocks are inadequate. Mini-epidemics of illness can mean a sudden demand for one particular item, and then we run out of stock. Careful thought has to be given to how to cater for the rare but serious conditions. Some items have to be kept in stock even though it is highly unlikely that they will ever be used. On the other hand, a decision could be taken not to cater for rarities and accept that a patient could die as a result.

The purchase of equipment has to be carefully thought out, as maintenance of sophisticated equipment is difficult and potentially very expensive. It is pointless buying sophisticated equipment if it cannot be maintained. Visiting specialists may not always appreciate this and may demand items that are wholly inappropriate.

Quality control in laboratories is a problematical area – just because the laboratory is producing results on paper does not mean that they are reliable. Laboratory machines are temperamental and require careful maintenance, but the technicians also have to be meticulous in their procedures. The only solution to this is to become a member of a quality control scheme such as the British National External Quality Assurance Scheme (NEQAS). This, in itself, has logistic problems about how to ensure that the samples arrive on time and that the results are dispatched in such a way as to be on time.

## Staffing

Remote medical organisations are generally smaller than the more centralised systems that one is familiar with. This means that a smaller number of individuals have to provide the whole range of care. In our experience it is necessary to have General Practitioners who have extended their range of skills. This creates both the challenge and the reward of working in remote areas. One can have the satisfaction of being involved in areas which would be the preserve of a specialist in a less remote setting. On the one hand the diversity of roles expected means that one can never be bored because every day is different, but on the other hand one must be able to accept the challenge of having to deal with unfamiliar situations and cope with the stresses that this can engender.

Recruitment of suitable staff can be difficult as the main drive of First World medicine is towards increasing specialisation and super-specialisation. In the field of surgery in particular, this is creating major difficulties for the remote areas. What is required is the old-fashioned general surgeon who could turn their hand to any surgical problem. A remote community may have a small population and therefore a surgical workload that barely justifies one surgeon let alone a whole range of surgeons who would have virtually nothing to do. There is no easy answer to this problem, although the issue is of major import to the remoter areas and there are also similar problems in the rural areas of Europe, Australia and North America. Unless the training schemes recognise this problem and address it, there will be increasing difficulty in sustaining the standard of surgical provision in remote areas.

## Training

The fading of skill and remaining up-to-date are problems that are relatively easy to resolve if there are sufficient funds available to provide adequate periods of study leave on a regular (annual) basis. One of the problems is that many courses are not appropriate for the remote doctor, either because they are too specialised or because they merely skim the surface and do not provide sufficient detail. However, I have always found doctors in the UK extremely helpful and very willing to assist in any way they can. The onus is on the remote doctors to create their own personalised study schemes.

It is also possible for training to be organised in the remote location. Individuals and organisations are often very excited at the prospect of providing training in a unique environment. As remote organisations tend to be smaller, it is possible for a greater proportion of the staff to have specific training. For example, here in the Falklands all the doctors are ATLS® trained, as are most of the nursing staff. Advanced paediatric life support (APLS®) is being run for all medical and nursing staff later this year, and it is hoped that an advanced life support (ALS®) course will be held within the next 2 years.

Maintaining nurse registration with the United Kingdom Central Council (UKCC) and medical registration with the General Medical Council (GMC) and the Royal Colleges and faculties is perfectly possible but requires more effort and forethought by the individual.

## Major Incident/Disaster Planning

Just because the location is remote does not mean that major incidents and disasters will not occur. For example, in the Falklands there is an international airport and a major aeroplane crash could occur. It is less likely than at Heathrow because there are far fewer flights, but the consequences of a crash for the rescue services would be significant. We also have large cruise liners bringing upwards of 25,000 tourists a year and a major ship fire would cause large numbers of casualties. The deep sea fishing fleet usually has one major incident a year (either a fire or a sinking). Further comments on cruise ships can be found in a separate section.

The relatively small medical services must have a realistic plan to cater for these eventualities. The staff need to be trained and must practice regularly and the equipment levels need to be carefully thought out, as do Medevac procedures and reinforcement/re-supply procedures. Although a major accident does provide serious difficulties for a small organisation there is one major advantage – the same people and organisations are always involved in every incident so we learn from every incident and lessons are not forgotten.

We have found that the ATLS® trauma training promoted by the American College of Surgeons and the Royal College of Surgeons of England is ideally suited to remote locations. ATLS® not only trains the individual, but also gives a clear framework for a major incident plan, including equipment requirements. In our case the equipment requirements were rationalised and this reduced costs significantly. Other courses exist such as BATLS, which adapts ATLS® to the military environment, and Primary Trauma Care, which provides a trauma management template for developing countries.

## The Falkland Islands Experience

A description of the medical services in the Falkland Islands is the clearest way to describe some of the unique features and the fascination of remote medicine, and I hope readers will forgive me for writing at some length about this subject.

The one surgeon is expected to perform all life- and limb-saving surgery, including emergency Caesarean sections. Specialists in such fields as gynaecology, orthopaedics, ophthalmology, urology and ENT visit as required (usually annually) and perform all of the elective surgery. Should a patient require more urgent treatment or more sophisticated investigation or complex surgery they are referred to the UK. Critically ill patients may be flown to Uruguay.

The General Practitioners (GPs) undertake all care that is not surgery or anaesthesia. This includes general practice, accident and emergency, in-patient medical care, obstetrics, paediatrics and geriatrics.

The GPs also provide a flying doctor service to the outlying farms and settlements. There is a daily telephone consultation time for people in the outlying farms to ring in for advice. Each farm or settlement has a "medical chest" which contains a reasonable selection of items to treat most acute conditions. Replacement items are sent through the post. We are often called to treat patients on board ship prior to their transfer ashore. This means going out on the agent's launch, sometimes in bad weather, and climbing the ship's rope ladder, which can be a character-building experience!

Seriously ill patients have to be flown into Stanley and this requires a good working knowledge of aviation medicine, as do the decisions involved in flying critically ill patients to Uruguay. Referral guidelines are helpful in facilitating this kind of decision-making.

The GPs also have a wide range of subsidiary posts and other activities that they are expected to undertake.

- Police surgeon, forensic medicine, advice to the coroner and other legal reports.
- Occupational health, which includes pre-employment medicals, advice on health and safety issues, and specialist medical assessments, e.g. aviation medicine, Merchant Marine medicals, and food-handling medicals for European Community (EC) fish import regulations.
- Public Health matters, e.g. Port Health including de-ratting inspections of ships, inspection of food-handling premises, and advice to the planning and building committee.
- Development of specialist services, e.g. diagnostic ultrasound, endoscopy, slit-lamp examinations, care of patients in the Intensive Care Unit or Coronary Care, and so on.
- The Chief Medical Officer also acts as the Head of a Government Department and therefore has a significant administrative role, including advising the Government on all health-related issues.
- Issues related to interdepartmental liaison and liaison with foreign governments regarding the care of foreign nationals.
- The Chief Medical Officer also has a key role in policy making and planning, which includes the development of a workable major-incident plan.
- The staff have to be able to deal with patients of many nationalities and cultures. It is not unusual to have six languages being spoken in the hospital! Not only are there difficulties with translation, there are problems with different cultures – this can mean that the patient has a totally different concept of their condition and different expectations regarding care. This can be particularly difficult with psychiatrically disturbed patients.

All the medical staff have to live within the community which they treat. This can cause problems both for patients and staff. It can be particularly stressful to have to cope with the serious illness or death of a close friend, but on the other hand it can be extremely rewarding when patients regard you as their friend and advisor as well as their doctor.

Conflicts of interest can develop because of the multidisciplinary role one is expected to undertake. For example, if a patient sees me as their GP, they may tell me something which could have an adverse affect on their employment, and as the Government's medical advisor I would have to advise the Government about that person's fitness to be employed. Whilst these issues are not unique to remote areas they certainly do crop up more often and one must think carefully how to handle each situation.

One of the major advantages of the small, remote medical service is that all services are integrated. There is no differentiation between primary and secondary care; social services and social security are also an integral part of the medical services. The dental service is also totally integrated, which leads to better care for the patients.

I hope that this has given the reader a flavour of the immense satisfaction one can gain from working in a remote setting, and has also demonstrated some of the pitfalls. One needs to be self-confident, enjoy new challenges and have a flexible attitude to all matters.

# Expeditions

Before concluding this part of the manual a few words on expedition medicine are appropriate, and this includes comments on being a ship's doctor at sea.

Expeditions, by their very nature, mean that the team is going to remote, often dangerous regions. The expedition will be far from civilisation and the logistics will be demanding.

The key to successful medical care for an expedition is meticulous planning and also developing a strong relationship with the members of the team, especially the leader and the head of logistics. At the outset there are a number of questions which must be answered.

- What type of expedition is it?
- Where is it going?
- What are the particular risks associated with the activity and location?
- What are the restrictions on size and weight of kit that can be transported?
- How isolated will you be, and for how long? What are the logistics for arranging a Medevac if required?
- Are there any local political or cultural factors to be aware of?
- What are the financial constraints?

All of these factors will play a part in determining the type and range of medicines and equipment required. They will also determine whether there needs to be a medical selection policy for team members. Expeditions where there are sub-groups who may be remote from the main group may need medical kits and appropriate training. The type of expedition and the climatic conditions may require the doctor to acquire specific skills or knowledge, e.g. tropical medicine, diving medicine, care of cold injuries, management of heat stroke, altitude sickness and so on. The increasing trend for "round the world" sailing rallies brings particular problems in that the yachts may be separated by considerable distances and radio advice may be necessary. Appropriate crew selection and training can ensure that there are some medical skills available on each yacht.

Each expedition will have its own particular logistic difficulties, but I think it is worth mentioning a few very particular points.

Climbing at high altitude is highly dangerous and is usually in very remote and inaccessible areas. Detailed planning and discussion with the local medical services, rescue services and military authorities will clarify what is and is not possible. Can the rescue services get to you rapidly, and can you communicate with them? In the Himalayas there is often the problem that rescue helicopters cannot fly above a certain altitude.

Expeditions that involve diving require careful consideration of how to deal with decompression sickness. Where is the nearest compression chamber and do you need to have one with the expedition?

Round-the-world rallies or other long-distance expeditions create a multiplicity of problems, as the logistics will vary according to the expedition location. The diseases and injuries that are to be expected will also vary according to location.

Psychological problems are common during expeditions, especially those which are hazardous and when things start to go wrong. This is where the pre-expedition planning and relationship building become crucial. If there is a medical catastrophe such as serious illness, accident or death, then the strength of the relationship between the doctor and the rest of the expedition will be tested. It is vital that the expedition leader has total confidence in the doctor's abilities and advice. It is also essential that the doctor's advice is clear, concise, practical and appropriate; the doctor must be assertive, but at the same time accept that the team leader's decision is final.

Climbing expeditions seem particularly prone to personality clashes. This is partly due to the difficulties faced in climbing at high altitude, but also to the fact that the personalities of successful climbers tend to be very dominant. The team leader often has a difficult choice as to which members should be in the summit team. The doctor can be of enormous moral support to the leader or can be very destructive.

Some expeditions require the doctor to be as fit as the other team members. There is also the risk that the doctor may become the patient! What contingency plans have you made for this? Are you emotionally strong enough to cope with the death or serious injury of a team member whom you will have become very close to during the expedition?

## Ships' Doctors

I intend to discuss only cruise liners and will make no mention of military ships. In my experience there are two quite distinct types of provision of medical services on board cruise liners. The larger companies have permanent medical staff, which may be supplemented by temporarily employed doctors. Smaller companies employ a succession of temporary doctors and generally do not pay them, but give substantial discounts on the holiday to the doctor and possibly their family.

It may be obvious, but I think it is worth stating, that once the ship is at sea you are on your own medically speaking and you have to deal with all emergencies with whatever facilities are available. Generally most of the passengers are elderly, as these seem to be the only people with enough money and time to go on cruises. Cruises can go to very remote areas; for instance there are upwards of 25,000 passengers sailing to the Antarctic every year and calling at the Falkland Islands. The average age on these ships is over 70, and 90-year-olds are common! There is no medical screening of potential passengers and many passengers are, in my opinion, wholly unfit for this kind of adventure. However, the ship's doctor is unlikely to have any say in passenger selection. Many of the passengers come from countries where the standard of health care is high, and also where there is a philosophy of litigation.

The equipment and medical supplies on board cruise liners can vary dramatically. At the one extreme the well-equipped ship will have a mini-intensive care unit with superb facilities including on-board laboratories, X-ray facilities and the ability to have telemedicine consultations with a medical centre of excellence. It is important to bear in mind, however, that sometimes the quality control of the laboratory equipment may be suspect. At the other extreme are cruise liners where the equipment is inadequate, broken, dangerous or just missing. Drugs may be out of date and critical drugs may be absent. These problems appear to be more common on the ships which use a succession of unpaid doctors who are having a subsidised holiday.

You may also be faced with drugs from foreign countries with which you may not be familiar. Passengers may not speak your language and may have wholly different expectations from yours.

Do check the situation regarding medical malpractice insurance and be very suspicious if the company makes vague statements that it will cover you. Make sure you see the insurance documentation and/or insure yourself with a reputable malpractice insurance organisation.

Remember also that once the ship is at sea it is too late to complain about the lack of facilities, so do try to get as much information as possible prior to the journey and also do go through the medical inventory very carefully when you board the ship. Mentally go through a checklist of what you will need for the most common emergencies – is it all there? If you are seriously concerned regarding the quality of medical facilities available you must make these concerns known to the captain and demand that they are rectified as far as possible prior to sailing. You may also have to communicate with the ship's owners and/or the tour organisers and express your concerns in writing.

Lastly, remember that once at sea the ship's captain is the boss! Normally the captain will listen to sensible medical advice, but sometimes weather or other factors may dictate a course of action which you, as the doctor, might disagree with. Be firm, clear, realistic and assertive, but having said all that accept the captain's decision with good grace.

This may sound like doom and gloom! Many doctors have had wonderful holidays as ship's doctors, but every now and then there is a disaster story. Forewarned is forearmed.

# Part C – Medicine at the Ends of the Earth
Iain C. Grant

| Objectives | • To give an insight into medical care in cold and remote environments. |
|---|---|

## Introduction

Very high latitudes probably provide the most remote settings in which a doctor can practise. Such settings are so unusual that they have been described as the "Fourth World". However, organisations that routinely deploy personnel to the Polar Regions demand a service that is as close to that of the First World as practicable.

Polar medicine derives it identity from the geographical location and the nature of the environment in which it is practised. There is no physiological process which makes polar medicine different from other branches of medicine, as there is for example in hyperbaric work. It is simply the remoteness, the hostility and the unforgiving nature of the environment in which man struggles to survive, let alone work, which makes polar medicine so challenging.

Even to define "polar" regions is far from easy. The Arctic and Antarctic circles lie at latitudes 66°33′ North and South, respectively, and at these latitudes, on at least one day a year, the sun does not rise or set. The 10°C isotherm (i.e. where the maximum temperature does not exceed this figure) correlates quite well with this defined area, but it is at greater latitudes and considerably more extreme temperatures that the British Antarctic Survey (BAS) and other organisations undertake the majority of polar science and exploration.

While both poles of the earth share common attributes of cold, dark and severe weather, the two ends of the earth are very different. The Arctic is a sea surrounded by land, while the Antarctic is a land mass surrounded by ocean. As a result, Antarctica is colder and considerably drier. The average winter temperature at the South Pole is almost 40°C colder than that at the North Pole. The Antarctic plateau is more similar in climate to Mars than to the rest of the earth. It is a frozen desert, much of it above 10,000 feet, where little in the way of natural life forms can exist.

There are indigenous people in the Arctic. Throughout Northern America, Europe and Asia, native peoples carve out an existence, living all year round in the area. Medicine among these peoples is like that in any other aboriginal population. In the Antarctic, however, the population is transient. There are scientists, explorers and tourists. Most of those who visit, and certainly all who stay for the long harsh winter, are young, fit and carefully medically screened before they are permitted to journey

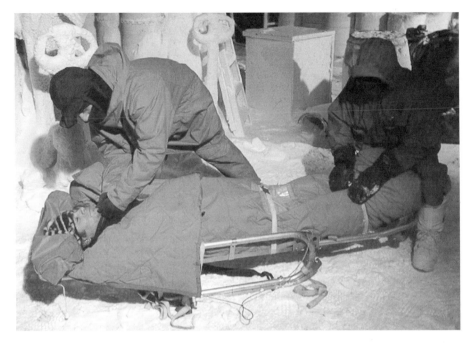

**Fig. 5.1.** Casualty handling at Halley.

south. Nevertheless, injury and illness do occur. In recent years tourism has steadily increased, the geopolitical importance of the polar regions is increasingly recognised, and more and more research takes place. NASA has recognised the analogies with space travel, which Antarctic isolation provides at a fraction of the cost of actual space flight. Polar medicine grows in importance with the "development" of the continent.

Perhaps, above all else, it is the isolation that makes polar, and particularly Antarctic, medicine unique. Anywhere else in the world it is usually possible to arrange a medical evacuation within at most a few days. At Halley, one of the British research stations, in winter, such an arrangement may not be possible for several months. A doctor practising polar medicine must be self-reliant. The welfare of the doctor, the patients and other base members depends upon it (Fig. 5.1).

Evidence on which to base medical decision-making in polar regions is extremely sparse. The principles of trauma care, environmental and occupational medicine, and of the management of emergencies undoubtedly apply to polar medicine as they do in temperate zones, but the detail of Western medicine does not necessarily translate well to the polar environment. The doctor needs to become more self-reliant, to develop clinical judgement and at the same time learn to depend less on investigations (which are simply not available). Prevention and preparation are both of increased significance in polar isolation where treatment may be more difficult.

Where lives are at stake, it is possible to argue that planning should be for the worse-case scenario rather than for likely events. This philosophy has to be tempered to some extent by realism as far as costs and benefits are concerned. This results in Antarctic bases which are equipped to an adequate but necessarily lower level in terms of therapeutic equipment than can be expected in a hospital. The doctor cannot be too specialised in approach; a broad knowledge and a wide range of practical skills are necessary to provide good polar medical care. In small bases, where fewer than 25 personnel over-winter, there is no room for the luxury of anaesthetists and surgeons, dermatologists and psychiatrists. These roles all reside with the same person.

Modern developments in communication and information technology help make the polar physician less isolated from advice and counsel, but it remains impossible to physically evacuate patients or provide specialist skills "in person" to a substantial proportion of the polar population for the majority of the year. The doctor is an important member of the polar team and must strive to maintain the highest practicable standards.

The "generalist" is a very rare medical animal nowadays. Increasingly, doctors become more specialised at an earlier stage in their careers. Therefore, recruiting Antarctic doctors is based more on the person than on their curriculum vitae. Training can help to provide the necessary knowledge and skills, but cannot produce the type of person who will participate and contribute in the widest sense in a winter community in an Antarctic station.

Doctors come from a wide range of backgrounds. In recent years, anaesthetists, general practitioners and emergency physicians have formed the majority of appointees. These doctors spend between 6 and 9 months preparing for deployment, during which time they acquire practical skills and specialised knowledge. Most BAS doctors undertake a diploma or masters degree in Remote Healthcare at the University of Plymouth during their preparation and deployment, and undertake research while deployed which can form the basis for a master's dissertation on their return.

## Antarctic Medical Problems

### Physical Health Problems

In British Antarctic bases, the vast majority of the work for the doctor is of a routine, relatively minor, nature (Fig. 5.2).

Many of the somatic health problems in Antarctica have to do with cold, altitude and trauma. In a midwinter setting, where a cup of tea thrown in the air freezes before it hits the ground, the dangers of cold injury are obvious. It has been estimated that in winter an inactive person in full "polar" clothing can have a drop in core temperature to life-threatening levels in less than 30 min. Cold injury is also frequent (if usually minor), and particular care is needed when handling liquids at low ambient temperatures where even a small accidental splash can mean instant frostbite.

It is not only patients who suffer from the effects of cold. Medical equipment is often not designed to function at these extremes of temperature; plastics become

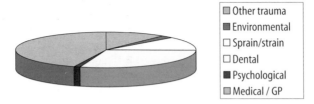

**Fig. 5.2.** Approximate breakdown of the medical workload in British Antarctic Stations 1995–1998.

brittle, metal is untouchable, fluids are impossible to keep liquid, and necessary clothing simply gets in the way. The unpredictability of the weather makes rescue difficult and sometimes dangerous, and rescuers and medical staff must be constantly wary lest they themselves become victims.

Much of the fieldwork in Antarctica is carried out at a relatively high altitude. Most bases are at, or close to, sea level, and ascents tend to be rapid as field parties are air-lifted straight onto the plateau. At the South Pole, a weight loss of 5 kg in the first week has been reported. This is attributable to resting tachypnoea and tachycardia, emphasising the physiological stress applied by such rapid ascent.

In summer, the combined effects of an ozone hole and reflection from snow with a ground albedo of 80–90% can rapidly become painfully evident to the unwary.

Nutrition has always been important in polar expeditions. Fresh food is at best available for the short summer season in limited amounts. For most of the year there is total reliance on dried, frozen and tinned foodstuffs. On expeditions away from base, the amount and type of food that can be carried is limited. There is therefore much reliance on dehydrated meals, which are lightweight and easy to prepare with limited equipment. Energy requirements are high, with the allowance on field trips being about 3,500 calories per person per day, but meeting this simple nutritional goal can be very difficult in the ill patient. Field rations and hard work can lead to considerable drops in body fat, increased high-density lipoprotein (HDL) cholesterol, increased overall strength and a paradoxical drop in aerobic power.

Vegetables are relatively scarce, but other sources of fibre and vitamins are available. Personnel need to be encouraged to take supplements, and medical officers should be alert for vitamin deficiencies. Shackleton (to many the greatest Antarctic explorer) was himself sent home from an early expedition suffering from scurvy. While theoretically this should not be possible today, sub-clinical vitamin deficiencies remain a possibility, especially in those who have undertaken two consecutive winter stays. Conversely, of course, with relative inactivity and the free availability of high-calorie diets, those who over winter have a temptation to eat too much and a tendency to gain weight. The doctor needs to be active in promoting healthy eating at all times.

There has been much speculation about the immunosuppressive effects of Antarctic life. There is evidence of leucopoenia and depression of cell-mediated immunity during winter isolation, but the clinical effects of this are not fully understood. Many current studies are attempting to explore apparent viral reactivation and the longer-term effects of possible immune suppression.

A number of studies have investigated the effects of constant darkness on circadian rhythms, melatonin and other hormonal mechanisms. Significant biochemical disturbances have been reported (e.g. the "polar T3 syndrome", where marked drops in free thyroxine were demonstrated in US over-wintering personnel), but the clinical significance of these findings remains uncertain.

## Environmental, Occupational and Public Health

Under the terms of the Antarctic Treaty, environmental pollution is strictly regulated, with responsible waste management being undertaken by most nations. However, the environment in Antarctica is extremely sensitive, and personnel must be ever vigilant to prevent personal inadvertent pollution by even minor spillage of toxins. At one stage there was a nuclear reactor at the American station McMurdo. Early problems prompted the removal of this particular potential disaster, but fossil fuel remains a requirement, and the potential for dramatic oil spillage exists and requires careful monitoring.

The mere disposal of clinical waste, so easy to get rid of in hospitals, needs careful thought in terms of how and where it can be stored, and how it can safely be removed from the continent for safe permanent disposal.

Trauma is probably the single most important medical problem in Antarctica. Although many injuries are minor, the potential for severe trauma exists and it is incumbent on the Medical Officer to help as far as possible in accident prevention. Interestingly, in several reports, the incidence of trauma has been higher during leisure than in work activities.

Adherence to strict occupational health guidelines may be more difficult at remote work sites. The availability of mechanical handling devices may be limited, and where these are present there may be practical difficulties in their use in certain circumstances. The potential for manual handling injuries is high, and the doctor must be vigilant in observing lifting practises and the technique of each individual. Noise pollution, over-use and repetitive work syndromes have all been reported.

Fire is a major hazard in Antarctica where, because of low humidity, wooden buildings become very dry, while the availability of water for fire fighting can be very limited. At least four major fires have occurred, thankfully with few deaths or serious injuries. However, the base members of the Russian Vostock station had to spend 8 months without a power plant to supply heat after a fire. When one considers that Vostock is the place where the coldest temperatures on earth have been recorded, the feat of endurance involved is almost incredible.

Air safety is also a serious concern. The majority of the deaths in the US Antarctic programme have been aircraft-related. The doctor must be vigilant for signs of stress and physical illness among aircrew, and may have to be quite forceful in resisting operational pressures to allow a sick pilot to continue flying. Pilots' hours are limited by law. In a busy Antarctic summer it is possible for a pilot to "run out of hours", and the doctor will be involved in an application to the Civil Authorities for an extension.

The expanding tourism industry in the area increases the potential for medical problems. Tourists are often elderly, have little or no medical screening before departure, and may themselves considerably underestimate the rigours of even a short trip on land in Antarctica. There is much debate about the responsibility of government-sponsored organisations to provide a medical response and care for tourists, and this poses interesting medico-legal questions. On this issue, the BAS position is to encourage self-reliance by tour operators. The BAS achieves this by supporting the policy of the International Association of Antarctic Tour Operators (IAATO) to maintain adequate levels of medical screening, cover and contingency planning.

## Psychological Health Problems

Psychological "problems" have been reported since the earliest polar expeditions. The lifestyle in Antarctica does put personnel under extreme pressure and minor adjustment problems are not infrequent, although more serious ones are thankfully rare. On most bases alcohol is freely available, and irrespective of advice from doctors and policies imposed by management, some base members will use alcohol as a coping strategy, sometimes to excess. This can lead to problems of competence at work as well as antisocial behaviour, aggression and personal ill health.

The effects of psychological stresses on the immune system are recognised but poorly understood, but it seems likely that further work will prove this to be an important factor.

The effects of social isolation, disillusion with the reality of Antarctic life when compared with expectations, the severity of the environment and the closed nature of the communities are all potential stressors which are encountered more frequently in polar regions. The doctor needs to have a basic understanding of small-group dynamics and should be aware of described "syndromes" such as seasonal affective disorder (SAD) although this may be no more prevalent in Antarctica than at lower latitudes) and the so-called "winter-over syndrome". Mood swings are common among personnel and do not necessarily imply maladjustment. The working group in human biology and medicine of the Scientific Committee on Antarctic Research (SCAR) has for many years been trying to identify and quantify "abnormal" adaptation to Antarctic life, but with only limited success. Most of the "symptoms" of maladjustment can be "normal", and it is a difficult task for the doctor to weigh often multiple factors in assessing an individual and deciding who actually needs help.

Many countries use formal psychological screening tests in the selection of personnel, especially for over-wintering posts, but there is no agreement as to which of the many available tests are valid in the Antarctic environment. There is currently little evidence as to whether these screening tests improve outcome, although research now underway may help to clarify this contentious issue. Some national programmes also undertake formal debriefing of Antarctic winterers, but again the benefits are unclear.

# Arctic Medical Problems

Healthcare in the Arctic has lagged behind that in other parts of the same countries, with higher infant mortality, shorter life expectancy, and a higher incidence of diseases such as tuberculosis. There remain problems with parasitic diseases, which reflect the lifestyle of the indigenous peoples, and at the same time increased contact with "civilisation" increases exposure to other infective disease, and industrialisation poses concerns over environmental health. Alcohol abuse is reportedly very prevalent, the problems of isolation cannot be ignored, and the incidence of seasonal affective disorder may be as high as 20%.

Polar medicine poses great challenges to the doctor. The workload is often low and remaining motivated, continuing education and maintaining skill levels can be difficult. The doctor is subjected to the same stresses as the rest of the population, yet is expected by peers to rise above this and be unaffected. A special type of person is required to succeed. My best wishes go with all who read this chapter and do embark on a polar expedition.

# Further Reading

Auerbach PS, editor. Wilderness medicine: the management of wilderness and environmental emergencies. Philadelphia: Mosby, 1995.

Dupont HL, Steffen R, editors. Textbook of travel medicine and health. Hamilton: Decker, 1997.

Health aspects of work in extreme climates within the exploration and production industry. The cold. London: Exploration and Production Forum, 1998; 6.65/270. The heat. London: Exploration and Production Forum, 1998; 6.70/279.

Health assessment of fitness to work in the exploration and production industry. London: Exploration and Production Forum, 1995; 6.46/228.

Health management guidelines for remote land-based geophysical operations. London: Exploration and Production Forum, 1993; 6.30/190.

Hobbs BC, Roberts D. Food poisoning and food hygiene. London: Edward Arnold, 1987.

Mark R, Tomlins M. Medicine in remote places. In: Greaves I, Porter KM, editors. Prehospital medicine: the principles and practice of immediate care. London: Arnold, 1999.

Standards for local medical support. London: Exploration and Production Forum, 1995; 6.44/222.

Stevenson D, editor. The control of disease in the tropics: a handbook for physicians and other workers in tropical and international community health. London: Lewis, 1987.

Stoy WA, Klein J. International first responder. London: Mosby Lifeline, 1998.

UK Offshore Operators Association Ltd. Guidelines for medical aspects of fitness for offshore work: a guide for examining physicians. Aberdeen: UKOOA, 1995.

# 6. Medical Interventions in Catastrophes and Conflict

Alan Hawley

**Objectives**

- To examine the concept of medical intervention in conflict and catastrophes.
- To discuss decision making.
- To describe risk assessment.
- To describe the problems associated with intervention.

## Introduction

In this chapter, the concepts of medical intervention in the event of a catastrophe or a conflict will be examined and analysed. A convenient starting point, therefore, is an understanding of the terms involved. A medical intervention is an action taken by an agency in order to remedy a medical shortfall or problem. As such it does not necessarily have to be purely clinical in nature. Rather, it must simply address a medical requirement in the target population. Its delivery may be undertaken by a variety of non-medical agencies such as food-relief programmes. Similarly, a catastrophe or conflict is an event which has produced an inability to cope with the extra humanitarian demands consequent upon the incident. Such a mismatch between demand and supply may be temporary, as in earthquake recovery in developed nations like Japan, or be long-term and seemingly intractable, as in many cases of internal conflict in Africa.

Whilst there are some clear differences between a natural disaster in a developed country and a post-conflict situation in a developing nation, there are also some similarities. Firstly, both events are likely to produce the same mixture of shock, bewilderment and loss amongst the affected population. Such a combination may at least compromise, if not render impossible, coherent and effective immediate responses from that unfortunate group. Thus additional assistance will almost certainly be required, and this may come from the national government and its agencies or from the international community. A myriad of possible helping hands can be proffered from the small non-governmental organisations (NGOs), through to the established international organisations (such as the International Committee of the Red Cross or Médecin sans Frontières) or even inter-governmental or international coordinated responses possibly involving the military. Equally, this scale of response will have been at least partially generated by the shared sense of shock and sympathy which cataclysmic events evoke in the global public. Such a response is likely to impel, and possibly compel, governments (particularly those of liberal democracies) to offer humanitarian intervention as an answer to the problem.

Such a reaction may paradoxically aggravate the problem. Hastily mounted expeditions to alleviate obvious human distress and devastation may themselves become part of the problem. Inadequate preparation, poor equipment, ill-focused priorities and sheer logistical non-sustainability may lead to the helpers needing help themselves and so detract from the main effort. In the maelstrom of an immediate response to a crisis, philanthropy is a poor substitute for professionalism.

Yet since the Berlin Wall came down, symbolising the ending of the Cold War, the need for humanitarian intervention has mushroomed. In many cases this has been due to the increased regional political instability that has accompanied the loss of surrogate control consequent upon the passing of the Soviet Union. In addition to this, there has been a more than usually high incidence of natural disasters as well as major industrial accidents such as Chernobyl and Bhopal. Governments and NGOs have responded to these needs with a varying record of success. All possible combinations of agencies have been deployed during these responses and much has been learnt. Working together under the difficulties of humanitarian relief has generated mutual understanding and respect between uniformed and civilian agencies. Preconception and prejudice are uncomfortable bedfellows with success in a multi-agency response to a clear human need. It is entirely likely that this process of coordinated response between all agencies will continue. Accordingly, it behoves all involved to ensure that both professionally and personally they are able to undertaken their part of the enterprise.

## The Decision to Intervene

Regardless of whether the projected humanitarian team is uniformed or civilian, a decision process will have to be followed prior to deployment. Naturally the process will be dependent upon the culture and standing operating procedures of that particular organisation. Equally, these will differ both within NGOs and between military and civilian agencies. However, the end point of the process will be to decide whether to deploy, and if so what to deploy. A key consideration will be the likely and foreseeable effects of deployment by that particular agency.

- Can they offer something worthwhile to the situation?
- If so, can this be delivered at an affordable cost?
- Will this cost be purely financial, or are there foreseeable opportunity costs (there will always be a potential for unforeseen opportunity costs)?
- Are there other predictable constraints?
- What are the consequences of deployment for the organisation?

This is a sample of the questions which an organisation will have to answer before committing itself to the rigours and challenges of a humanitarian operation. Many of these questions are hard-nosed issues of cost–benefit analysis. Disquieting as this may be to pure humanitarians and philanthropists, it reflects the reality that resources are finite and the decision to commit them needs careful consideration and justification.

Responses to human need in catastrophes and conflict are essentially concerned with facets of the human condition. These are at heart people decisions made by people for people. Care is an intensely human concept with profound ethical and practical underpinnings. At the centre of all decisions to commit humanitarian resources to a specific operation is this commitment to care. Yet in the rush to actually deploy, the continuing requirement to care for the deploying team may be missed. The pace of events, the excitement and the anticipation may cloud the normal approach to the duty of care. This is the commitment which all organisations must have to their individual members. Not only is there a clear moral basis for this, but increasingly there is also a legal requirement. In order to ensure its correct application, the example of risk assessment familiar to many in occupational medicine is a suitable approach to adopt.

First, two small definitions to aid the application of risk assessment methodology. A *hazard* is a substance (or for our purpose an exposure) which has the potential to cause harm to individuals. A *risk* is a measure of the probability of harm actually resulting from an exposure.

Although originally designed for application within the Control of Substances Hazardous to Health legislation, this process of analysing risk is very useful when applied to all exposures which are likely to be encountered. The method is shown in outline in Table 6.1. This shows the initial stage as being the identification of a hazard. Following this, an estimate of likely exposures is required which, when taken in conjunction with hazard identification, allows some sort of assessment of the risk. Risk management follows risk assessment, which process allows a number of different techniques to be tried. These include hazard elimination, containment of the exposure, limiting the duration and concentration of exposures to individuals, and finally complete protection of the personnel. Some imagination is required to adapt the process to the requirements of humanitarian operations, but a suitable context can be derived from the methodology.

The types of hazard normally considered are shown in Table 6.2. They are conveniently considered as a set of separate types of hazard. However, experience shows that operations will invariably involve more than one type of hazard in each scenario. Equally, individual susceptibilities will vary as a result of biological variation as well as:

- previous operational experience,
- past medical history,
- family and social circumstances,
- earlier exposures to hazards.

All these will need consideration and due weighting must be accorded.

Prior to deployment to Rwanda in July 1994, this particular process was followed by the British Army contingent deploying as part of the United Nations force

**Table 6.1.**  The risk assessment process in outline

Hazard identification
   Physical: heat, light, cold, radiation
   Chemical: gases, vapours, dusts
   Biological: animal, plant, bacterial, viral
   Mechanical: lifting, posture
   Psychosocial: stress, isolation, lack of support

Risk indentification
   Which of the hazards actually exist and in which form?

Risk assessment
   High, medium or low risk, dependent upon degree of exposure
     to risk and individual vulnerability

Risk management
   Avoid exposure
   Control exposure
     Rotate individuals through exposures
     Substitute harmful substances/procedures with lower risk
       options
   Protect individuals by other means
     Personal protective measures
     Vaccinations

Surveillance
   Health surveillance relevant to risk
     Routine examinations
     Blood markers
     Psychological support

**Table 6.2.**  Types of hazard

Physical: heat, cold, climate, light, dryness, wetness, electricity, other
   radiations, vibrations, noise
Chemical: gases, vapours, solids, dusts, solvents
Biological: large animals, smaller animals, plants, bacteria, virus,
   fungi, other microbiological entities
Mechanical: lifting, loading and unloading, pulling, pushing, trips,
   falls, dropped objects
Psychosocial: stress, bereavement, isolation, fear, uncertainty

(UNAMIR). All potential hazards were identified and possible corrective actions considered. As a result, a plan for the management of foreseeable risk was put together as well as the beginnings of a health surveillance plan for the eventual return to the United Kingdom. This process is shown in detail in Table 6.3. Points of particular note include the significance of the biological and psychosocial aspects. Whilst most people will be familiar with the biological hazards of refugee work in tropical Africa, the psychological aspects are rather more covert and provide a suitable example to demonstrate the risk assessment tool.

**Table 6.3.**   Risk assessment process for the UK military contingent to Rwanda 1994

Hazard identification
Physical
  Climate (dry season followed by wet season halfway through deployment)
  Light (sub-equatorial Africa)
  Heat (sub-equatorial Africa)
  Trauma (conflict)

Chemical
  Usual range of solvents and preservatives in workshops

Biological
  Insects (biting and local lesions)
  Range of disease entities including cholera, dysentery, typhus, malaria, rabies, HIV, tuberculosis, meningitis

Mechanical
  Usual activities involved in loading, unloading, moving and deploying a unit

Psychosocial
  The unknown
  Genocide and war
  Separation from loved ones
  Stress of working in refugee camps

Risk identification
As per hazard identification

Risk assessment
Some of the elements of the force were more likely to be exposed to some risks than others. Thus, the medics were more
  likely to be exposed to the full range of biological and psychological risks than those involved in supporting the operation from HQ. Equally, some groups have a traditional closeness and support mechanism enabling them to cope with
  risks better than others. Notable in this regard were the Royal Engineers, who have a tightly knit organisation with a
  strong support ethos.

Risk management
Fit for deployment, including personal circumstances and social relationships
Safe food and water
Vaccinations against all the major biological hazards
Malaria prophylaxis (including covering up at biting times, use of mosquito nets, insecticides, no standing water etc.)
Open attitude to stress and its management, briefings to all (including loved ones), monitoring of all personnel through-
  out deployment, regular contact with home through telephone and mail, adequate breaks from duties in refugee
  camps, follow-up on return to UK

Surveillance
  Regular monitoring of all personnel throughout deployment
  Ready access to medical and psychological assistance in the deployment
  Psychological follow-up by questionnaire and personal consultation
  Random stool sampling

The psychosocial hazards were split into a number of separate specifics: separation, apprehension, problems dealing with refugee populations, problems dealing
with orphans, difficulties with death, genocide and murder, and finally dealing with
unexpected incidents of maximum stress.

Next, an assessment of the susceptibility of different components of the force to these hazards was made, so that the engineers and medics were expected to be maximally exposed to them whilst it was recognised that all components were exposed to some degree. This had to be further refined to identify susceptible individuals within the components since such qualities vary greatly within populations. Having achieved this stage, it was then necessary to develop a risk management strategy. The initial step was a full briefing given both to members of the contingent and to their families. This explained the nature of the deployment and the likely tasks and conditions to be met. The psychological aspects of the operation were covered so that there was complete transparency of the possible difficulties. The responsibilities of team leaders to ensure the health and safety of their personnel were emphasised, and the channels of support within the unit for both the leaders and the other individuals were rehearsed. In the case of the problems in dealing with refugees, orphans and the consequences of genocide and murder, the total elimination of exposure was impossible by virtue of the humanitarian task to be undertaken. Instead, a policy of controlled exposure on a rotation basis of working in refugee camps was employed, along with a focused and active leisure time programme. In addition, a welfare strategy allowing frequent contact by letter and telephone with loved ones in the UK helped to support everybody in the trying circumstances of the camps. Such a policy helped those left behind at home to continue to play their part in supporting the deployed force. An important element of this process was the production of weekly videos, which were sent back from Rwanda and showed the contingent at work. Prior to return to the UK at the conclusion of the deployment, all individuals took part in re-patriation groups where the accumulated experience of months work in Rwanda could be put into context with the normal pressures and tensions of home life. Simultaneously, the families of the deployed force received leaflets explaining the circumstances under which the tour had been completed and the normal range of reactions to be expected. On returning home, the entire contingent worked as usual for 3 weeks whilst staying together, and then going on leave. Lastly, there was a follow-up of personnel by questionnaire, with referral to psychiatric assistance as identified by this means or by medical attendants. Such a complete programme of psychological risk assessment and management is unusually detailed and full. This was partly due to the inclusion of a consultant psychiatrist as part of the contingent, as well as a high index of suspicion of the psychological aspects of the operations that was entirely in keeping with the accumulated experience of the force. Psychological aspects are discussed further in a later chapter. However, this process of risk assessment is required of any command element about to commit its personnel on operations of whatever kind. Failure to follow it, or something like it, constitutes a neglect of the duty of care.

## The Act of Intervention

Essential questions, which must be posed and answered before the deployment, are listed below.

- What is our aim?
- What are we trying to achieve?
- Why are we trying to achieve it?

Again, these fundamental concepts can be overlooked in the race to respond rapidly to an actual or an emerging humanitarian crisis. However, they are crucially important, since they define the ethical and practical context of the proposed action. In essence, what is required is *a mission statement.*
A mission statement gives the task and its purpose.

*"You are to provide such and such in order that this may be enabled."*

Again considering the British Contingent in Rwanda in 1994, the initial deployment saw the medical element, with some engineering and communications support, being deployed to the northwest of the country. They were told to provide medical support to refugees in that region. Since the situation was extremely fluid, with over 1 million refugees living at Goma Camp just over the border in Zaire, and with sporadic continuing violence in the area, this mission was re-interpreted as:

*"To provide humanitarian assistance in the northwest of the country in order to encourage Rwandan refugees to return from Zaire."*

This statement gives a clear task (to provide humanitarian assistance, note not just medical support) and an equally clear purpose (to encourage Rwandan refugees to return from Zaire). Accordingly, a basis for planning and prioritisation has now been provided. All actions can be measured against this mission. Anything which does not assist its successful completion should be disregarded. Conversely, success can be assessed by how far this mission is met.
In the case of Rwanda, the British contingent treated 4,500 people in 10 days (as well as repairing hydroelectric facilities and water supplies). At first sight this is a good return on the investment. However, closer inspection revealed that none of those treated were refugees; they were local people. Whilst there was an undoubted medical need, it lay outside of the mission statement. At the same time, in the south west of the country, the French military were preparing to withdraw from the humanitarian protection zone (HPZ) that they had established earlier in the year. In the HPZ were an estimated 1.5 million internally displaced people (IDPs). These were overwhelmingly Hutu people who had fled their homes on the advance of the Rwandan Patriotic Army (RPA). This was a largely Tutsi dominated army and was victorious in the war which had followed the genocide of Tutsis and moderate Hutus. The occupation of the HPZ had led the RPA to stay outside its borders. As a result, the Hutu IDPs had been reassured by the overt French military presence, which was taken as a guarantee of their continued safety from Tutsi revenge attacks. The projected withdrawal of the French now threatened to undermine that confidence, with the consequent fears that the IDPs would follow the troops into Zaire and the catastrophic problems of Goma would be repeated. In order to prevent this, the British element in the northwest was redeployed to the HPZ. Its mission was re-cast as follows:

*"To provide humanitarian assistance in order to persuade the IDPs to stay in Rwanda."*

Again, a clear distinction between task and purpose can be seen. Using this mission, a new plan was developed which recognised the changed circumstances of the new location and its political, demographic, geographical and humanitarian factors. It was also useful as an audit measure. Within 1 week of deploying and operating in the HPZ, the British contingent had the satisfaction of seeing the exodus of IDPs fall from 20,000 a day to zero. The mission was being accomplished, and in so doing untold thousands of lives were being saved by the avoidance of inadequate humanitarian provision in Zaire.

The mission statement goes a long way towards answering the fundamental questions of how and why. There will remain other queries about what. Any major catastrophe or conflict will produce many different needs. It is understandable that medical personnel will see these needs as being largely medical in nature. After all, it is precisely this dimension in which health care professionals have been laboriously and expensively trained. However, rather than resorting to a default-type response, a dispassionate view of the circumstances is required. *An ability to provide a specific capability is not a necessary justification for actually employing it.* Rather, there needs to be an actual requirement on the ground. As has previously been pointed out, most of the need (even if not actually medical) has significant health implications and consequences. We are, after all, considering the needs of a population in distress. As such, it is useful if health care professionals always keep in the back of their mind the different elements which comprise the usual range of human needs. In extremis, human needs focus on food, shelter, water, sanitation, security and health. Health needs and interventions will be considered in the next section. The others will be discussed below.

Security is an underpinning requirement, especially in post-conflict situations. Even in natural disasters there may be elements of opportunistic criminality. When all has been lost and a sense of shock and bewilderment surrounds everything, the need for a sense of personal security can be enormous. Naturally this requirement extends to the other members of a family or similar tightly knit group. Equally, in many conflict and post-conflict situations, security may only be guaranteed by the presence of some sort of law enforcement capability. It must also be remembered that a uniformed presence may not always be reassuring to a displaced population, particularly if similar armed groups have been responsible for the refugees' plight. So security is more than a situation of law enforcement. It is a perception and belief that the needs of the individual and the social group are met, including the requirement for personal safety. It is the aggregation of all the factors and dimensions together which comprise a sense of well-being and fulfilment. The usual enabler for this circumstance is an acknowledged and accepted rule of law. Sadly, post-conflict situations, particularly civil wars, frequently result in the complete tearing up of the social fabric and all the corresponding instruments of law and order. In such a time of human despair and shortage, it is hardly surprising if some elements take advantage of the situation to gain some advantage. However, the evidence suggests that this is a relatively infrequent occurrence; most people respect the social norms as regulators of conduct.

Insecurity and violence affect not only the refugee or displaced population, but may also directly impinge on the operations and safety of the humanitarian workers. There has been a steady and tragic loss of life amongst the humanitarian community. Violence against them has become a perennial feature. This may result from a sense of the political implications of their work, particularly if they are being successful. This is especially relevant in the confused but heightened political tensions accompanying a conflict. In such circumstances, humanitarian assistance may make the difference between life and death for many people. This presents a clear opportunity for the application of power and leverage over a target population. After all, in starvation conditions, food is power, food is life. The control of these resources has an obvious political attraction. Such a situation prevailed in the refugee camps set up in the northern region of the former Zaire following the 1994 Rwandan genocide and war. The Hutu militants attempted to control the provision of humanitarian assistance in the camps as a vehicle for political organisation and control over the Rwandan Hutu refugees. This posed a real ethical dilemma for many of the NGOs, since to continue the delivery of aid would be to assist the establishment of the political legitimacy of the perpetrators of the genocide. Without such assistance, many of the refugees would suffer further. This is truly a dilemma whose resolution needs consideration of the ethical, legal and security factors.

Therefore, security can be increased by the usual techniques of providing law and order. Existing and acceptable organs of law enforcement may be reinforced or assisted, depending upon the legitimacy and degree of popular support. Care may need to be exercised to ensure that any external forces brought into the country do not arrive with any residual or historical connotations. Thus, some nations with a long or bitter history of mutual antagonism and mistrust would hardly be appropriate either to receive or provide security elements. There has to be some sort of acceptance by the population of the right and ability of an external force to act. Impartiality and adherence to an accepted corpus of law are crucial foundations for this relationship. Clearly, trust between all sides is an ideal. At the very least there should be some sort of acceptance on behalf of the displaced population. An example of a successful use of soldiers in resolving a problem with violence was seen in the British Army's deployment in the north of the HPZ in Rwanda during 1994. In this area, two of the camps were proved to be the targets of violence, intimidation and attack by militia groups. Reasonably enough, the civilian NGOs assessed the situation as being too uncertain for their personnel to operate there. Accordingly, the military deployed a mixed force of medical staff, engineer resources and infantry. By virtue of their presence, the militia were deterred and the threat was removed, so that within 3 weeks the civilian agencies returned to the area and restarted their work.

Conversely, there are times when the military may not be helpful or successful. Thus, in the demanding and confused political cocktail of Somalia in 1992, the initial success of the military in support of humanitarian efforts quickly changed into a bitter and unhelpful conflict situation. In humanitarian terms, the military became part of the problem rather than the vehicle for greater efficiency in humanitarian relief. The UN may also have a role to play by deploying additional professional policing capabilities from other member states with recognised expertise and no history that might offend susceptibilities. Recently, this has increasingly been recognised as a crucial enabler for nation-building, and hence the creation of a stable and peaceful situation.

Nevertheless, whilst uniformed elements may be necessary, they are not sufficient. A full sense of security can be reached only by meeting all the needs for human fulfilment. This requires all the components of a state to be provided. Thus, economic, educational, health and social systems require attention. Again this will be especially pressing after a civil war. Quite clearly, such events have often led either to the overthrow of an existing social system, or a degree of damage to it such that its operation is compromised to some degree. It is this endeavour that demands the full participation of all the agencies in the area. There will also be a corollary, since the very profusion of these agencies will similarly require coordination. That leads to another set of concerns about leadership and legitimacy. Fortunately, recent operational experience has seen a much closer integration of all elements in situations of need. Such joint approaches are vital to the creation of a real sense of security. Even so, it may be an extended period of time before real and substantive progress is achieved. In the meantime, other requirements will need to be managed and met. Security is a critical enabler of the entire humanitarian effort.

*Shelter* is an important element of well-being and health. It provides physical and psychological reassurance to a displaced and dispossessed population. Naturally, the better the shelter then the better the effect achieved. Equally, there is a clear link between the provision of shelter and the sense of security engendered. A sense of ownership and the possession of an anchor in a changing and threatening situation is an important underpinning of stability. Accordingly, there are different ways to achieve an appropriate level of shelter.

Climatic factors are self-evidently important drivers of the type of shelter required. Thus, in cold or mountainous regions the needs are markedly different from those in desert or tropical locations. The more adverse the conditions, then the more demanding is the logistic bill for shelter. At the same time, there is a smaller margin for failure, since the climate will be more unforgiving of shortfalls in provision. Such vulnerability amongst the displaced population will inevitably be increased by the very fact of displacement. Adversity is a multiplicative process in a displaced people, since climatic, nutritional, disease and security dimensions all seem to conspire against the population. An important start in redressing the balance can be made by tackling the shelter requirement appropriately and with dispatch.

Usually, a displaced population will move to another place with a pre-existing infrastructure and people. Accepting that difficulties between the indigenous society and the newcomers can be resolved, the central question then concerns the ability of the location to absorb the influx. Naturally enough there is a correlation between the numbers and needs of the displaced population and the state of development, investment and circumstances of the existing community. The ability of a rural society employing subsistence agriculture methods to accommodate a sudden, large inflow of needy people is likely to be severely constrained. Such a circumstance could reduce both communities to desperation and destitution. In such unhappy straits, the situation can rapidly disintegrate into conflict and strife between two needy peoples. Such was the experience in northern Zaire in 1994 after the arrival of one and a half million Hutu refugees from Rwanda. Such a massive influx completely swamped the ability of the local Zairian community to cope. Inevitably, conflict followed as competition for scarce resources occurred. The international attention that the needs of the refugees attracted, and also resentment at the presence of armed Hutu militia amongst the refugee population, fuelled this hostility between refugees and locals. Clearly, the lesson of this unhappy episode is that the needs of the total population at risk (refugee plus local) must be considered as part of the aid package.

However, if these tensions do not exist and the needs of the displaced people are modest, then the most effective and efficient solution is for them to be absorbed into the local community. Such a process is greatly aided if there are ethnic links between the two populations. Again the Rwanda crisis furnishes examples of successful aid from the local population to the refugees. In the southwest of the country, in the HPZ, many small villages took complete families of refugees into their homes, sharing all their facilities with the newcomers. Accordingly, many of these villages became small camps with no hint of conflict between the two populations. This process was largely possible because of the identification of the local Hutu people with the plight and difficulties of the displaced Hutu population. It was the shared ethnic foundation and heritage that made the process possible. Equally, a policy of village improvement and assistance was instituted by the British military in order to encourage the assimilation and so avoid the unhappy experience of similar refugees in Zaire.

Should the local infrastructure be incapable of receiving the incoming people, additional assistance will be necessary. Frequently this requires the planning and provision of camps with associated individual shelters. Whilst shelters themselves may be improvised from locally available sources, they are often supplemented by other means such as the UNHCR shelter materials. Such means have to be tailored to the rigours of the climate and need to be easily erected and maintained. Happily, the process of improvisation lends itself to both these requirements. Indeed, the act of building a shelter may be of considerable assistance to the sense of well-being amongst a refugee population since it represents evidence of self-help and a return to responsibility and hence dignity. Such initial positive outcomes are clearly dependent upon other factors such as the previous circumstances of the migrants. Thus, an educated urban elite is likely to find the harsh realities of temporary shelters in a mass of similarly dispossessed people much harder to endure than would people from a background of subsistence farming. For the latter, the hardship of a refugee camp may not be far removed from the experience of normal life.

Refugee camps are frequently the consequence of mass population movements. Such migration patterns often end at the first convenient location regardless of its suitability for any extended occupation. As a result, these camps are often unsustainable without considerable external assistance. The sudden imposition of 100,000 needy people in an area will understandably lead to eventual resource depletion and exhaustion. Thus, aid in providing shelter is an initial imperative. This will serve to stabilise the situation and allow the population movement to be controlled. However, such dependence may soon become a two-way street, since not only does the refugee population rapidly become reliant upon external aid, but the providers of that assistance become trapped into that commitment by the continued deprivation and need amongst the migrants. This dual dependence may serve to confuse the existing situation since it sets up its own political dynamic. Thus, refugee camps always run the risk of becoming centres of political and military action. Nor is this process restricted to the indigenous population and security forces. The experience of living in a camp may act as a powerful source of political unrest as a sense of injustice and exasperation grows. Consequently, refugee camps may not provide the ideal method of dealing with the problem of shelter provision. The permanence of many such concentrations has served to aggravate existing political uncertainties and conflicts so that their successful resolution becomes increasingly difficult. Examples of exactly this unhappy situation abound in the Middle East, where Palestinian refugee camps have become spawning grounds for the young disaffected and nurture an increasingly hostile and militant outlook against the Israelis, who are seen as the agents of the Palestinian misfortunes. Such a cycle of a sense of grievance and injustice, violent action, violent counter-action, an increased sense of grievance and injustice, heightened violent action and heightened counter-action is the pernicious and tragic outcome of permanent refugee camps existing in a political vacuum. It is a possible outcome for many such camps.

Nevertheless, for the migrant population, such concentrations of their own people has an obvious appeal. The shared experience of dispossession, migration and hardship acts as a bond which links them together. Thus, it is entirely understandable that by living together in unfamiliar (and possibly hostile and dangerous) circumstances some degree of reassurance and comfort is achieved. Such are the strengths of these psychological imperatives that refugees will willingly run the risks associated with camps (e.g. disease and food shortage) in order to live with their own people. For the humanitarian worker, then, shelter as part of a refugee camp is likely to be a given in the complex patchwork of human need in a migrant population.

*Water and sanitation* (which are covered in detail in later chapters) are critical requirements for displaced populations. Many enteric and vector-borne diseases may be avoided or ameliorated by adequate provision of safe water and appropriate sanitation. Similarly, the supply of safe water may allow the stabilisation of an uncertain situation, thus going some way to meeting a psychological need in migrant populations. However, ensuring safe water and effective sanitation is not without problems. The initial difficulty is to estimate the water requirements of a community based upon average consumption rates. Having established the total required volume, it then needs to be produced, which is dependent upon the local resources.

Water is necessary for bathing, cooking, washing and sanitation, as well as for drinking. The total requirement is clearly an aggregate of these subtotals. However, the climate and geography of the location will further define the volume which needs to be produced. Thus, hot climates will need more water than temperate climates. A useful rule of thumb is 20 litres daily per person in hot climates, but this may be halved in cold temperate conditions. These totals may be revised and prioritised in the face of a water shortage, so that drinking and cooking may take preference over washing. Equally, water-recycling measures may help to reduce the total required.

In addition, the quality of water necessary for each activity varies. Hence, drinking demands a much higher level of microbiological scrutiny and survey than water for cooking or cleaning. This difference in water quality may help the supply of water since higher levels of purification need more expertise and sophistication. The means of purification may range from the ultimately safe but very energy-intensive reverse osmosis methods to the simple chlorination of a supply. Clearly, assessments have to be made as to the suitability and sustainability of the chosen technique. In addition, there is the question of the acceptability of some methods. For instance, the residual chlorine taste commonly experienced with some methods of drinking water production may be unacceptable to a community which is suspicious of chemical agents following attack by such weapons. In order for a strategy of water production to be successful, some measure of cooperation with the population needs to be established. By such means, a degree of trust and sustainability can be forged. In these circumstances, a partnership between provider and receiver is most helpful.

The same considerations surround the institution of an effective sanitation plan. Custom, modesty and convenience all impinge on the utility of a sanitation and sewage-disposal process. The techniques available vary from permanent or semi-permanent structures based upon the principles of sedimentation and purification which underpin such systems in developed situations, to the cat scratch or temporary latrines of austere field conditions. The choice of approach will depend upon the projected lifetime of the camp, whether it is a new camp or an absorption of the displaced people within an existing infrastructure, and the religious sensibilities, social customs and mores of the population, as well as the availability of resources. It is impossible to be prescriptive when there is such a wide set of variables. The only certainty is that lack of attention at the earliest possible stage to the requirements of sanitation will cause a greatly increased risk of avoidable disease.

*Food* provision is of fundamental importance to migrant peoples. The lack of adequate nutrition is a recognised accompaniment to the hardships of mass population movement. Thus, evidence of malnutrition is frequently found in such circumstances, as are the more extreme manifestations of starvation. A deficiency in energy and protein will also render an individual more susceptible to other afflictions such as infection and disease (particularly measles). This means that a food strategy will need to meet a variety of needs ranging from therapeutic feeding to normal daily nutritional requirements whilst being sensitive to the political dimension of food delivery in certain post-conflict situations. It will also require a calculation of the total requirements in order to inform the considerable logistic effort that normally underpins such programmes. As with many such humanitarian ventures, a hard-nosed assessment of need and the matching of resources provide the basis of success.

Some assessment of need is a vital initial step. Widespread protein-calorie deficiencies will be obvious to all. In such circumstances a complete therapeutic feeding campaign may be necessary, although such a venture is very resource-intensive and complex. Repeated drought aggravated by conflict has seen such tragic situations in the Horn of Africa over the last 20 years. More usually, malnutrition is experienced in specific vulnerable groups of a migrant population, at least initially. Such depravation may subsequently become more general. Those elements of a community that are especially at risk include the young, pregnant and lactating mothers, and the elderly. The young always attract much attention. Within this group, weight/height ratio and mid-upper arm circumference are two indices commonly used to assess nutritional status. Of these, the weight/height ratio is the more reliable and is assessed by reference to standard tables. Generally, if the young are well nourished then the population will tend to be sufficiently resourced.

Therapeutic feeding programmes are complex and require detailed collaboration between a number of agencies to ensure success. There is an initial nutritional assessment, followed by a specialised logistic effort and augmented by a medical supervisory role. All of these elements are crucial at the beginning of the programme. Subsequent success and future needs have to be addressed by continued surveillance and audit. The intention of a therapeutic programme should be to correct the nutritional imbalance as quickly and effectively as possible in order to allow the victims to return to normal feeding and hence life activities. Accordingly, a therapeutic (or supplementary) feeding programme is a short-term intervention.

Frequently used combinations of foodstuffs are corn–soya milk (CSM), wheat–soya blend (WSB), dried skimmed milk (DSM) and fish protein concentrate (FPC). The exact combination will depend upon cultural, religious, financial and logistic factors. Commonly, a number of these factors will be acting simultaneously. A system of surveillance should be instituted on the commencement of a therapeutic feeding programme. Such a system of surveillance will necessarily focus on the groups most at risk, and will require a sound sampling strategy. An important element of this process will be a medical review of nutritional deficiency as revealed in clinical cases.

## Medical Interventions

The medical needs of a displaced population may well be both huge in scale and complex in detail. This poses considerable challenges to both logistics and actual medical care. As a result, it is depressingly easy to be confused and even paralysed by the task. The pressures of decision making are compounded by the almost universal goad of time. Complicated actions frequently have to be initiated against a backdrop of an elevated mortality rate and a climbing morbidity rate. In such circumstances, clear thinking is at a premium. An essential foundation for this process is information.

*Information* usually exists but may not be easily available. Equally, the sources of the information may be variable in terms of both reliability and quality. Hence, some care needs to be applied in evaluating the information. However, the incidence and prevalence of disease is clearly a critical element of the information requirement. The World Health Organisation (WHO) will normally be able to provide reliable indicators of disease incidence and prevalence in particular regions. According to circumstances, this information may be both accurate and up to date, particularly when attention has been focused on the location for some time. Equally, reliance upon official government statistics may not be well placed. Sadly, accuracy in such data may be difficult to achieve because of administrative shortcomings, or may be compromised by political expediency. After all, the admission of endemic disease and an under-resourcing legacy may not be helpful or profitable in all circumstances. Consequently, official government sources may need to be interpreted with caution.

Other agencies may well be able to provide reliable data. Such sources include NGOs operating within the area as well as UN agencies. Help may also be available from relevant academic units such as schools of tropical medicine or academic departments dealing with particular groupings. In any event, the collation of such information from as broad a range of sources as possible within the available time will prove invaluable in the initial planning of an operation. Hazards, risks and priorities can all be initially assessed at this stage.

Equally, any information will need to have caveats applied prior to deployment. These caveats can be confirmed or revised once information becomes available on deployment. This requires a strategy for data collection and collation within the operational area. Naturally, collaboration between all the agencies working in an area will greatly enhance the utility of the data. However, this approach brings with it all the complications of an agreed set of clinical definitions and diagnoses. Despite the apparent simplicity of this requirement, it can prove difficult to institute such a system given the disparity in resources, expertise and motivation which may exist in the humanitarian community. In such circumstances, the best should not be allowed to become the enemy of the good, and a reliable but partial solution should be accepted. Thus, the majority of the humanitarian agencies could provide clinical and epidemiological data which would be adequate to inform decisions on prioritisation and resource allocation.

*Priorities* will usually have been allocated prior to deployment using the best available information. These priorities will have to be constantly reassessed in the light of additional information that will follow deployment. Such a regular review of tasks and their relative importance is not a sign of weakness. Rather it is evidence of a sensitive and realistic approach to disaster planning and action. Nevertheless, the key to effective assistance in a disaster situation is a clear list of priorities and a sequencing of measures to implement them. Equally, the temptation to use a set template for all situations must be resisted. Each situation is different in detail from the preceding ones, and indeed will posses its own set of dynamics and drivers. These have to be recognised in the setting of priorities. In addition, priorities may well vary within a locality, reflecting different sets of local circumstances and needs. Hence, the whole process of priority setting is both complex and dynamic; it is never completed.

*Medical intervention* may take the form of therapeutic or preventive measures. Thus, the preventive measures may include a suitable vaccination programme tailored to the threat and its incubation period. Often this is a difficult judgement, since the data on which decisions to initiate vaccination programmes are based are themselves invariably imperfect and incomplete. Yet the commencement of such a programme may represent a substantial commitment of resources in material, human and financial terms. The common vaccination programmes encountered in many refugee situations include measles and meningitis. Whilst the organisation of the programme may take time, it is a relatively simple process. Nevertheless, whilst it is simple, it may not be easy. The requirement for cool storage to protect the vaccines and the actual organisation of the human resources, both medical and refugee recipient, are potentially fraught. Hence, a simple but robust plan to achieve the purpose must be adopted. Complicated planning will invariably be a hostage to fortune in the uncertainty and organisational maelstrom of a displaced population.

Frequently, the widespread use of the displaced population itself in the organisation and delivery of the programme achieves the best results.

Therapeutic interventions will also be determined by the nature of the problems and the resultant needs. Clearly, there will need to be a balance between surgical, emergency and medical provision, as well as age- and sex-specific programmes. Areas in which conflict has been, or continues to be, a concern are likely to need continuing trauma care. Equally, tropical zones are likely to generate considerable numbers of medical cases from endemic disease. In addition, enteric disease is an ever-present danger in displaced populations regardless of geographic zone and climate.

A frequent finding in displaced populations is the special vulnerability of some groups. Thus, the young, pregnant and lactating mothers, and the elderly are particularly vulnerable. They may require specific medical support and expertise in their reduced circumstances. The provision of paediatric, midwifery and geriatric services will have to be addressed in some form so that those needs may be both effectively targeted and managed. Failure to accommodate these groups within the overall plan would be to exclude those with the greatest need.

All people involved in a disaster situation are likely to be subject to a degree of psychological stress. Self-evidently, the greater the stress, the greater the likely psychological reaction. Thus, genocide and expulsion are generally likely to cause more psychological stress than an industrial spillage in a confined area. This psychological dimension may be overlooked or inadequately resourced, particularly in the acute phase of a disaster. Necessarily, any attempt to offer support or psychiatric attention needs to recognise cultural and religious sensitivities. Whilst this is true of all therapeutic interventions, it is particularly apposite to psychiatry, given the cultural determinants of many behaviour types and coping mechanisms. This transcultural dimension of psychiatric care in refugee situations is particularly demanding. A mixture of in-patient and community care approaches may be required in order to achieve effective intervention. Necessarily, a reality check will need to be applied so that the clinically ideal is tempered with what is actually feasible. There are likely to be difficult and distressing decisions with no obvious clear basis for decision making. Yet, psychological well-being is critical to the creation of some stability and hope for the future. This general hope may be underpinned by effective psychiatric provision at the individual level. Accordingly, the psychiatric care of a displaced population is a crucial component in the overall effectiveness of the intervention.

Another area of difficult therapeutic intervention is with the problem of sexually transmitted disease. This may be difficult for religious, social or medical reasons. However, the incidence of sexually transmitted disease in displaced populations may be very much higher than the pre-disaster level. Nor should this be a surprise given the degree of disruption that the society may have undergone. Social norms, even the social fabric, may have been entirely lost in the trauma of genocide and displacement. Given a reservoir of pre-existing sexually transmitted disease, desperation and destitution may lead many into part-time prostitution in order to eat or provide for their families. Trying to quantify the size of the problem is likely to be impossible in a refugee situation. Equally, the difficulties of confidentiality, contact tracing and continuity of treatment complicate management. At the same time, the spectre of HIV has to be managed, since exposure to a sexually transmitted disease must raise the possibility of infection with HIV as an accompanying risk. It is unlikely that sufficient resources will be available for any meaningful intervention against HIV to be made in any refugee situation. Thus, an emphasis on education and prophylactic measures will almost certainly be required.

Reference has been made in the above discussion to cultural aspects. These are important elements in any plans for disaster relief since they will define the acceptability, and ultimately the success, of specific measures for the target population. There may well be a range of factors which have to be considered, including religious, social, ethical and historical dimensions. The relative importance and significance of these will need assessment and accommodation. Such measures as modifying dietary provision to reflect religious practice, or special provision of clothing and personnel for intimate medical examinations, especially of females, may need to be implemented. At all times the plan for disaster relief must be culturally appropriate.

Another aspect that needs early recognition is the disaster–development continuum. This is a theoretical construct that seeks to show the relationship between disaster relief and development. The response to the acute phase of a disaster is nakedly utilitarian; the greatest good for the greatest number. It should also reflect the need for cultural appropriateness. This combination requires some forethought in order to avoid initiating interventions, both preventive and therapeutic, which are not sustainable. Equally, the relief strategy must not use techniques and methods that may skew or compromise subsequent development. An example of this might be the use of external fixators in refugee situations where there was no previous use of these techniques and no possibility of imminent acquisition of them. The commitment of resources in the acute relief stage must recognise the realities of subsequent development potential. This is aided by using the disaster–development continuum as a working model. Simplistic though it is, it serves to ground decisions on interventions on a bedrock of reality (*see also Ch. 21*).

# Conclusions

The decision to intervene in a natural or man-made disaster is not one to be undertaken lightly. The range of medical needs in any displaced population will be almost infinite. Thus, there is no place for a prescriptive answer; one size does not fit all. Instead, there must be a dynamic approach to priority and task-setting. In the light of particular and changing circumstances, planning must reflect reality against a background of constant change. It is the common approach which is crucial, not the common answer.

# 7. The Players

## Part A – The Humanitarian Aid Organisations
Cara Macnab and Deborah R. Aspögard

| Objectives | • To describe the agencies and organisations involved in medical care in hostile environments.<br>• To distinguish between international, national and non-governmental organisations.<br>• To provide a broad classification.<br>• To direct readers to appropriate web sites and other resources dealing with the topic. |
|---|---|

## Introduction

A volunteer deploying on a humanitarian mission can expect to encounter fellow aid workers from a bewildering variety of agencies. Increasingly, there will be a mix of military and non-military personnel working side by side, not always harmoniously.

Even among the strictly civilian agencies there is, at times, confusion, misunderstanding and even rivalry. Further, on the civilian side, the number of agencies is vast and increasing. The question that may reasonably be asked is: "Who are all these players?"

This two-part chapter attempts to address these questions. Part A considers the civilian agencies and players; military involvement is considered in Part B.

### Humanitarian Aid Agencies

By convention, humanitarian aid agencies are divided into three types.

• IGOs: intergovernmental or international organisations.
• GOs: governmental or national organisations.
• NGOs: non-governmental organisations.

Full lists and descriptions of these diverse organisations can be found in the Resources section of this handbook. Interested readers should browse through the classifications and be directed to gateway and individual web sites. The aim in this chapter is to provide an overview, to differentiate between the agencies and to illustrate the types with a small number of case examples.

## Intergovernmental Organisations (IGOs)

IGOs are organisations or institutions created and joined by governments. Their members are states which give them the authority to make collective decisions to manage particular problems on the global agenda.

They may be universal, such as the United Nations, or regional as in the case of the European Union. The aims of these organisations may vary from a military alliance (NATO) to health care (United Nations agencies.) Larger organisations have multiple purposes and areas of interest, and consist of organs, specialised agencies and autonomous organisations. The United Nations web pages illustrate this graphically (see Resources section)

### *The United Nations*

The United Nations (UN) was founded in 1945 and is the best-known international organisation. Its aims are to promote international peace and security, and to develop international cooperation in economic, social, cultural and humanitarian problems. The name United Nations was coined by Franklin D. Roosevelt, then President of the United States of America, and was first used in the "Declaration by United Nations" on 1 January 1942, when representatives of 26 nations pledged that their governments would continue fighting together against the Axis powers.

Representatives of 50 countries at the UN Conference drew up the UN Charter on International Organisation at a meeting in San Francisco from 25 April to 26 June 1945. The delegates deliberated over proposals drafted by representatives of China, the Soviet Union, the United States of America and the United Kingdom at Dumbarton Oaks from August to October 1944.

The representatives of those 50 countries signed the Charter on 26 June 1945. Poland, which was not represented at the conference, signed it later and became one of the 51 original member states. The UN officially came into existence on 24 October 1945 when the Charter was ratified by China, the Soviet Union, the United States of America, France and the United Kingdom. By 1994, the original 51 states of the United Nations had grown to 185, and United Nations Day is still celebrated on 24 October each year.

When states become members of the UN they agree to accept the obligations of the UN Charter. The Charter expresses the fundamental purpose of the UN and sets out a basic framework for international relations. The UN is intended as a centre for the-harmonisation of the actions of nations. The signatories to the UN Charter agree to:

- maintain peace and security,
- develop friendly relations between nations,

- cooperate in solving international problems,
- promote respect for human rights.

The UN is composed of five main bodies which are based at the UN Headquarters in New York, USA.

- The General Assembly.
- The Security Council.
- The Economic and Social Council.
- The Trusteeship Council.
- The Secretariat.

The judicial arm of the UN, the International Court of Justice, is located in The Hague, The Netherlands.

### The General Assembly

All member states are represented in the General Assembly. The Assembly acts as a parliament of nations that meets to discuss the world's most pressing problems. Each member state has a single vote. It is important to realise that the UN is not a governmental or legislative body. The objective of the UN is to help to resolve problems, and all member states, independent of political stance, size or economic power, have an equal voice in the formulation of policy.

The General Assembly does not force action by any state. It serves as a barometer of world opinion and represents the moral authority of the community of nations. When the Assembly is not in session, the UN Secretariat carries out its work by the other main committees and subsidiary bodies.

### The Security Council

Helping to preserve world peace is a central purpose of the UN. With that aim in mind, the UN Charter gives the Security Council responsibility for maintaining international peace and security. Under the Charter, member states may agree to settle disputes by peaceful means rather than by using threats or force against each other. The Security Council will try to broker a ceasefire in the event of conflict, and is able to send a peace-keeping force to maintain a truce and keep opposing factions apart.

The Security Council can take measures to enforce decisions made by the UN by imposing economic sanctions and applying an embargo on arms sales. It has a mandate to use all necessary means, including armed force, to see that its decisions are carried out.

The Security Council has five permanent members (China, the Russian Federation, the United States of America, France and the United Kingdom) and ten other members at any one time. The ten temporary members are elected for 2–year terms by the General Assembly. Decisions of the Security Council require a majority of nine out of ten members, but each of the permanent members of the Council may apply a veto.

*The Economic and Social Council*

The Economic and Social Council is under the authority of the General Assembly, which elects each of the 54 members to 3-year terms. This Council meets for 1 month each year and serves to discuss and define international and social issues, and foster cooperation to aid the development of nations. It consults with non-governmental organisations (NGOs) to help maintain links between the UN and civil society. The executive arm of the Economic and Social Council includes the Commission on Human Rights that monitors the observance of human rights throughout the world.

*The Trusteeship Council*

This council was established to provide international supervision for 11 Trust Territories, which are administered by seven member states. The purpose of the Trusteeship Council is to groom Trust Territories for self-governance or independence.

*The Secretariat*

The Secretariat's role is administrative, and it is composed of departments and offices with a staff of nearly nine thousand people from 160 countries. The offices are in UN Headquarters in New York, Geneva, Vienna and Nairobi. The head of the Secretariat, the Secretary-General, provides overall administrative guidance and is often the public face of the UN.

*The International Court of Justice*

This body is also known as the World Court and is the judicial organ of the UN. It is composed of 15 judges elected by the General Assembly and the Security Council. Its purpose is to provide judgements to the General Assembly and the Security Council on disputes between countries. Participation by member states is voluntary, but if a state agrees to participate then the rulings of the World Court are held to be binding.

*The International Criminal Court (ICC)*

On 17 July 1998, in Rome, 160 nations established a permanent international criminal court in response to the horrific events in Rwanda and the former Yugoslavia. Although *the UN Security Council had established ad hoc tribunals*, international interest identified the need to establish mechanisms to try individuals for offences such as genocide, war crimes and crimes against humanity. A permanent court was recognised as having the ability to react more quickly than ad hoc bodies and would act as a strong deterrent. The court is situated in The Hague in The Netherlands, but the authority of the ICC can be used to try cases at other venues when necessary.

*Specialised Agencies*

The International Monetary Fund, the World Bank, the World Health Organisation, the International Civil Aviation Organisation and ten other independent organisations are known as "specialised agencies" and are linked to the UN through co-operative agreements. These organisations are autonomous bodies created by inter-governmental agreements

Within the UN system there also exist a number of UN offices, programmes and funds, for example the Office of the UN High Commissioner for Refugees (UNHCR) and the UN Children's Fund (UNICEF). These agencies work to improve the economic and social conditions of people around the world, and report to the General Assembly or the Economic and Social Council.

## Governmental or National Organisations

A number of countries, in addition to belonging to and participating in IGO and NGO activities, have developed their own national aid agencies. While the aims and objectives of these agencies mirror those of many IGOs and NGOs, governmental agencies also have as their aim the advancement of national interests. Two agencies are briefly described.

### Department for International Development (DFID)

The DFID is the United Kingdom's national humanitarian aid agency. Formerly known as the Overseas Development Agency (ODA), DFID is charged with carrying out the British Government's aid and development efforts. It achieves this either by deploying its own personnel to carry out its tasks, or by employing and funding specialist agencies within the NGO network.

The DFID has a number of recognisable activity streams. These are:

- missions to reduce extreme poverty overseas;
- conflict-reduction activities;
- direct humanitarian assistance activities;
- measures to enhance the safety of humanitarian aid workers.

DFID has an extensive web site; the address is in the Resources section.

### US Agency for International Development (USAID)

USAID is an independent federal government agency that conducts foreign assistance and humanitarian aid to advance the political and economic interests of the United States.

USAID's history dates back to the reconstruction of Europe under the Marshall Plan and Four Point Program. USAID was formally created by President J F Kennedy in 1961.

As with DFID, USAID receives direction and foreign policy guidance from the National Government. The agency works within six definable areas:

- economic growth and agricultural development;
- population, health and nutrition;
- environment;
- democracy and governance;

- education and training;
- humanitarian assistance.

USAID also works with non-government partners in many of its missions. Its web site is listed in the Resources section.

## Non-Governmental Organisations (NGOs)

Non-governmental organisations (NGOs) are composed of individuals with shared interests and goals. Their work may be paid or voluntary, and they are able to take direct action in their sphere of interest or intervene politically to influence governments and other NGOs.

In the context of this book, NGOs are considered to be concerned with health, welfare and humanitarian matters; however, NGOs may also concern themselves with the actions of multinational corporations, religious groups or political movements.

Even within purely health-related NGOs there is a huge diversity, as they range from small groups of concerned individuals to professionally led, multi-million-dollar organisations. NGOs may be aligned to one side or another, or they may be politically neutral and adopt an advocacy role, exposing and publicising injustice or the abuse of human rights. Thus, each NGO has a political stance and philosophy that encourages or dissuades individual sponsors or volunteers from becoming involved. Examples of NGOs include the Red Cross and Red Crescent Movement, Oxfam, Médécin-Sans-Frontières and the Save the Children Fund. We describe only one agency in detail by way of illustration.

### The Red Cross and Red Crescent Movement

Although it is international, the movement is clearly non-governmental in structure and philosophy. Established by Henri Dunant in 1863, the Red Cross and Red Crescent Movement is the largest humanitarian network in the world. The movement is guided by seven fundamental principles: humanity, impartiality, neutrality, independence, voluntary service, unity and universality. All Red Cross and Red Crescent activities have one central purpose: to prevent and alleviate human suffering, without discrimination, and to protect human dignity.

The movement is composed of the International Committee of the Red Cross (ICRC), National Red Cross and Red Crescent Societies, and the International Federation of Red Cross and Red Crescent Societies.

The International Committee of the Red Cross (ICRC) is the movement's founding body. In addition to carrying out operational activities, it is the promoter and custodian of international humanitarian law. It is the guardian of the fundamental principles and, in cooperation with the federation, it organises the movements' statutory meetings.

The ICRC is impartial and independent of all governments. Its work is guided by empathy for the victims of conflict, and it remains detached from all political issues related to conflict. By applying these principles, the ICRC is able to act as an intermediary between parties to armed conflict and to promote dialogue in situations of internal violence, with a view to prevent a worsening of crises and even at times to resolve them.

The ICRC reminds all military and civil authorities involved in armed conflict or internal violence of their obligations under international humanitarian law and the other humanitarian rules by which they are bound. In all societies and cultures, the ICRC endeavours to promote international humanitarian law and the fundamental human values underlying that law.

The ICRC directs and coordinates the international work of the Red Cross and Red Crescent movement in its involvement with armed conflict and internal violence. There are now more than one hundred and sixty National Red Cross and Red Crescent Societies around the world. National Societies act as auxiliaries to the public authorities in their own countries, and provide services ranging from disaster relief, health and social assistance to first-aid and child-care courses. In time of war, the first-aid staff are incorporated into the army medical services. All National Societies must be recognised by the ICRC, and subsequently they may become members of the Federation, the National Societies' umbrella organisation.

The Federation works to inspire, facilitate and promote humanitarian activities carried out by its member National Societies. Founded in 1919, the Federation co-ordinates international assistance from National Societies to victims of disasters, whether natural or man-made, outside conflict areas. It encourages and promotes the establishment and development of National Societies, e.g. helping them to plan and implement disaster preparedness programmes and long-term projects designed to reduce vulnerability and contribute to sustainable development. It acts as a permanent liaison body for the National Societies.

### Birth of Humanitarian Law

To put the concept of the protection of the wounded and their personnel during hostilities into practical effect, the cooperation of governments was vital. The founders of the Red Cross persuaded the Swiss Government to lend their support to the text of an international treaty.

The Diplomatic Conference met in Geneva in August 1864. There, the representatives of 12 states signed a brief international treaty which included ten articles. The articles bore the title "The Geneva Convention of August 22, 1864, for the Amelioration of the Condition of the Wounded in Armies in the Field". The first "Geneva Convention" was a great historical step forward in the protection of victims involved in armed conflict and the personnel responsible for their care.

## Other NGOs

There are over 5,000 NGOs in existence, not all concerned with humanitarian assistance. Information on the major humanitarian NGOs can be found in the Resources section at the end of this handbook. Readers can access the organisations by using one of the gateway sites or go directly to an individual NGO web address.

# Conclusion

Humanitarian assistance is a growing activity. It is also becoming complex and complicated, with many agencies, groups and individuals involved. A prospective volunteer could be forgiven for not knowing where to begin in a quest to become involved. We hope the forgoing may give some sense of structure and direction.

## Suggested Further Reading

Moorehead C. Dunant's dream: war, Switzerland and the history of the Red Cross. London: Harper Collins, 1998.

Hegley CW, Wittkopf ER, editors. Universal and regional intergovernmental organisations (IGOs). Non-governmental actors on the world stage. In: World politics: trend and transformation. London: Macmillan, 1999; 145–205.

# Part B – The Military – a Player, a Facilitator or the Cause of the Problem

David Morgan-Jones

**Objectives**

- To describe the changing role of the military in the developed world.
- To discuss the use of the military as a humanitarian aid agency.
- To describe the impact on non-military aid agencies.
- To discuss military capability.
- To outline the advantages and disadvantages.

# Introduction

The last decade has seen considerable changes with the rapid collapse of the Former Soviet Union, and therefore of the stability and certainties of the "cold war". The use of proxy wars and the ruthless suppression of "member" states has left a legacy of increasing intra-state conflict resulting in considerable loss of life and associated human tragedy, and this has been fuelled by the relatively easy access to the surplus weaponry no longer required by superpowers. In response to these global changes military organisations, particularly across Europe and North America, have also undergone significant downsizing as government treasuries have grasped considerable savings opportunities. Partly as a process of self-survival and partly due to external demands, the Western militaries have changed from large static forces providing a defensive capability to smaller more flexible forces designed to be of a more expeditionary nature.

Whilst military organisations can be viewed as highly capable systems with significant potential to assist in humanitarian operations, it needs to be understood that the military is an extension of the political will of a given country. The main role of the armed forces in the latter half of the twentieth century has primarily been in territorial defence and protection of strategic interests requiring the use of a combat force. During the last decade, these aspects have been demonstrated by the Gulf War in 1991, which principally concerned the preservation of oil supplies to the West, and by the intervention of NATO and Russian forces in the Kosovo crisis in 1999, which has resulted from an attempt to minimise internal conflict spreading across borders into Macedonia and Albania. In the latter example NATO troops were initially deployed as a combat force, but with the imminent destabilisation of the Macedonian Government through the impact on the country of the large number of Albanian refugees, they were tasked to undertake a humanitarian aid role by building and running refugee camps. However, once the aid agencies started to mobilise in greater numbers, this role was handed over to the UN and NGOs.

However, the ability of the media to influence the political will can be considerable, and this was partially responsible for the deployment of Western forces into Rwanda in a belated attempt to minimise the effects of genocide, and of Australian Forces into Papua New Guinea following the effects of a massive tidal wave. However, this is not a function for which the military is particularly well suited as it is large, slow to mobilise in strength, expensive and does not necessarily have the appropriate expertise and flexibility required to operate effectively as a disaster relief organisation.

History has shown that the use of the military can have diametrically opposed outcomes. On the one hand military deployment can result in the cessation of conflict, while on the other it can be the cause of significant human suffering as seen in the use of military force intent on controlling a state, which increasingly seems to involve the removal of other ethnic groups within that country (Rwanda in 1994 and the Balkans in 1990—1999).

# The Evolving Nature of Catastrophes Caused by War

## The Changing Role of the Military

Part of the remit of the UN is to mediate and manage conflict between warring states. The recent increasing involvement in intra-state hostilities has introduced new operational concepts into the military lexicon such as peace enforcement and peace support. Yet these concepts are only an extension of using military force to maintain or enforce a semblance of stability within a warring state. As involvement becomes more widespread, these new concepts are evolving as both Government and the military learn from experience. These aspects have already been raised in earlier chapters The requirement for increasing military involvement in humanitarian operations has been accepted by international bodies such as the UN, which has issued

Guidelines on the Use of Military and Civil Defence Assets in Disaster Relief, thereby acknowledging that the military element will integrate closely with relief organisations and host-nation assets. In the UK, this change of attitude has been expressed within the Military of Defence by accepting humanitarian operations as one of its grand strategic level tasks. This will be carried out at:

- the military strategic level by coordinating foreign humanitarian and civic assistance, together with the provision of support for, and cooperation with, NGOs;
- the mission level through the provision of service support for disaster relief and humanitarian aid outside the UK;
- the tactical level (on the ground) by using the command and control systems to engender effective working relationships between the military, local inhabitants and NGOs.

## Impact on the Aid Agencies

Recent conflicts have demonstrated an increasing trend by lawless elements to rob, take hostage or even kill aid agency workers. Therefore, the provision of security for aid agency workers in areas of conflict is becoming a factor that needs to be considered. However, there remains significant antagonism from some of these agencies towards the military for the reasons given below.

- They feel that a military presence has the potential to compromise their ability to work as neutral agents within these environments. However, recent experience has helped to soften this view as direct military assistance to NGOs seems to be appreciated in a variety of areas such as effective command and control, flexibility of manpower, the resources available, integral logistic and medical capability, and general self-sufficiency.
- It is perceived that military involvement is a cynical move on the part of affluent nations to contain the world's poor and dispossessed.

## Military Capability

When deployed, the military can provide a wealth of capabilities that extends from the provision of large amounts of well-organised and disciplined manpower, to highly sophisticated command, control and communications facilities. An overview of these is given in the box below.

In general, the military now tends to perform two major functions.

- The provision of a secure environment within which humanitarian work can be undertaken by the aid agencies.
- Logistic support, including the use of engineering and medical support assets.

- Command
- Security:
  - Effective policing or military force
- Communications
- Engineering:
  - Infrastructure repair to power stations and water supplies
  - Repair of internal and external communication systems such as roads, railways and airports
  - The building of temporary or permanent shelters
  - Disposal of explosive ordnance such as bobby-traps, mines and unexploded ordnance
  - Mounting environmental clean-up campaigns
- Sophisticated logistics support systems:
  - Supplies of water, food, clothes, fuel and equipment
  - Environmental protection (shelters etc.)
  - The provision of significant transport by land, sea and air
- Medical
  - Advice to both the population and aid agencies on environmental, public and occupational health
  - Primary care and specialist secondary care

## Advantages and Disadvantages

From the points listed above it can be seen that the military tends to provide only those skills which it inherently requires to carry out its own specific combat functions. However, like any tool, if used imaginatively it can provide a capability outside its original design specifications! When attempting to define the advantages of using the military for humanitarian operations, for every positive factor there is a negative example to contradict it. For example, it is generally assumed that the military will be used for short-term operations, and yet a military presence has been required in Bosnia for most of this decade. The general advantages and disadvantages are listed below.

### The Advantages

- *Neutrality.* The military are normally tasked on a specific mission and therefore have no hidden political or commercial agendas.
- *Security.* The military can provide security for both the aid agencies and the local population. This can be seen in the creation of:
  - *safe havens,* which are circumscribed areas where the displaced can seek protection and sustenance close to their homes. (The Economic Organisations of West African States Military Observer Group (ECOMOG) provided a safe haven for both the population and aid agencies in Liberia. However, on three occasions, in 1992, 1994 and 1996 during periods of ECOMOG instability, the

situation became insecure and resulted in a partial or complete withdrawal of UN agencies and international NGOs from this country.)

- *safe zones* which protect the victimised population in its usual location.
- or the complete *"occupation"* of a failed state. (However, to be effective military forces need to be deployed in considerable numbers in order to provide the overwhelming strength required to suppress the factional fighting.)

- *Coordination and facilitation.* As military organisations gain increasing experience from humanitarian operations they are developing sophisticated skills in mediating between and coordinating the efforts of aid agencies.
- *Self-contained.* The military arrive with their own integral logistic and medical support, whilst many of the aid agencies rely heavily on other organisations.
- *Multipurpose.* Increasingly, military organisations need to be flexible and responsive to different needs. They can adopt an overt military war-like posture, an internal policing role or the simple provision of engineering and logistic support.
- *Rapid response.* The military are capable of responding rapidly, e.g. the parachuting of Australian medical support into Papua New Guinea following a massive tidal wave, and the movement of US medical staff to Ecuador in 1996 following the crash of a civilian 707 cargo jet. However, these rapid responses tend to be limited in terms of both capability and duration.
- *Controllable.* Military organisations tend to be highly controllable and rapidly respond to the requirements of the situation and to political direction. However, this is not always the case, as was seen in Liberia when elements of the ECOMOG mission were involved in attacks on the National Patriotic Front of Liberia.

## The Disadvantages

- *Mission orientated.* The military are generally tasked with a specific mission. This aspect has been described in the chapter on medical intervention. This can lead to a perceived inflexibility by civilian agencies.
- *Cost.* Owing to its size and relatively complex management structure, the use of the military is often perceived by Government as an expensive option. As in all organisations, the major component of the budget is the salaries of those it employs. Service personnel will be paid irrespective of whether they are in barracks or deployed on humanitarian operations. However, there is a tendency for the civil secretariat to include salaries as a major part of the costings.
- *Size.* The sheer size of the military can overwhelm the NGOs and other UN agencies, and when they depart it can leave a significant vacuum which the aid agencies can find difficult to fill.
- *Short duration operations.* Owing to the cost and operational overstretch, and in a bid to ensure that long-term strategic defence is not compromised, governments are loath to commit the military to long-term operations. Therefore, there is a general assumption that armed forces will tend to be used for short-term operations such as the deployment to Rwanda. However, this does not always happen, as is currently being seen in Bosnia.
- *Inflexibility.* Whilst aid agencies can be light, small and highly responsive to emerging situations, the military response generally tends towards the opposite.

# Conclusions

The role of the military in the last years of the twentieth century and the beginning of the twenty-first century is continuing to undergo significant changes in response to wider political needs, reflecting the increasing occurrence of intra-state wars, with their associated human suffering. However, in all conflicts, whether they are inter- or intra-state, military force will play a causative role. The military has been used as a "player" in Rwanda through the provision of direct humanitarian support, and as a "facilitator" in Bosnia and Kosovo by enforcing peace within these failed states. It has the ability to provide effective support rapidly to help ameliorate the effects of natural catastrophes within the emergency relief phase of a disaster. However, the main mission of most Western militaries will be to continue to provide an effective combat force for the provision of national defence both territorially and strategically.

## Further Reading

Outram Q. Cruel wars and safe havens: humanitarian aid in Liberia 1989–1996. Disasters 1997;21:189–205.
Stockton N. Defensive development? Re-examining the role of the military in complex political emergencies. Disasters vol. 20, No. 2:144–148.
Sutherland NA. Reconstruction in Bosnia – winning the peace. Br Army Rev 120:19–28, 1998.

# SECTION 2

## The Process and Related Issues

# 8. The Process

Steve Mannion, Eddie Chaloner and Claire Walford

**Objectives**

- To consider the motivation behind getting involved.
- To indicate the importance of personal and professional preparation.
- To give general advice on travelling and arriving.
- To consider the implications of returning home.

## Introduction

When questioned, many a medical student or nursing student will profess a deep desire to work in the field of international humanitarian aid overseas at some time in their future career.

In practice, for a variety of reasons, only a small proportion ever get to realise this ambition. Some will accrue family and financial commitments which prevent it; others will feel that such work may be detrimental to their career progression; yet others may perceive that the personal safety risks associated with such programmes are too great.

Even for those who maintain their enthusiasm and ambition for such work, getting a first foot in the door can be a difficult and daunting prospect. This chapter aims to examine some of the issues associated with making this first step and tries to offer some practical advice.

## Part A – Getting Involved

This part of the work is concerned with how to get started and how to begin working in the field of medicine in a hostile environment, be that working in the field of humanitarian medicine overseas, or in other hostile environments such as the oil and gas industry.

## Motivation

Before embarking on the quest for an overseas post it is wise to consider your own motivation for doing so. These may include the points listed below.

- Altruism – a determination to help needy populations.
- Religion – medical missionaries undertake this work as an expression of their religious faith.
- Career – to gain experience that will help NHS practice and advancement.
- Adventure – the chance to see and do unusual things.

In practice most people undertake aid work for a complex combination of these factors and others [1].

It is perhaps unwise to pursue this work purely out of disaffection with NHS practice. Only a small proportion of expatriate doctors will find their true long-term vocation in aid work [2]; the remuneration is often poor, living conditions are difficult and there is no security of tenure. The majority, therefore, will be obliged to return to a NHS practice which, if they found it to be unsatisfactory prior to departure, will no doubt be more so following their return.

Care should also be exercised with regard to one's personal life [3]. In crisis situations, it is rarely appropriate for aid workers to be accompanied by their partners and children. With the minimum duration of a first mission for many agencies being 3 months or longer, the strain of separation needs to be considered. Where partners can live in the country, their needs should also be addressed. For example the difficulties of social isolation can be reduced if your partner is professionally qualified; some agencies will offer dual appointments at one location if both parties hold appropriate qualifications.

## Qualifications and Skills

Increasingly, aid organisations are demanding greater levels of experience and qualification from their candidates for overseas posts [1]. This is appropriate, as the expatriate must be able to contribute significantly to the programme concerned.

Most agencies will not consider newly qualified or immediately post-registration house officers (in a medical role; people with additional qualifications in, say, logistics may be suitable for other roles). The minimum is usually 2 years post-registration experience including senior house officer (SHO) work in accident and emergency, paediatrics, and/or obstetrics and gynaecology.

There are additional courses and qualifications that make the candidate more attractive to potential employers. These include the DTM&H (Diploma in Tropical Medicine and Hygiene, a 3–month full-time course offered by the London and Liverpool Schools of Tropical Medicine), the DMCC (Diploma in the Medical Care of Catastrophes, a modular diploma qualification run by the Society of Apothecaries of London) and Masters degrees in aid-related subjects such as public health, international community health and epidemiology. (Further details of courses and institutions can be found in the resources section.)

The requirements for specialists (such as surgeons and anaesthetists) are more exacting. Médecins sans Frontières (MSF) looks for a minimum of 2 years experience at Specialist Registrar (SpR) level. The International Committee of the Red Cross (ICRC), who recruit for their surgical programmes via Red Cross National Societies, usually look for people at Senior SpR/consultant level.

The prospective first-time candidate cannot be expected to have direct experience of humanitarian aid work, but previous overseas trips (such as a medical elective or independent travel) are well looked upon by employing agencies. (Student electives are considered in Ch. 10 in this section).

Most of the employing agencies offer some form of further training before sending anyone into the field. MSF run a Preparation Primary Departure (PPD) course. The British Red Cross runs a week-long introductory course for potential delegates. These courses cover aspects of professional skills, general skills and the individual agency's health care and aid philosophy.

# Integration of Overseas Experience with an NHS Career

In 1995, a circular from the NHS Executive [4] drew the attention of NHS Trusts to the potential professional development obtained by staff who participate in humanitarian aid work overseas. The document sought to encourage trusts to develop schemes whereby staff could be allowed time off to undertake such projects, with a guarantee of re-employment on their return (current procedures for the mobilisation of reserve military personnel include such agreements with employers). Similar sentiments have been echoed by a royal patron [5].

While some trusts have made local initiatives, it still remains difficult to integrate overseas work with mainstream career progression. This situation contrasts sharply with that in many other European countries, where time off for aid work is encouraged and facilitated.

## So, How to Combine Aid Work with Career Progression?

Discuss your plan with mentors and referees. It is helpful to have someone within the system who understands what you are doing and why, and who can explain it to their colleagues and support job applications.

At SHO level it is possible to engineer a 3- or 6-month gap between appointments (ideally arrange a job to come back to in order to avoid losing time searching on your return or having to take an unsuitable position).

For specialist registrars it can be more difficult. Particular times may be more suitable for taking time out, such as after successfully passing a membership or fellowship examination. Negotiate with the local Director of Training and College Tutor. They and the trust will need time to adjust the training rotation allocations in your absence and arrange internal cover or appoint a locum.

The possibility of doing research during the mission may also help your negotiations with the NHS. Talk to people who have recently been in the country to see what projects are running or could be set up. The best options are to carry on a project that is already running, or have people in the country begin preparations before you arrive (it is also important not to be too ambitious, and to remember that many field projects cannot be completed due to a multitude of different factors so do not be too disappointed if this happens).

Unfortunately, owing to minimal/absent levels of supervision, overseas aid work is unlikely to count towards higher surgical or medical training (although some specialities do permit up to 3 months for professional development or specialist military medical training if agreed in advance with the relevant training authority), and accreditation dates will probably be put back by an appropriate period. Another possibility is to combine annual and personal study leave allocations, but this will only allow limited durations of deployment.

For consultants and general practitioners, contracted sabbatical periods are a good way of participating in overseas missions [6]. A number of senior people realise their overseas aid work ambitions after retirement.

## Which Organisation?

There are an ever-increasing number of non-governmental organisations (NGOs) employing health care professionals in aid projects. Each will differ in a number of aspects, such as:

- type/duration of project;
- qualifications required;
- pre-deployment preparation and briefing;
- pre-deployment medical/vaccinations (and who pays for these);
- salary (or no salary);
- living conditions in the field;
- insurance;
- communications (to and from the field);
- medical evacuation in the event of illness or injury.

These factors are *critical* to the individual deploying. Talk to people who have worked for the organisation(s) you are considering and ask if their expectations were met. This will be considered further in the preparation section below. Find out if the organisation adheres to the "People in Aid Code of Best Practice in the Management and Support of Aid Personnel".

After deciding which organisation(s) you would prefer to work with, the next step is to make contact and register with them. This is often an interview-based process, after which references will be taken up. For some organisations a successful interview leads to a further assessment and training course before a decision on your suitability for working with them is made.

Appointments to a programme depend on a number of factors. If you are multi-skilled and available for an unlimited period at short notice, you are likely to be placed quickly. If your availability is more limited or for short periods and your skills are specialised it may be more difficult. Keep in regular contact with the organisation's head office/personnel department so they will consider you when vacancies arise.

International Health Exchange (IHE) is an organisation that helps to recruit, train and retain health workers for relief and development projects. IHE maintains a register of health workers who are interested in working overseas, produces Health Exchange magazine, runs courses and advertises available posts in the magazine and a job supplement (see resources).

# Part B – Preparation

Once appointed to an overseas programme, gather as much information about the country and programme as possible.

A good organisation will assist by providing briefing sheets, including post-mission reports from previous volunteers.

Speak to someone who has recently returned from the same programme to discuss the nature of the work and get recommendations regarding personal clothing and equipment.

Read guide and travel books about the area you are going to.

Prior to the war, Afghanistan was very popular on the overland route to India. Many travel authors wrote interesting accounts of that country.

Remember, however, that areas and routes recommended before a conflict may not be safe or usable during and after a conflict.

Look at internet sites, particularly those of reliable news services working in the country.

One delegate's report is worth reiterating:

> I was due to deploy with an NGO but read in The Economist that the place I was going was back in rebel hands. The organisation could not confirm this but did admit they were having difficulty contacting their people on the ground. I decided not to go.

Decide in advance what degree of personal risk you are prepared to accept.

## Dealing with Families

There is a degree of risk of injury, illness or death in most worthwhile activities. Not all overseas missions are fraught with danger, but some are. You will have to judge for yourself how much to discuss with your partner and family, although for many a rational and realistic discussion is far more reassuring than leaving them wondering and filling in the blanks for themselves. Emphasise how much you will rely on them when you are away for moral support, mail and just knowing that matters at home have been left in capable hands.

Leave your partner/family/solicitor a list of:

- contact names, addresses and telephone numbers for the employing organisation (both UK and overseas);
- contact names, addresses and telephone numbers of your employer in case your plans change while you are in the country;
- bank details;
- passport number/photocopy of passport;
- travel plans/photocopy of travel documents;
- location of important documents (e.g. the car may need taxing in your absence; insurance premiums may need to be paid; General Medical Council (GMC) registration must be maintained).

Make a will and leave it with someone who will be notified in the event of your death. Give the employing NGO the contact details for this person.

## Medical Preparation

A good organisation will assist with pre-deployment medical preparation. The independent worker should consider contacting specialist organisations such as Interhealth, the Travel Clinics run by Hospitals of Tropical Medicine, or those run by travel companies (see Resources section).

Below is a list of areas to consider.

- General health advice for the country or area you are travelling to.
- A dental check-up.
- Vaccinations and supporting certificates (remember – if a number of vaccinations are required they may need several separate visits to the clinic).
- Yellow fever vaccination certificates are required at the port of entry in many African countries.
- Personal medical supplies (enough for the duration or until the next guaranteed re-supply).
- Anti-malarial precautions and prophylaxis.
- Check that the medicines you are taking will be allowed into the country.
- Consider the purchase of a traveller's IV pack, which contains needles, syringes and IV cannulae: most countries will let you bring these in provided the seals on the packs are unbroken.

Possession of recreational drugs carries life imprisonment or the death penalty in many countries.

If you have a pre-existing medical condition (such as asthma, diabetes or ischaemic heart disease) discuss this with the organisation or their medical service. It can be very difficult to manage even mild medical problems when working in the field. If your health deteriorates you may put yourself and others at risk. Remember that the health service in a conflict area or developing country may be limited or non-existent.

Ask what arrangements the organisation has for medical treatment and evacuation (both in-country and for repatriation) and if pre-existing illness is covered. (Aspects of in-country care are considered in the chapter on emergency medical systems (EMS) in Sect. 3).

Keep copies of the relevant policy documents and contact telephone numbers to hand.

## Insurance

There are two main types of insurance – for yourself and for your personal effects. Again this should be provided by your employing agency, but find out. Check that the level of cover is suitable for your needs and that the type of work you are intending to do is covered.

Contact details for insurance and repatriation agencies are given in the Resources section.

## Passport and Visas

Your passport must be up-to-date with at least 6 months to 1 year until expiry.

Visas and travel arrangements should be handled by the employing agency.

Keep photocopies of the key pages of your passport in case it is lost or stolen as this helps the local embassy if a replacement is needed.

If you are travelling independently remember it takes time and effort to get visas.

Special visa agencies can be employed to do the queuing and leg work.

Visas may be needed for transit countries, especially if you need to stay overnight before travelling onward.

Check the political situation regarding existing stamps and visas in your passport. (At the time of writing, entry to Syria or Lebanon will be refused, even with a valid visa, if there is an existing Israeli stamp in your passport.)

Once in-country, travel permits or local identity papers may be needed. Having extra (about 20) passport-size photographs with you speeds this up.

## Travel Documents

Travel in the developing world and in conflict areas is subject to disruption and delay. Transit through isolated or dangerous areas is unpredictable. A competent NGO will plan your travel arrangements accordingly.

Check tickets when you receive them.

Check that accommodation is booked for overnight transits and stays.

Check that connecting arrangements are satisfactory and that there is adequate time between connections.

Ask if you are being met at the airport or other point of entry to the country and by whom.

Take photocopies of travel documents in case the originals are lost or stolen.

## What Clothing and Equipment to Take?

Here is another quote from an experienced delegate:

> In 1992 I set out for Afghanistan to provide medical support for the HALO trust, a mine-clearing charity. It was my first trip abroad in the "aid game". I was, however, confident I could look after myself in Afghanistan. Unfortunately when I arrived in Kabul airport my rucksack was still on the tarmac at Heathrow and still at Heathrow when I got back 3 months later. All I had was my hand luggage and duty-free. I learned never to put all my eggs in one basket, how few items you actually need to survive and the trading value of duty-free.

What to take depends on the type of job you are going to do, the duration, the likelihood of re-supply, the quality of your living conditions, the security situation, the climate, access to communications, luggage allowances and whether or not you will have to carry everything around in-country on your back.

The organisation you are working for should brief you on these points. Travel light if possible. There is a 20-kg weight restriction on most aircraft and you will probably want to bring souvenirs back, so leave space.

In most places there will be shops (of some sort).

In most circumstances you will get the chance to wash yourself and your clothes.

If you are not deploying with the military, DO NOT take clothing or rucksacks that look even vaguely military (particularly olive green, camouflage or with military insignia and patches) or you may be mistaken for a mercenary and killed.

Remember the local culture and customs where you are going, and that revealing clothes may cause offence, particularly around religious sites.

# Luggage

Luggage will get rough treatment by baggage handlers, by being dropped from vehicles and by being squashed under other loads or people.

Options include strong trunks, suitcases or rucksacks. A trunk is good for working in a static location, but take a suitcase or rucksack if lots of moves/carrying belongings are expected.

All should be lockable but easily opened by you for customs inspections and checkpoints. Rucksacks can be protected by lockable covers or metal meshes.

A small day sack is useful for hand baggage and day trips in-country.

# Clothing

Additional clothing can usually be bought in-country if needed. Clothing needs to be practical, hard wearing, easily washed in a bucket and NON-MILITARY in appearance. Several layers that can be put on/taken off according to the climate are practical.

Some suggestions are given below.

*Boots:* Robust good-quality lightweight boots (broken in before hand) that can be worn all day but are suitable for difficult terrain if necessary.

*Training shoes.*

Flip-flop-type *sandals.*

*Trousers:* light-weight walking or climbing trousers with lots of zipped pockets.

*Thermal vests:* silk or polypropylene.

*T-shirts/cotton shirts.*

*Shorts/Tracksuit bottoms* (Ron Hill type very hard wearing).

Good quality *fleece jacket* or (if very cold) down jacket.

*Waterproof clothing* (depending on the area of work).

*Sun hat.*

*Sun glasses* (prescription ones are useful).

Individual *mosquito net* (although most organisations set them up in the residences, the ones in hotels/transit areas may be full of holes).

Some people use ops *waistcoats* with lots of pockets, but these can look military.

Surgical *scrub suit(s)* and *shoes* (if not supplied by the organisation).

Coordinators/delegation heads may need a *jacket* and *tie* (or the female equivalent.)

# Personal Kit

This can make all the difference between comfort and misery. Remember that personal kit is just that – personal so it is your choice. Here are some suggestions.

*Wash kit.* Soap/shampoo/shaving kit. Soap can be purchased/bartered for in most places.

*Sleeping bag.* Depends on the quality of accommodation in-country.

*Glasses.* Take spares and a copy of the prescription (and leave a copy of the prescription with family/partner).

*Contact lenses.* Remember that working conditions may be unhygienic and dusty, and a new supply of contact lens fluids cannot be guaranteed.

*Books/journals.* Check that these are not banned in the country of destination (some medical texts are). Books and journals are of two types – those specific to your task and those for leisure. In the Resources section there is a list of medical books that contributors have found essential. The rule with paperbacks for leisure is take as many as you can, they can always be left in-country and if you don't read them some one else will.

*Torch.* Take a high-power head torch. Power supplies are frequently erratic. A head torch can also be used to operate by when the theatre lights fail.

*Radio.* Get a good quality compact short-wave radio (cost around £70) that will pick up the BBC World Service. (Any Briton working abroad can testify to the morale boosting effect of hearing Lillibullero belting out before the world news.)

*Camera.* The use of cameras will depend on the organisation's rules and the security situation. For medical workers, photographs are the key to presenting your work on your return (and impressing the medical establishment so they will let you or a colleague do this work again in the future). A quality single-lens reflex (SLR) camera with a versatile 80–200-mm zoom lens and a decent flash is good for clinical pictures, and a compact lightweight pocket-sized camera is good for more general work. Slide film is best for presentations; 200 ASA is versatile and 400 ASA is useful for low light conditions. Disposable cameras are of variable quality but it is worth taking one (with its own built in flash) in case the other cameras fail/run out of batteries.

*Batteries.* May or may not be available in-country. Think of batteries for your camera(s), radio, personal CD/cassette player, torch (and laptop computer for the discerning/well-paid aid worker).

*Personal stereo.* Great for delays/waits/periods of isolation/mentally recharging after a hard day.

*Personal computer.* Good for data collection and e-mail (although modems are not permitted in some places), but risk damage or theft. Some electrical items are subject to import taxes in some destinations unless the original receipts can be produced. (Check with the employing agency.)

*Dictation machine/tapes.* Good when compiling reports or making rapid comments when assessing the scene of a disaster or major incident.

*Airmail paper/envelopes/address book.* Even if there is no local postal service, other expatriates will take letters out for you and post them when they get home.

*Sewing kit.*

*Nail clippers* (especially for surgeons).

*Inflatable neck pillow.*

*Swiss Army Knife*/Leatherman or equivalent.

*Games.* Travel chess/backgammon/cards.

*Gifts.* Tea/coffee/chocolate/cheese/processed meats/wine/recent video releases/recent newspapers. Any or all of these will start you off well with your new colleagues. Small gifts of sweets/pens and pencils/cigarettes may be useful en route.

*Postcards/photographs* of your home area (if appropriate) to show local people how and where you live.

*Money.* Travellers cheques in dollars or sterling can be exchanged in most major cities although they have very limited use out in the field. The US dollar is widely accepted (even in places hostile to America). Take small-denomination notes for taxis, tips and other expenses (see section on arriving). Some Eastern European countries (much of the former Yugoslavia) prefer Deutschmarks. Most organisations will provide pocket money in local currency and money spent as dollars/Deutschmarks will usually get change in local currency. Beware of local rules on using moneychangers. Take a credit card for emergencies (such as needing a night in a hotel if flights are delayed or cancelled). Do not carry all your money in the same wallet/pocket or bag.

*Communications.* Find out in advance what communications facilities are like. If you are taking a mobile phone, check that the area concerned is served by your network. E-mail is rapidly becoming available in many locations. There is further discussion about communications in Sect. 3.

## Packing

Lay all the kit out on your floor and prioritise it. Try packing the rucksack/case and see what will and what will not fit in.

Pack your pockets, bum bag and hand luggage with essentials (e.g. travel documents, passport, medical kit, essential books, camera, film).

Assume hold luggage may be delayed or at worst lost en route, so pack this with items that are desirable but not essential (at least for the first few days).

# Part C – Arriving

Arriving and negotiating ports and airports can be a tedious and trying part of the mission. Here are some more quotes from experienced delegates.

> At Freetown's Lungi airport, 10 dollars got me past the immigration police, 20 dollars in fives smoothed my way through beaming customs officers without a bag opened, and I was feeling quite pleased with myself till the local fixer arrived just as I was leaving the terminal. She was late, but made it clear at once that I should have waited for her. She started shouting and made such a scene that the officials I had just bribed began to take an interest again, seeing the chance of further handouts. The last thing I wanted was for them to search my baggage. Quickly I paid her another 10 dollars to shut her up. Mollified she calmed down and ushered me from the terminal, as if her magic alone was responsible. This was normal; this was Africa. (Reproduced with permission from Once a Pilgrim by Will Scully, © Headline Book Publishing, 1999, ISBN 0 7472 6096 6.)
>
> I don't smoke but I buy cheap cigarettes at the airport as they are useful to give as presents. When you pack your rucksack leave a couple of packets on top of all the stuff. If you get searched at the other end the guard will often just pocket the fags and let you through without rummaging through your other stuff. (Ed C, medical aid worker.)

Individual organisations will have their own advice and policies for how they want their employees and representatives to negotiate their way through customs and immigration. Generally this boils down to just show your ID and explain who you are working for; they know us and you will have no problems. Sometimes this works. Most state officially that you must not offer presents however hard the officials press you, but in practice may acknowledge privately that small-denomination dollar bills or cigarettes are an unofficial arrival and departure tax. If this is the case, do not be too generous as people coming through after you will get pestered all the more.

Ideally the organisation should send someone to meet you, and it is a major bonus if they can meet you before customs and immigration with a translator to smooth your arrival.

It is valuable to question co-workers and returnees in detail about what to expect and what procedures need to be followed at your destination. Check with up-to-date travel guidebooks or internet groups.

## General Advice

- Always be polite and very patient. Do not rise to any provocation. Do not ignore official's questions. Answer clearly and precisely, backing what you say with documentation if available or necessary. Do not be over friendly, but do not appear cold and arrogant.

- Always be ready to have your property searched and have keys to cases readily available.
- Keep a vigilant eye on your property while you are waiting.
- Talk with your companions quietly and do not laugh loudly or shout to avoid drawing unnecessary attention to yourselves.
- As soon as possible make contact with your organisation's local representative.
- Check that nothing is missing from your luggage before you move on to your accommodation.

# Part D – Coming Home

If you take mail out for your friends when you leave your mission it is a *sacred duty* to post it as soon as possible. It is also helpful to ring the relatives of your friends to let them know everything is OK. Do not take mail out for strangers or carry packages when you do not know what they contain.

The return home from an overseas mission can be traumatic for some volunteers. Initial euphoria on being reunited with family and friends often gives way to a feeling of mild depression and a desire to return to the overseas project. Having a job to come back to undoubtedly helps in this regard, enabling the individual to refocus their efforts on new tasks and challenges. However, there is the potential for psychiatric morbidity among returned volunteers, and this is considered further in Ch. 12 of this section. Adjusting to coming home may be aided by a debriefing process organised by the employing agency. MSF has the psychological support (PS) network under which returned volunteers are contacted by a member of the network (who has previous field experience) so that emotions and concerns can be discussed confidentially with someone who has insight into the types of situations that have been encountered. Note that the British Red Cross runs "Homecoming Seminars".

In the first part of this chapter, the question of combining aid work with career progression was considered. Presenting clinical cases and a summary of your experiences to colleagues on your return to the UK helps make this work acceptable to the medical establishment and may even inspire others to undertake something similar.

A small proportion of returnees go on to pursue careers in the field of international healthcare. Whilst no defined career path exists, this may involve further missions with the same or other non-governmental organisations, progressing to become a location manager or country project manager, working in a head office and maybe obtaining a paid position with a governmental or international organisation [7].

# Conclusions

International medical humanitarian aid work has the potential to be very challenging and professionally rewarding. Very few of those who engage in such projects regret doing so, and there is increasing recognition of the potential benefits of having undertaken such work to one's First World medical practice [8].

The degree of experience and qualifications needed to participate in these programmes is increasing.

It is difficult to integrate this work with standard medical employment and career progression, but with determination and single-mindedness it can be achieved.

Overseas work has its down side. It can be very hard work, living conditions are Spartan, and there may be risks to personal health and security.

The chance to make a real difference in a challenging environment is very worthwhile.

# References

1. Johnstone P How to do it – work in a developing country. BMJ 1995;311:113–5.
2. Banatvala N, Macklow-Smith A. Integrating overseas work with an NHS career. BMJ 1997;classified supplement 24 May.
3. Chaloner E, Mannion SJ Working overseas – salvation or suicide? Surgery Scalpel supplement 1995;July.
4. NHS Executive. Overseas work experience and professional development. Leeds: NHSE, 1995; EL 9569.
5. Christie B NHS staff should work in the developing world says princess. BMJ 1995;311:77–8.
6. Abell C, Taylor S The NHS benefits from doctors working abroad. BMJ 1995;311:133–4.
7. Easmon C. Working overseas. BMJ 1996;classified supplement 5 October.
8. Banatvala N, Macklow-Smith A Bringing it back to blighty. BMJ 1997;classified supplement 31 May:2–3.

# 9. A Guide to the Medical Student Elective Abroad

Jane Zuckerman

| Objectives | • To address the particular problems faced by medical personnel in hostile environments.<br>• To highlight the importance of preparation.<br>• To discuss the risks and safety.<br>• To discuss avoidance strategies. |
|---|---|

## Introduction

Medical students training in the United Kingdom have an opportunity in their final year to experience medicine in a setting which is different to that of their medical school and its associated satellite district general hospitals. During a period of 2–3 months, medical students may choose from an array of destinations (commonly with the clear objective of studying a specific speciality of personal interest during this time). As travel has become so much easier, with ever shortening times needed to reach far-flung destinations, so the possibility of experiencing medicine in exciting, sometimes hazardous and completely different situations has increased. This finding was confirmed recently by a study, which reviewed both the destinations as well as the hazards associated with the medical student elective. A nationwide survey which included medical students throughout the United Kingdom demonstrated that 97% of students choose to travel abroad, with 69% visiting developing countries, with southern Africa being the most popular [1].

## Preparation

The objectives of the elective period should be clearly defined. Most obviously, the student will have an opportunity to experience the provision of health care in a different country, and this is often associated with different cultural beliefs as well as being more basic in its delivery and its setting. Consequently, students often return from such experiences with a greater understanding of the social perspectives of medicine, including the variation in standards of provision of equipment or availability of therapeutic agents used in a health care setting. Many return more mature and responsible as a direct consequence of their visit, often because they were placed in a position of responsibility not previously encountered (for example undertaking a surgical procedure). Several papers have already described the opportunities and challenges realised in these situations [2, 3].

The importance of ensuring the well being of a medical student during the elective period must clearly be considered and carefully balanced against the rewarding experiences that may be gained at the chosen destination. The suitability of the destination raises issues of both occupationally acquired and travel-related risks of exposure to a variety of hazards, both infectious and non-infectious [4]. It is essential that a dedicated period of time is spent with each student discussing every aspect of their plans, both occupational and travel, in order to identify any potential problems [5]. The importance of such an interview cannot be emphasised enough, as this is an opportunity to minimise exposure to occupational or travel hazards by ensuring that the student understands the methods of preventing such exposure.

In general, medical students choose to gain work experience during their elective period abroad, and the destinations vary from the United States of America, Canada, Australia and New Zealand to developing countries including sub-Saharan Africa and the Indian sub-continent. Many issues should be considered, including environmental hazards and health, security and safety abroad, and the preparations involved when travelling. The initial point of discussion must be the purpose of the elective from the student's perspective. The important points around which the discussion should be based include:

- destination;
- mode of travel;
- duration of travel;
- risk of exposure to disease – both occupationally as well as travel-related.

Each destination and setting requires specific consideration in terms of risk assessment. Some students choose to experience health care in a rural setting, while others may choose a university teaching hospital. The setting, risks and learning experience will be quite different in each location and students must be aware of this.

Before travelling for long periods of time, it is advisable to have a dental and medical check-up so that medical or dental treatment while abroad may be avoided as far as possible. It is strongly advised that comprehensive travel and health insurance is obtained and that this provides cover for accidents, medical treatment abroad and medical repatriation.

# Safety

## Blood-borne Diseases

It is of overwhelming importance to ensure that the student is able to observe universal health precautions. The paucity of medical resources in some settings in developing countries may place the medical student at an unacceptably high risk of occupational exposure to blood-borne viruses by failure to implement universal precautions. The risk may be enhanced by the expectation of the host for the medical student to undertake medical or surgical procedures in which the student may not have a wealth of experience. Finally, the seroprevalence of blood-borne viruses in some developing countries such as southern Africa may be as high as 25% for HIV, resulting in a high risk of nosocomial transmission of HIV in such countries. A recent study confirmed that this risk is real, with five out of eight doctors experiencing a needle-stick injury while treating an HIV-infected patient during an attachment at a rural district hospital in southern Africa, which is equivalent to 0.75 exposures per doctor per year [6]. Medical students, being less experienced, are at an even greater risk of exposure, as demonstrated by a survey of medical students at a London teaching hospital. In this study, two-fifths of students were unaware of the high prevalence of HIV infection in their chosen destinations for their elective. Three out of four students experienced a percutaneous or permucosal exposure to potentially infectious body fluids while on elective in an area of high HIV seroprevalence [7].

It is important to emphasise that the risk of exposure to hepatitis B and hepatitis C is greater than for HIV. Although the majority of students are protected against hepatitis B, a small minority may be non- or hypo-responders to the currently licensed vaccines and so remain susceptible to infection. Conservative estimates of 350 million chronic carriers of hepatitis B virus world-wide, with a risk of seroconversion of 30% if exposed to highly infectious blood in an accidental needle-stick exposure, confirms that the risk of exposure may be high. The seroprevalence of hepatitis C is approximately 170 million, which is several times less than that for HIV. An accidental needle-stick exposure to hepatitis C infective blood carries a risk of seroconversion of 3% [8]. There is currently no available vaccine against hepatitis C and no post-exposure prophylaxis, unlike hepatitis B or HIV. Therefore the risk of exposure to all blood-borne viruses must be carefully considered and discussed with each student individually so that the methods of transmission are fully understood and the methods of prevention are followed to avoid accidental occupational exposure to all such viruses.

### Sexually Transmitted Diseases

Medical students going on their elective should be advised about sexually transmitted diseases and blood-borne viruses in a travel-related setting. Students must be advised to avoid casual sexual contacts, and to use latex condoms correctly with every sexual contact. It should be emphasised that blood-borne viruses may be transmitted by the sharing of needles or syringes, and also by the use of unsterile equipment during ear-piercing, tattooing and acupuncture, particularly in developing countries. Sometimes an accident may require medical intervention with the use of blood and other volume expanders, as well as the use of medical equipment. Where possible, it is advisable to avoid a blood transfusion unless absolutely essential, and if blood products are required, it is advisable to ensure that they have been adequately screened before transfusion. It is always useful to know one's blood group in advance since this may be of great assistance in a medical emergency. In non-emergency situations, it is strongly advisable to request repatriation.

Students travelling to developing countries where the provision of health care may be basic are strongly advised to travel with a sterile medical equipment pack and also to take a small first aid kit, which should contain antiseptic cream, dressings and plasters, anti-fungal powder, anti-histamines, antibiotics, analgesics, anti-diarrhoea agents, insect repellent and scissors (see information in the Resources section).

## Anti-retroviral Kits

An area of controversy surrounds the provision of an anti-retroviral medical kit for students going on an elective to a country with a high HIV prevalence. United Kingdom guidelines do give a recommendation that health care workers with a high risk of exposure to HIV should be advised to take a supply of triple therapy that is currently available [9]. However, the provision of such a pack does have some limitations. First, there may be an element of false security in having such a kit, and complacency with regard to universal precautions must be avoided. Clear instructions would need to be provided on the use of these drugs, whose side-effects are well documented. These problems may become compounded in a foreign setting. Most importantly, the necessary drugs are very expensive, and at present no medical school provides such a kit for elective students. It could be argued that the onus of responsibility should fall upon the student who has chosen to undertake an elective in such a country and therefore they could purchase such a kit. The provision of advice for elective students and the necessity of an anti-retroviral medical kit is under discussion on a national basis, and at present if an accidental exposure should occur to a student while aboard, they are advised to seek immediate local advice as well as contacting their own medical school. If necessary, repatriation can be arranged, and elective students are advised to ensure that they have a comprehensive travel insurance, including repatriation, before they travel abroad.

## Medical Indemnity

It is also important to discuss the arrangements regarding indemnity. Indemnity for clinical practice undertaken during the elective period must be in place. Some medical schools (the employer) do provide this as part of the overall training for each medical student. If this is not the case, any of the medical defence organisations will arrange the appropriate cover for its members. Rarely, the host employer or physician will accept liability on behalf of the student, but it is strongly recommended that each student ensures that they are indemnified for their medical practice during the elective period.

## Other Hazards

Once the occupational risks of exposure have been addressed, it is then important to consider other difficulties and hazards associated with travel. Many students on their elective will take the opportunity to travel within the country or region. It is therefore essential to discuss the associated risks in this context. These include the possibility of culture shock, language difficulties and loneliness. Some students may get carried away with the high expectations associated with their elective plans and not consider these potential problems. Other areas of concern include environmental hazards such as extremes of climate, and venomous bites and stings, as well as accidents. Most importantly, appropriate advice must be given regarding immunisations, anti-malarial prophylaxis and other general methods of prevention of illness while abroad. Where possible, the provision of written advice for the students to read and have readily available is advisable [10].

# Specific Disease Risks and Avoidance Strategies

## Malaria

Malaria remains the single most important disease hazard. Anti-malarial prophylaxis should be discussed, particularly regarding areas of chloroquine resistance and the use of mefloquine or alternative prophylaxis. It is important to point out that prophylaxis remains essential for those who have lived or previously visited endemic areas as they will not have retained immunity against malaria. It must be emphasised that anti-malarial prophylaxis does not confer 100% protection, and the following principles of prevention must be explained.

1. Be Aware of the risk.
2. Prevent or reduce Bites by wearing long sleeves and trousers, especially after dusk. Use insect repellent, especially in the evening and in certain other circumstances, mosquito nets and nets impregnated with insecticide.
3. Full Compliance with chemophylaxis.
4. Seek advice about Diagnosis and treatment promptly if unwell.

Anti-malarial drugs other than mefloquine should be started 1 week before departure and finished 4 weeks after returning. If mefloquine is prescribed appropriately, it should be taken 3 weeks before departure in order to identify any side effects. On return home, any student who develops symptoms of a flu-like illness, or is in any way unwell, must seek medical advice and be tested for malarial infection, which may occur up to a year after return from an endemic country.

Malaria is not the only disease transmitted by the bite of an insect. Other mosquito-borne diseases include dengue fever, for which there is no available vaccine or prophylaxis.

## Immunisation

Depending on their destination, most students will require routine immunisations including hepatitis A, typhoid, tetanus, diphtheria and polio. These should be commenced at least 8 weeks prior to departure. Other recommended vaccines, include rabies, Japanese encephalitis, tick-borne encephalitis and meningococcal meningitis, should be considered depending upon the risk of exposure to disease. Yellow fever is a mandatory vaccine for visits to defined countries in sub-Saharan Africa and South America.

## Tetanus

The risk from tetanus exists throughout the world. All students should maintain protection by receiving booster doses of tetanus vaccine every 10 years.

## Poliomyelitis

Vaccination against polio is recommended for most destinations, and particularly in a health care situation where there will be prolonged and close contact with the indigenous population. If you have never been immunised, a primary course of three doses of vaccine should be administered at monthly intervals. A booster dose is recommended every 10 years for travellers.

## Diphtheria

Since 1991, diphtheria has re-emerged particularly within the former Soviet Union and Eastern Europe. Health care workers should be protected, as transmission may occur in a health care setting when working with the local population. A student who is not immune to diphtheria or tetanus should received three doses of tetanus/low-dose diphtheria vaccine, given 1 month apart. For previously immunised students, a single booster dose of low-dose diphtheria should be given, or where appropriate, tetanus and low-dose diphtheria should be given.

## Hepatitis A

There is a risk of infection with hepatitis A in countries outside North America, North Western Europe, Australia and New Zealand. A complete course of immunisation given on Day 0 and again 6–12 months later will confer protection for up to 20 years.

## Typhoid

This food- and water-borne disease is prevalent in countries with poor sanitation and hygiene. Typhoid vaccine is usually administered by a single injection which affords protection for 3 years. A booster is required every 3 years for those at repeated risk. An oral vaccine is also available, with three doses administered on alternate days and with which an annual booster is recommended.

## Hepatitis B

Health care professionals are required to receive hepatitis B vaccine as part of their employment. Where appropriate, a rapid schedule of vaccination may be administered, after which the antibody response should be measured. For those who have not fully responded to the hepatitis B vaccine and remain at risk of infection, any accidental exposure to blood or body fluids should be reported so that the necessary measures can be taken, including a booster dose of vaccine and/or hepatitis B-specific immunoglobulin.

A bivalent hepatitis A and B vaccine is now available, which is given on Day 0 and at 1 and 6 months later. This will give protection for 5 years against hepatitis B and 10–20 years for hepatitis A. The administration of booster doses using the monovalent vaccines may be considered where appropriate.

## Yellow Fever

Yellow fever vaccine is mandatory for travel within sub-Saharan Africa and South America or for those arriving from infected areas. Immunisation must be documented by an International Certificate of Vaccination, which is valid for 10 years from 10 days after vaccination.

## Meningococcal meningitis

Meningococcal meningitis vaccine is mandatory for anyone visiting Saudi Arabia during the Hajj, and is otherwise recommended if travelling rough, or living or working with local people, and for longer visits to sub-Saharan Africa and areas around Deli, Nepal, Bhutan and Pakistan.

## Tuberculosis

Health care professionals are at increased occupational risk of tuberculosis. Immunisation is recommended for anyone who has not previously been immunised or who is tuberculin-skin-test-negative, and with no evidence of the characteristic BCG scar.

## Rabies

Rabies vaccine is recommended for travel in enzootic areas, particularly if medical help is some distance away. Intradermal immunisation should not be used concomitantly with chloroquine.

## Cholera

Although present in the Far East, Africa and South America, WHO does not recommend the use of cholera vaccine, and immunisation is no longer an official requirement for entry into any foreign country. General food and water precautions are advisable to prevent infection. Cholera exemption certificates are available in certain defined circumstances.

## Japanese Viral Encephalitis

This vaccine is recommended for visits to rural areas of South East Asia and the far East for longer than a month.

## Tick-Borne Encephalitis

This insect-borne disease, which causes meningoencephalitis, is endemic in forested areas of Europe and Scandinavia. Vaccination is recommended for anyone trekking or camping in these areas.

## Hygiene

Other methods of prevention must be discussed as not all vaccines provide 100% protection against disease. Up to 50% of all travellers contract diarrhoea during their trip, with contaminated food and water being the most common cause. It is strongly advised that travellers eat freshly and thoroughly cooked foods and avoid cold platters, salads and shellfish. They are advised to eat easily peeled fruit and vegetables such as tomatoes. Bottled water with an intact seal should be drunk, and ice cubes and non-pasteurised milk should be avoided. There are methods of purifying water including purification tablets and other more complex kits. The phrase "boil it, cook it, peel it or forget it" is a handy way of remembering the principles of food hygiene, especially when travelling.

## Accidents

Unfortunately accidents are a common cause of morbidity and mortality in all travellers, and medical students on their electives fall into this group as well. It is important to ensure that they are aware of the hazards of consuming alcohol and drugs, which can result in uninhibited behaviour and avoidable accidents such as diving into shallow water. They should avoid using motorcycles and travelling at night, especially in rural areas where the road-worthiness of vehicles as well as the standard of the road itself may well be very low. All available safety equipment, including seat belts and helmets, must be used where possible.

## Climate

The use of appropriate clothing will provide protection against exposure to extremes of climate, particularly the sun, as well as providing protection against bites and stings. Sunglasses, an appropriate hat and loose-fitting clothing will provide protection against exposure to the ultraviolet rays from the sun which can adversely affect the skin as well as the eyes. Protective footwear is particularly important in rural settings, both during the day and particularly at night when walking barefoot may result in bites and stings from animals and insects.

## Coming Home

Some students may return unwell from a variety of causes ranging from malaria to amoebic dysentery to schistosomiasis. Medical students and health care professionals in particular should ensure that they obtain medical advice if they return unwell in order to avoid transmission of infection to close family and friends as well as in a health care setting.

# Conclusions

There are many issues which require detailed discussion with medical students going on their elective. By careful planning and seeking advice in advance, many of the hazards, both occupational and travel-related, may be prevented [11]. Medical students must be fully aware of the occupational risks associated with both their chosen specialty and their destination. It may be appropriate for those providing advice in these situations to suggest that it would be inappropriate for the student to undertake an activity deemed to be particularly hazardous and which may result in accidental exposure to blood-borne viruses in an occupational setting [12]. Such a decision needs to be carefully balanced, and often a compromise may be reached so that the medical student still benefits from an exciting and important experience during their training. Although the medical student elective may be considered hazardous from both an occupational and a travel perspective, the majority of students do enjoy a safe and healthy elective and gain experiences which they may not have an opportunity to encounter again.

See also Ch. 17 for further advice.

# References

1. Moss PJ, Beeching NJ Provision of health advice for UK medical students planning to travel overseas for their elective study period: questionnaire survey. BMJ 1999;318:161–2.
2. Personal view. BMJ 1998;316:1466–7.
3. Elective report. Student BMJ 1998;6:32–4.
4. Cossar J, Reid D, Whiting B, Allardice G Health surveillance of Glasgow medical undergraduates pursuing elective studies abroad. Abstract No. 201, 5th International Conference on Travel Medicine, 1997.
5. Westall J, Zuckerman JN. How to plan a clinical attachment abroad. Student BMJ 1998;6:5.
6. Gilks C, Wilkinson D Reducing the risk of nosocomial HIV infection in British health workers working overseas: role of post-exposure prophylaxis. Br Med J 1998;316:1158–60.
7. Gamester CF, Tilzey AJ, Banatvala J Medical students risk of infection with blood-borne viruses at home and abroad: questionnaire survey. BMJ 1999;318:158–60.
8. Zuckerman JN, Clewley G, Cockcroft A, Griffiths P. Prevalence of hepatitis C virus antibodies in health care workers. Lancet 1994;343:1618–20.
9. Department of Health Guidelines on post-exposure prophylaxis for health care workers occupationally exposed to HIV. London: UK Health Departments, 1997.
10. Zuckerman JN Electives: an essential guide for students. 1997. ISBN O 902 094 645.
11. Wilkinson D, Symon B Medical students, their electives and HIV [editorial]. BMJ 1999;318:139–40.
12. Banatvala N, Doyal L Knowing when to say "no" on the student elective [editorial]. BMJ 1998;316:1404–5.

# 10. Avoiding Trouble – Cultural Issues

C.J. Blunden and Campbell MacFarlane

| **Objectives** | • To advise a deployed person on keeping out of trouble.<br>• To raise some of the less obvious issues.<br>• To heighten awareness on issues surrounding religion and gender during deployments. |
| --- | --- |

## Introduction

Most travellers understand that "avoiding trouble" in a foreign country in which they are travelling will include issues that may affect personal safety and security, for example such obvious things as avoiding being present during a gunfight between warring factions within the country, not engaging in espionage, not being caught smuggling drugs through customs etc.

While these obvious examples are valid, avoiding trouble includes a whole range of less obvious aspects, and medical aid workers deploying abroad can find themselves in potentially difficult situations, particularly if the country or cultural environment is unfamiliar. If time permits, workers should therefore try to read up on the country of deployment in advance, noting areas where difficulties might be encountered. Verbal reports from workers who have been in the region are of great value, and clarification of important issues during any handover/takeover is essential.

Assimilation of information, observation, talk, understanding and consideration can go a long way towards avoiding trouble. Probably the single most important factor is attitude. The loud-mouthed, arrogant, disparaging Westerner who is dismissive of the local scenario and culture and will only do things his or her way is looking for trouble, even when involved in humanitarian activities. Insults given, either consciously or subconsciously, or through simple ignorance or failure of understanding, or failure to respect cherished customs and symbols can result in reprisals.

Cultural, religious and gender matters relate not only to relationships with the community involved and patients, but also to relationships with medical aid workers from other groups, relationships with fellow team members and personal behaviour.

The objective should be to show sensitivity, goodwill and a willingness to conform to local customs.

# Culture and Religion

In encountering different cultures for the first time, it is important for medical aid workers to keep an open mind and balanced approach. It is wise not to be disparaging or openly display shock. It is to be remembered that foreigners, even those who are there to help, are guests in the country. There must be respect for national symbols and institutions. In certain Middle Eastern countries the lack of such respect, for example making fun of the national flag, is treated very seriously.

Culture and religion are often interwoven. Therefore both aspects must be taken into consideration simultaneously when trying to establish the dos and don'ts of a particular area or a specific group within an area.

## Culture

In general, respect is shown in Western cultures in various ways, e.g. a firm handshake when greeting people, raising one's hat/cap as a form of greeting, looking someone directly in the eye when speaking to them, standing up when a superior or a lady enters the room etc. Furthermore, it is also expected that men stand back for their superiors and ladies, i.e. allow these persons to precede them through doorways, etc.

In Africa, these Western signs of respect may be misinterpreted. In many African cultures a firm handshake may be interpreted as a sign of aggression. Looking a superior directly in the eye would be a sign of great disrespect. Standing up when a superior enters the room would be totally unacceptable, as having one's head higher than that of a superior is disrespectful. Men precede women through doors to protect them from potential danger.

Some cultures do not shake hands at all when greeting, but show respect in different ways, e.g. Japan (bow, the depth of bow depends on the importance of the person being greeted), China (slight bow), Thailand (slight bow, hands together, fingers pointing up), India (hands together, thumbs against forehead) etc. Europeans, all the way across to Russia, may hug and kiss on the cheeks (usually both cheeks) when greeting. This can come as quite a shock to the unprepared American, British, Australian or South African male. Fortunately, many of these people will include the Western handshake in their greeting ritual so as to put you at your ease.

In certain cultures ritual or actual washing of hands is necessary before eating. A host may offer the guest a certain component of the meal, which is considered a local delicacy, at the beginning of a meal. This should not be refused, even if it is not appealing. To accept a meal invitation and not to eat is also insulting. In conservative Moslem countries the right hand only is used for eating, the left being used for personal cleanliness. In barren desert, with a minimum of water, it is easy to understand how this has evolved. It is wise to express appreciation for the meal at the conclusion. This may include "burping". Be guided by the others. In Middle Eastern countries, introductions may include hand shaking and ritual kissing. It is customary for greetings and introductory small talk to last a considerable time. It is considered rude to get down to business straight away. In conservative Muslim countries it is not appropriate in such small talk to enquire after the health of wives or female family members. Negotiations are likely to be interrupted by other persons barging in and conducting a voluble, animated dialogue with the host. Do not be irritated by this. Negotiations may take the form of bargaining as in the bazaar.

Body attitude is important. It is highly insulting in Arab society to display the soles of the feet to another person; therefore care must be taken to avoid this, especially when sitting on the floor.

In many of these cultures a person who is offended may not show it at the time, but may react at a subsequent opportunity.

## Dress

It is important to understand local dress customs. Women may have to cover themselves appropriately, especially when wearing Western-style clothing. It may also be offensive for men to wear shorts or to discard shirts. Bathing in the sea, rivers or pools may require covering dress also. An aid worker wandering about in miniskirt, halter top and bare midriff off duty could paralyse the work of the team. Cultural realities should be assessed in advance or be rapidly adjusted to in the early stages of deployment.

## Interpreters

It is to be remembered that interpreters may put things their own way and that there can be confusion. It is worth remembering that the other party, although working through an interpreter, may understand varying amounts of English. Apart from words, facial expression and body language can speak volumes in total silence. Care is needed!

## An Example – Sub-Saharan Africa

Culture has been influenced by the colonial period in the past as well as by urbanisation and the advent of radio and television. The original culture of a group may be more visible in rural areas. Since there are many different ethnic groups and languages, all with different cultures, beliefs and value systems, no single description will cover all circumstances, but some general observations may be of use.

Respect for elders is very important. In Africa especially, do not make the mistake of underestimating an old, seemingly unimportant person sitting in the dust in front of a hut. Home life is based on the extended family. This can create some unexpected misunderstandings. For example someone working for you may request time off to attend the funeral of his mother. Some time later he may once again ask for time off for his mother's funeral. While this may be an outright lie, it is more likely to be due to the fact that in the extended family more than one person may be regarded as the mother, e.g. the biological mother and the woman who actually raised the child while the biological mother was away earning money. This same worker may also request time off, possibly several days on each occasion, to attend funerals of aunts, uncles or cousins, which may seem somewhat excessive from a Western point of view with its emphasis on the nuclear family. Be tolerant. The funeral process is also usually much longer than in Western society and may take some days, including travelling time.

Show respect for the local "medicine man/woman" even if you do not think much of his or her bedside manner or seemingly primitive medical skills. Remember that he or she is held in high esteem by the local population and will probably be the only person in the area with any medical skills whatsoever once you leave. Furthermore, these medical skills will be strongly interwoven with the local religion and will have a very strong psychosomatic effect on the patient. This "medicine man/woman" will therefore very often obtain surprisingly good results (which the Western doctor will, possibly somewhat cynically and not necessarily correctly, attribute to the placebo effect).

Do not think that members of the local population will automatically think that your Western medical knowledge is superior to that of your local counterpart. You may find that once you start taking a history or doing a general examination, the patient loses all respect for your ability. The local "medicine man/women" will not take a history or do a Western medicine type of examination, but will, during the course of the consultation, gradually tell the patient what is wrong, where the pain is, who or what is to blame for the patient's current problems and what remedial action is required.

Women usually have a subservient role in their families and do not play prominent roles in the community, even though it seems as if they do the bulk of the manual labour in their households.

Circumcision, both male and female, is still practised widely in Africa despite international opposition especially to female circumcision. If you are going to an area where this may be an issue, before going, decide how you intend handling the situation should you be faced with it, and make sure that all of the members of your group understand the complexities of the problem and are in agreement as to how the group should react.

Punctuality is not a strong point in many areas in Africa. Make allowances. Remember that many people do not own watches, distances are great, public transport is often unreliable, private transport is very expensive (seen from the local inhabitant's point of view) and walking takes time.

## Other Cultures

There are many other cultures across the world, each with its own particular mores. For example in some areas in Japan and China, blowing one's nose and then placing the handkerchief in one's pocket is offensive, the caste system in India places certain restrictions on some people and may affect their relationship with you because of contact that you may have with members from another caste, etc.

Remember that even when you are going out of your way to be accommodating in all cultural and religious matters you are bound to make mistakes or overlook things. Do not despair. If you observe closely you will probably find that your hosts, especially in those situations where humanitarian aid is concerned, are making an even bigger effort to accommodate your (to them) strange Western religious and cultural idiosyncrasies. Very often, what is most important is not the fact that you have mastered every local religious or cultural detail, but the fact that it can be seen that you are making an effort to be accommodating and respectful of matters that are important to your hosts.

# Religion

It is very difficult to describe what would be "typical" behaviour shown by every member of a specific religion, as every individual does not necessarily practice his faith to the same degree as all other members of that faith. The descriptions given below must therefore be regarded as guidelines only and each situation must be assessed individually.

Try to avoid a preconceived negative attitude to religions other than your own. When travelling in areas where the religious beliefs and customs are radically different from your own, be polite and friendly, but above all mind your own business. Do not be judgemental. Do not try to convert anyone to your own religion. Do not mock or be openly derisive of customs or practices which you regard as primitive or amusing. Respect all local customs. Behave with proper decorum at all religious sites. Be aware of local dress etiquette and do not wear clothes which may give offence. Avoid wearing any religious insignia which may cause controversy. Treat all religious objects (no matter how trivial from your point of view) with respect. Be aware of religious periods of significance to the local population and respect the spirit and customs of these periods.

While Sunday is considered the holy day for most Christians, Muslims regard Fridays and Jews regard Saturdays as their respective holy days.

Some religions frown on the drinking of alcohol. Respect this and do not serve alcohol in the presence of members of such religions. Be especially careful not to sell alcohol-containing beverages to members of these communities who approach you "discreetly" with such requests.

Ensure that you understand the male/female roles in a particular culture or religion and how you, as a stranger, should conduct yourself.

Avoid obvious potential religious conflict, e.g. it may not be a good idea for one of the Jewish faith to be travelling through a fundamental Islamic area.

Be aware, especially if you are left-handed, that the left hand is considered unclean in some religions and should not be used for eating, for passing objects to other people or for touching holy objects.

Taking photographs of people may be unacceptable. Always ask permission first and do not insist if permission is refused. Do not try to take "sneak" photographs.

If allowed into places of worship or homes, it is often customary to remove shoes. Do not ogle the women if any are visible. If no women are visible, do not ask why the women of the household are not present or enquire after their health.

There follow some comments on the more common religions which you may come across. These comments are by no means detailed, and are in fact only some very general pointers to those things which may have an influence on the way the local inhabitants interact with you.

## Christianity

The attitudes of practising Christians can vary from ultra-conservative to ultra-liberal, with most being somewhere in the middle of the spectrum. There are also some variations of the Christian faith which may be overlooked, for example some sects regard Saturday as the holy day of the week, Quakers will not fight under any circumstances, and Jehovah's Witnesses will not permit blood transfusions.

## Islam

The Muslims believe that Allah is the one true God who created heaven and earth. The prophets in the Old Testament, Abraham, Isaac, Jacob and Moses, are also regarded as prophets of Allah, as are Jesus and the last prophet Mohammed. Muslims are in general conservative. Modesty in dress is expected. The following points should also be borne in mind.

- Visiting aid workers should dress appropriately and avoid revealing or tight-fitting clothing.
- Muslims are required to pray five times a day.
- Each of these prayer sessions may take up to 20 minutes.
- In some Moslem countries it is customary to close shops, interrupt TV programmes, etc. during these prayer times. It is necessary to become accustomed to this.

Friday is the holy day of the week. Government departments in Muslim countries will be closed. However, Muslim businesses in non-Muslim countries will usually still be open on Fridays although they may close for 2 hours at midday.

During the month of Ramadan, Muslims will fast from sunrise to sunset. Ramadan is the ninth month of the Islamic calendar, but note that this calendar is based on the lunar month, which is shorter than the Western calendar month – the month of Ramadan therefore shifts gradually through all of the seasons. Do not invite a Muslim to lunch during this period. An invitation to dinner, which starts after sunset, is acceptable. It is also courteous to avoid giving parties during the first month of the Islamic year (because Mohammed's grandson was murdered in that month).

Muslims eat Halal food, i.e. meat from animals slaughtered in a specific way. Muslims do not eat pork or a combination of dairy products and meat. Alcohol is taboo.

Muslims will want to bury their dead on the same day that death occurs, with the right-hand side (and the face) turned towards Mecca. Bear this in mind when you are required to issue death certificates or do post mortems.

Men and women usually pray separately. If women do come to the Mosque, they usually pray in a separate area or stand behind their menfolk. A woman should never greet a man by hand.

In conservative Muslim areas it is always better to have female members in a medical team to treat Muslim females. Male doctors may find that they will not be able to examine their female patients. Indeed, they may not even see their female patients, but may have the woman's husband describing his wife's problem, answering any questions, and then taking the resultant medication and advice on its use home to give to his wife.

## Judaism

Those of the Jewish faith vary from ultra-conservative Orthodox Jews who practice their faith in very strict accordance with the dictates of the Torah, to the more liberal members of the faith who have adapted many of the traditional ways to fit in with modern Western culture. Do not overlook the question of kosher food. Dietary laws specified in the Torah and followed by Orthodox Jews include the following: animals must be slaughtered in a specific way and the carcass drained of blood; meat and dairy products may not be eaten together and separate sets of crockery and cutlery are used for this purpose; pork may not be eaten; only animals which chew the cud and have cloven hoofs may be eaten; only fish with scales and fins may be eaten; etc.

If any potential team members are Jewish, establish exactly what their dietary requirements will be and whether these requirements can reasonably be met in the area to which you are going. If not, find out whether the team member is prepared to adapt to the local conditions, before he or she is finally accepted as a team member.

The Sabbath extends from sunset on Friday evening to sunset on Saturday evening. When planning duty rosters make allowance where possible.

## Hinduism

Hinduism is a many-sided faith. There is no single supreme deity, but rather a pantheon of Gods which has developed over thousands of years while absorbing and assimilating many religions and cultural movements over this time. Followers of this faith are usually vegetarians and usually do not take alcohol. The essential spirit of Hinduism seems to be live and let live, and it is thus very tolerant of other religions and cultures. Hindus believe in reincarnation, and that performing good deeds during one lifetime will result in birth at a higher level in a subsequent lifetime.

Women have a subservient role and are usually dependent on their fathers, husbands or sons. Women's rights are, however, gaining momentum.

## Other Religions

There are many other religions practised throughout the world. Make sure that you are at least superficially acquainted with those which are practised in the area to which you are going.

# Gender

Female team members are increasing in numbers. They have shown themselves to be outstanding in the field. Many females work more efficiently than males and have better powers of concentration; many have greater emotional resistance in adversity than males and greater physical endurance (as opposed to muscular strength). Recognition of these factors is resulting in more and more women finding their rightful place in many areas previously considered unsuitable. Even the military, traditionally conservative, has recognised this. The presence of women in the team invariably has a beneficial effect by increasing capability, introducing a civilising and caring ethos, and being of particular value in the handling of women and children in conservative countries where males examining or treating females is frowned upon. On the other hand, women freely mixing with males, and examining and treating male patients, may be considered unacceptable.

With regard to females in command, women are increasingly finding their rightful place in this situation, and because of long-held prejudices, this may be a particularly difficult task, requiring tact and understanding, but also strength and determination. Any male team member who has a problem with this should come to terms with it or leave the team prior to deployment. In the military it is easier; the commander, irrespective of gender, is the commander. Team members should be selected on their individual characteristics, with their individual strengths and weaknesses being taken into consideration, irrespective of gender. End of story!

These sentiments, however, are not universally held. The concept of a female in command may not only be unheard of, but also be totally unacceptable in certain conservative societies, especially if it involves authority over local males. Such a command structure may be considered an insult to the host country and lead to the undermining of the team's work or even a demand for its withdrawal. Realities such as this must be taken into consideration by the planners when configuring the team.

### Sexual Relations

Sexual relations between team members may or may not be a problem. Already established relationships, particularly within marriage, may strengthen the team by providing mutual support to team members providing this does not result in unfair division of labour or favouritism. Relationships outside marriage may be unacceptable to local culture. It is in the nature of humankind that people working together in close proximity and under conditions of stress may develop relationships with each other. This may be totally harmless and indeed beneficial for those involved, but if it results in work being affected or unacceptability in the prevailing culture, there is the possibility of trouble. The situation needs to be watched carefully. If one or other or both parties are married to other people, this creates more problems. Quite apart from the moral aspects this could create tensions in the team and outrage in certain communities. The knowledge that such events occur could prevent team members from deploying in the future because of spouses refusing to allow them to go. It is recommended that the moment such a liaison between married members comes to light, the team leader should counsel those involved. If warnings are ignored, one or other or both parties should be returned to home base at the earliest opportunity.

Sexual relationships with the local populace in the area of deployment are to be firmly discouraged. They can be a recipe for disaster. There may be cultural problems, the possibility of abduction or blackmail, allegations of sexual assault or improper behaviour, and, of course, potential health problems (*see also Ch. 9 and 11*).

The issue of HIV and post-exposure prophylaxis was discussed in the previous chapter on medical student electives.

## Political Sensitivities

Be aware that the political situation can change at the drop of a hat. Up-date your information regularly. Observe neutrality, and ensure that your conduct is such that accusations of taking sides cannot be made against you or any of your team members. Do not get involved with competing local groupings. Do not attend "discreet" private meetings with individual rival local warlords.

Avoid politics and political arguments as far as possible, and do not try to convert those around you to your point of view.

### Gifts and Bribery

Bribery is the normal way of getting things done in many developing countries and can take many forms, varying from an outright demand for money to hints (and nothing gets done if the hints are not taken) that require you to hand over a small gift, e.g. your watch or your pen. Find out in advance what can be expected in the area to which you are going and then comply appropriately, always with a smile on your face. In this kind of area it is especially important to be accompanied by a reliable local official (who may also require a "gift", but will at least ensure that the "gifts" that are handed out will be within reasonable limits). Where this practice is anticipated, ensure that you have sufficient money (American dollars, small denominations) or an adequate supply of pens, cheap watches and pocket knives.

# Conclusions

Avoiding trouble involves pre-planning, orientation and familiarisation, common sense, and the development of standing operating procedures. Great tolerance should be shown towards all religious and cultural matters, especially those which the medical aid team members may find strange or unsettling.

Even though the medical aid team members are in an area to render humanitarian aid, they can still be killed or injured in traffic accidents or during criminal acts committed by members of the local population who do not really care who gets in their way. The onus is thus on each and every member of a medical aid team to take all reasonable precautions to ensure the safety of all of the team members and thus also the ultimate success of the particular medical aid mission.

## Recommended Reading

Robert Young Pelton. Fieldings: The World's Most Dangerous Places. California: Fielding Worldwide, 1998. This interesting book covers all of the world's trouble spots in great detail. It is a very comprehensive book of essential information for the traveller going virtually anywhere off the beaten track. Quite apart from the invaluable advice and factual information, this soft-cover book will provide fascinating reading for those quiet times on your travels.

# 11. Dealing with Trouble – The Wider Issues

## Jeff Green

**Objectives**
- To inform the aid worker about safety issues.
- Specifically, to deal with common problems surrounding security and safety.

## Introduction

Conflicts and catastrophes, natural or otherwise, do not only visit themselves on the people living in the areas they hit. They can also have a profound effect on people who specialise in helping to sort out their aftermath.

Aid workers who go overseas as part of relief missions or to help set up or run medical stations and the like can find their personal safety at risk. Some of the dangers in a war zone are obvious. There is physical danger from military attack, deliberate or accidental.

On top of this kind of hazard come others that may occur in the wake of war or disaster. The political instability that results from conflicts or the breakdown of central control brings with it possible trouble. Police forces, the army and local militia can all become laws unto themselves.

Weapons become available to parts of the population that would not normally be armed. If this is the case, then aid workers may find themselves almost routinely in contact with people who are armed but have either no training or no inclination to exercise discipline.

Economic dislocation can be a recipe for banditry, and it is no great surprise that kidnapping hostages to hold them for ransom can quickly become a growth industry.

Regrettably, being there to help does not necessarily afford any protection at all. Medical aid workers will have things that other people want: transportation, money and food.

Aid workers can often find themselves in hostile environments where their presence is simply not wanted by some groups. A good example of this would be medical aid workers who find themselves tending the wounded of one particular faction in a civil war. They may be able to argue that they are non-partisan and are working in a particular spot through chance, but the other side in the conflict may simply decide that the aid workers are giving succour to their enemies.

Even nationality can be an issue. It is not uncommon for foreigners overseas to be taken captive, and one particular nationality is then singled out for harsh treatment. Often it is Americans who are the unfortunate victims of this kind of behaviour, but grudges can be held against any country or ethnic group.

However, there are a number of basic precautions you can take, both before you go abroad and when you get there. A great deal of this is common sense and involves making proper preparations, staying alert and not taking unnecessary risks.

## Preventative Measures

It is always better to avoid trouble in the first place rather than having to find a way out of it once it has happened. This starts at home with preparations before you leave the United Kingdom. Once you have arrived, there are a number of basic steps you can take to minimise any risks against you both immediately on arrival and through-out your stay.

The country or region you will be working in is likely to be unstable as a result of the conflict or natural disaster you are going there to help deal with. It is impor-tant to find out as much as you can about that area.

Unfortunately, the Foreign Office is not a great deal of help in this. It tends to issue blanket warnings for UK citizens not to visit an area it considers potentially dan-gerous. This is fine as a warning for tourists, but not a great deal of use to aid workers whose jobs it is to go there and clean up the mess the government is warning about.

However, you can contact some of the private companies that deal with just these kinds of security issues, and they can give you and your organisation information about the region you will be travelling to as well as practical tips to help when you get there.

Do remember that it is not just the current situation you need information on, but the local laws and customs too. Much ignorance of these last two accounts for most of the problems aid workers encounter. Some of these aspects were considered in the previous chapter.

A little bit of history can go a long way, too. Is the country a former colony, and if so, is there any continuing antagonism towards its former colonial masters? The same is true with regard to any former conflicts. If it is the case that there is a strong sentiment against the UK, then you need to question whether it is sensible to send a UK national there in the first place.

The choice of local help can be a sensitive issue. If there is a history of ethnic violence, it may be a mistake to employ members of one grouping when dealing with another.

Find out the locations and telephone numbers of the UK embassy or consulate along with those of friendly countries. You should also be issued with a plastic card with important contact numbers written on it. This should be in the language of the country you are visiting.

When you arrive at your destination, take the time to familiarise yourself with the area you will be staying in. Use local knowledge to find out where the local hot spots are. Certain areas may be controlled by particular groups. This could be a particular tribe prone to kidnapping to force concessions out of central government, or local centres of political influence in unstable countries.

The reliability of the local authorities is an important point. Can the local police or militia be trusted, or are they in cahoots with local criminals and kidnappers? It is not unknown in Latin America, for example, for local police to double-up as kidnappers.

It is a good idea to deal with the local authorities in a given area rather than the police. If there is central authority in the region, they will represent it and should therefore have some degree of control. In some countries or parts of countries, protection provided by law enforcement agencies can be construed by groups as co-operating with the "hated" authorities thus putting aid workers at greater risk.

Local consulates and embassies should also be able to provide some practical help in these areas. Again some private security firms will be able to help.

Look like an aid worker, do not dress like a soldier. You can usually assume that as part of a relief effort, your presence will be welcomed by most of the local population. Try as clearly as possible to identify yourself as an aid worker. Military clothing may be practical to wear, but it makes you look like a soldier and therefore a potential threat in people's eyes.

Be vigilant, notice what is going on around you. If something strikes you as odd or sinister talk to your colleagues about it and ask them to look out too. Just being aware of a trap being prepared can be enough to stop it being sprung.

- Find out about the country you will be working in before you leave the UK.
- Contact firms specialising in security issues.
- Try to find out how reliable the local authorities and police force are.
- Have full documentation and identification.
- Be aware of what is going on around you and if there are any likely threats forming.

## Arrest and Detention by Legitimate Authorities

Most problems experienced by aid workers when they come into contact with local police, army or militia groups is the result of ignorance or problems beyond their control.

The value of finding out about your destination before you leave for it cannot be over-stressed. Possession and consumption of alcohol is illegal in many Muslim countries. Find out if this is the case in the region you will be going to. If it is illegal, then do not do it.

Arrest and detention may be as a result of something beyond your control. For example, it is not unknown for workers to be detained because their employer has not fulfilled a contract, and then released when it has.

Work on the assumption that your general presence as an aid worker is welcome and be sure that both you and your vehicle are properly identified as part of a humanitarian aid group. This should help ease this kind of situation.

Whatever the reason, the first thing to remember is not to panic. Keep calm and try as quickly as possible to communicate your whereabouts to your colleagues and, very importantly, the British consulate. If there has been a misunderstanding or your arrest is the result of over-zealous behaviour by officials on the spot, they should be able to apply extra pressure to sort it all out speedily.

This may be done for you by the authorities holding you. If it has not been, then assert your right to do so. If this is the situation, be firm, but do not be haughty. You may have to rely on their goodwill, so there is no point in alienating them.

This is often easier done by insisting on talking to the officer in charge of the situation who may be more aware of the need not to antagonise your agency or employer. Go as high up the chain of command as you can as soon as you can.

It may also help to have someone with you who has local knowledge. They should be able to smooth out misunderstandings and get you on your way. They should certainly know what your rights are in such situations and how far you can push them. This will also help if a small gift or bribe is needed to speed things up.

As ever, try to talk to the local authorities rather than the police in these situations and make sure you have proper identification as well as contact numbers with you.

- Find out about local laws and customs.
- Do not offend local dress codes.
- Contact your organisation or the nearest British consulate as soon as possible.
- Insist on dealing with senior personnel.
- Use a guide or helper with local knowledge.

## What to Do at Road-Blocks

Road-blocks are an ever-present feature in conflict and disaster zones, whether they are there to restrict the flow of people and traffic to make relief work easier, or for one group or faction to exercise control over a particular area.

The people controlling or manning a checkpoint will not necessarily represent the legitimate authority in a particular area. It may be a police or army checkpoint, but it may also be manned by local militia or other factions.

Do some groundwork. The agency you work for should already have found out what the political situation is on the ground. Local authorities – not necessarily the police – should also be able to give further information on the ground. Since it is your job to go to these areas, being told simply not to go there because it is too dangerous may not be an option. Being prepared in advance may save a great deal of time and trouble later on.

If there is a risk that you may encounter an armed road-block, prepare for this. Do not wear military-style clothing. It may be comfortable and practical, but it also marks you out as a potential target.

If it is at all possible wear blue clothing, as this shows you are not military personnel. In particular, try to get hold of blue, rather than green or brown flak jackets.

The vehicles you travel in can also mark you out as a target. Once again, do not use vehicles that are painted in military colours, and mark your vehicle very clearly as one being used by an aid agency.

When and if you do encounter a road-block, the personnel manning it will often be very aggressive. There is also a good chance that they will be untrained, undisciplined and possibly intoxicated.

Do not make any aggressive movements that are likely to put the people manning the road-block further on their guard. Make sure you have proper documentation saying who you are, who you work for, why you are there and the authorities that have given you permission to travel in that particular area.

Local knowledge can be invaluable, so if at all possible travel with someone who knows the local area, the political situation and speaks any local dialects. This can help avoid or diffuse what can be potentially dangerous misunderstandings.

However, having bodyguards is impractical at best and at worst can make a non-aggressive situation explosive. Travelling with an armed escort automatically increases the tension at a road-block when the people manning it are also armed.

They may end up being shot at or, as they are often badly paid, either turn on you or simply make themselves scarce if trouble starts.

Do not let the age of any gunmen on a road-block put you at your ease. You need to assume that anyone carrying a gun is perfectly capable of using it, irrespective of age.

The people manning the road-block are likely to be junior in their organisation. Insist on talking to someone in authority as soon as you are able to. Go as far up the chain of command as quickly as you can and get away from the more trigger-happy and nervous junior personnel.

In this be firm, but don't be haughty. You will be in a situation where the person with the gun can decide your fate, so it is a bad idea to antagonise them.

Since you are an aid worker and are there to help people, establish your credentials as such as quickly as you can. You are there to help people and this is one of your greatest assets, so make full use of it.

There is a chance that the gunmen will demand either money or some of the aid – food or medicine – that you are carrying. If this happens, you really have no choice but to hand it over. They are the ones with the guns and the ability to imprison you.

On the other side of this coin, a small present or bribe may also help to oil the wheels and get you through a road-block faster. Do take care when you do this, and relying on someone with local knowledge here is preferable.

- Find out where the local hot spots are.
- Do not dress like a soldier.
- Mark vehicles clearly as ones working for an aid organisation.
- Be firm, but not aggressive and insist on talking to the officer in charge.
- Hand over money if it is demanded.

## Kidnapping

There may often be a serious risk that you could be abducted in the area you are working. This can be for a variety of reasons – straightforward ransom demands of money, demands for central authorities to improve conditions, political statements or outright revenge for perceived injuries.

Once again, being prepared for the worst happening in advance is important. Before you go to the conflict or disaster area, find out who to contact. Make sure you are issued with a plastic card that has all the contact numbers for your organisation on it. The sooner the kidnappers are able to make contact and make their demands known, the sooner the process starts that will end in your release.

If the worst does happen, don't panic. The vast majority of kidnappings end with the hostages being released unharmed. Deaths or injuries are usually the result of pre-existing medical conditions, heart problems for example, or botched escape or rescue attempts. You must also assume that everything is being done to secure your release.

Once in captivity, accept all food you are given and eat it, no matter how unappetising it may seem. You do not know when you will be getting your next meal, and the onus is on you to look after your health as far as possible.

Similarly, try to exercise each day. This may be difficult in cramped surroundings, but it is important both physically and mentally that you do so. If you do have a medical condition, tell your kidnappers. This could improve your treatment. A dead hostage is a bad bargaining chip and they will want to keep you alive.

Your stay with your kidnappers may be protracted. Often kidnappers will not claim responsibility for an abduction for a number of weeks. The aim is to sow confusion, uncertainty and panic in the minds of the people who will ultimately be working for your release. Try to play down your importance; stress that you work for a charity which, unlike a multinational corporation, is non-profit making and does not have lots of money. Explain that you are there to assist the local community and this type of action can only harm this assistance.

Try to establish some kind or rapport or relationship with your kidnappers. If you are able to build a relationship with them it will make it that much harder for them to mistreat or ultimately kill you. Note the box below on the Stockholm Syndrome.

Do not try to escape unless you are absolutely sure of success. Failed escape attempts make up much of the 10% or so of kidnappings that end with the death of a hostage. Unless the opportunity to do so is overwhelming, just don't.

Rescue attempts can also cause problems and account for many of the other deaths in captivity. Assume that your aid organisation and its advisers will be working for your release by negotiation.

### The Stockholm Syndrome

This is a recognised psychological reaction in hostages who come to relate closely with their captors and has variable outcomes for all parties. The syndrome is most likely to develop when the hostages and captors share the same conditions, live in close proximity and share a common language, and where hostages do not refute their captors' views.

In this "syndrome", hostages develop feelings of friendliness towards their captors and negative feelings towards the authorities outside. This is reciprocated by the captors. Such feeling can improve your situation and potentially diminish the likelihood of your being killed, so it is of potential use to you to empathise with your captors, but the consequences of such action following release are unpredictable.

However, look around you for the safest areas in the complex you are being held in. If there is a rescue attempt, then seek shelter by a solid wall or in a ditch or depression.

In the event of you being contacted to be told that one of your co-workers has been kidnapped, do not attempt to negotiate with the kidnappers. Professional hostage negotiators will do the job far better than you can and will understand far better what the kidnappers are trying to achieve.

It is also vital that when first contacted, you do not promise the kidnappers anything. This may come back to haunt you as a broken promise, or it may simply weaken your bargaining position at the outset.

You should also think very seriously about whether it would be a good idea to pull the rest of your personnel out of that area until the hostage crisis has passed. This may seem like an abdication of responsibility by aid workers, but it is not. Hostages cannot administer relief.

- Always carry identification and contact numbers with you.
- Eat any food that is given to you.
- Exercise daily.
- Build a rapport with your captors.
- Do not try to escape.

## Munitions

Working in war zones will bring many aid workers into contact with munitions. This can be as obvious as an armed military presence in an area, to armed road-blocks, minefields and booby traps.

If you know that an area has been mined in the past, then stick to well-used paths. The road itself may have been cleared of mines, but there is every chance that the verge or fields at the side have not been cleared.

Never go off for a wander in the woods or a field, and overcome embarrassment when it comes to toileting. This may have to be done in the open where there is no danger from mines.

When travelling in convoy, always drive in the tyre tracks of the vehicle in front where you know there are no mines. If the vehicle you are in or the one in front of you hits a mine, try not to jump out of the side of a vehicle. As far as is practically possible attempt to scramble over the back and then walk in the tyre tracks already made that are mine-free.

Beware of booby traps as well. These are often concealed amongst military equipment or dead bodies, so exercise maximum caution if you have to try to move them.

- Do not wander off.
- Always stay on marked tracks, even for personal functions.
- Drive in the tyre tracks of the vehicle in front.
- Beware of booby-traps when moving either military hardware or dead bodies.

# Conclusions

Much of the advice which aid workers need to minimise the danger to them when working in conflict or disaster areas is common sense. Be prepared before you leave the UK, and contact local authorities when you get there.

Find out about local laws and customs so you do not break them unawares. Check what the local political situation is and where the dangerous hot spots are located.

Always carry identity documentation with you and approach potentially difficult or dangerous situations with a firm but non-aggressive attitude.

If the worst happen and you are held by local authorities or kidnappers, remember that people will be doing their best to secure your earliest possible release. The overwhelming majority of hostage takings end with the victim returning unharmed.

Above all, keep in the front of your mind that you are there to help the local population. That very fact will be a passport to better treatment.

The main points are:

- Good pre-deployment briefings.
- Reliable communications.
- Good passage of information about developing situations.
- Clearly defined guidelines as how to react in risky situations.
- Identification of, and liaison with, influential people in the area.
- Be seen to be impartial.
- Be easily identifiable as an aid worker.

EDITORS' NOTE – See also the Resources section at the end of this manual.

# 12. Psychological Aspects of the Provision of Medical Humanitarian Aid

Ian P. Palmer

**Objectives**

- To raise issues about the pre-deployment phase.
- To discuss psychological problems arising during deployment.
- To heighten awareness of problems arising in the post-deployment phase.

## Introduction

The psychological aspects involved in the provision of medical aid in hostile environments relate to general issues and those specific to the location to which you deploy, as well as the phases of that deployment.

- Pre-deployment – preparation.
- Deployment – separation.
- Post-deployment – repatriation, reunion and readjustment.

Any deployment leads to a *constriction* of your world that creates a unique experience for those involved, the importance of which becomes clearer on your return home. Your experience may be positive, negative or anything in between, and will change you.

## Deciding to Go

This may seem an odd issue, especially if you have already bought this book AND read this far, but it is the key to the psychological aspect of the whole process.

Remember – any deployment leads to a *constriction of your world*. You will be spending time with people you may not know and may not like, but with whom you have to coexist and, at times, even rely on.

Emotions can run high and interfere with missions – remember isolation brings out the best and worst in humans! So ask yourself about the motives, drives and personalities of those with whom you are going, and whether you share a common agenda.

Try to assess what you hope *realistically* to achieve, as the reality on the ground may be vastly different from your expectations pre-deployment. Understand and accept from the outset that you (along with everyone else) will be changed by undertaking this work. Despite the hardships, unpleasantness and difficulties encountered, most people find it a positive experience. It may lead to a deeper understanding of humanity, the workings of the world and your place within it, yet for a minority the experience will be less positive.

---

**Why Am I Going?**

Be clear and honest in your mind as to your reason for going. Is it: to do something worthwhile; to utilise your skills; to "put something back"; to take a risk; to "escape" from something? (But don't forget that the something will generally be there on your return!!)

---

**Who Am I Going With?**

Organisation – what are its goals; are they trustworthy?

Others – what are their motives, ambitions, drives and personalities? Do we share a common agenda?

**What Information Have I Sought?**

What sources? Media, non-governmental organisation (NGO), friends, work-mates etc.

What ever you do, get as much information as possible in order to answer all your questions.

**What Are my Expectations of the Mission?**

How different will the reality be? Generate a picture of reality.

---

# Preparation – Pre-deployment

## Preparation for Separation

Your *aim* is to deploy in good physical and mental health in order to complete your mission.

Your ability to perform well on a mission is diminished if you are preoccupied with worries about home (money, legal, relationships etc.) and compounded by the boredom inherent in many deployments, which will lead you to ruminate about them. *So, sort things out now!*

## Systems

Deployment will lead to changes in your social *system*. The moment you decide to go, preparation begins in order to accommodate to your *loss* from this system.

Your exit may be supported, wished for, resented or not desired, but whatever the reason, a degree of emotional distancing in relationships is bound to occur. This may be reflected in quarrels or disagreements, a less than satisfactory sexual life and so forth. It is important not to misrepresent events or words at this time – full and frank discussion is the best way to deal with the situation.

Whilst you are away life goes on as normal, but those left behind will change during your absence. There is a natural tendency to hold a *fixed* view of life at home as a place that will be the same on your return. Whilst this is helpful *during* the deployment, it can cause problems afterwards if it is not reality-based.

There may be many frustrations before you even leave your country of origin. If possible, it is important to have a departure deadline after which you will actually leave, as numerous farewells are upsetting for all involved, especially children.

### Partners

It is important to share your thoughts, knowledge and opinions of the proposed endeavour with your partner. Will you have any concerns or worries about their ability to cope in your absence and vice versa? Can, or should, you reconcile their wants, needs and desires? It may prove helpful to work through a few vignettes, e.g. about how they will cope in your absence with various important events such as illness, financial problems and the deaths of family members. The possibility of your being taken hostage or your death should also be addressed, and you should include the NGOs policy in such circumstances in your discussion. Dependable lines of communication will allay many fears. Access to them should be clearly understood by everyone.

### Children

If you have children, it is important to get them involved from the outset with your decision to go. If they are old enough to understand, they may well support your decisions wholeheartedly, but the younger they are the more difficult this may be. It is important to answer any questions they may have honestly but without causing needless anxiety. Whether or not they understand, it is important for them to be made part of what is happening.

They need to be reassured of your return and that frequent communication by letters, videos and telephone calls will occur. Each child should be written to individually.Give them something of yours to care for and look after, and ensure that the family does not forget you in their discussions on a daily basis, for example children should have photographs of you in their room and bedtime rituals should include you.

Whilst potentially stressful and difficult, it is important that proper farewells should *always* occur. Young children have very little concept of time, so a calendar of your deployment is extremely important. The children's school should also be informed.

Underpinning all of this is an avoidance of too much change in the children's routines, which would unsettle them.

### Relatives

Don't forget your other relatives. Wherever possible, draw on the support they can provide for you, your partner, children and friends. Maintain contact with them to ensure that they do not become reliant on the media, as this may increase their anxieties.

Do take time to discuss with family and friends their concerns as well as your own *before* you leave; uncertainty is very stressful for *all* concerned.

## Deployment

### Work-related Issues

#### Interpreters

If you do not understand the language in your country of deployment it is essential to have good interpreters. Working with interpreters, especially in very hostile areas, can be very difficult and stressful for all concerned. In some situations the interpreter can become the focus of anger, aggression and even violence; protect them as best you can. You are likely to develop close relationships with them, with all the attendant benefits and drawbacks that entails.

#### Stressors

Different situations and work practices provide differing stressors. You may find yourself questioning your involvement from the outset. Have you been properly prepared for this work you propose to undertake? How flexible are you or can you be, and what are your strengths and weaknesses? Is your skill base up to the job given the constraints that you will encounter in theatre? How comfortable do you feel with the moral and ethical dilemmas of work such as triage where the "greater good" may disadvantage the individual, or the expenditure of finite resources on individuals will lead to greater suffering for the majority?

Remember, however, that for the vast majority of aid workers, their experiences add to their knowledge, skills base, confidence, insight and ability to cope generally.

#### Cultural views of illness

It is important not to impose your own illness beliefs on others and to try to understand how local populations view illness. The emotional way in which societies and cultures deal with illness, pain, suffering and death can compound or relieve the stress of your working practice. Some of those you treat will be refugees, displaced persons and involuntary migrants. Some will have been persecuted and even tortured, and some of those you treat may have perpetrated atrocities.

Do not forget the psychological aspects of their plight, and wherever possible help them to find support from their communities who have shared the same experiences, if they have not done so already. In the field of post-traumatic mental distress, attend to social therapies above medical ones, and be sensitive to the fact that simply talking about their experiences with you will be inadequate and possibly damaging.

## Types of Patient

Do not assume that everyone who presents themselves with physical complaints has a medical disease. Across the globe, patients present with symptoms that are impossible to explain medically. This is termed somatisation, and is a universal and common presentation of psychological distress. Remember that wherever you practice, patients attend medical facilities for physical, psychological or social reasons (or a mixture of all three) and if you do not accept or realise this you can become very frustrated. If individuals keep coming back with the same physical complaint it may be they are coming for psychological and/or social reasons which are of course extremely valid given the situation they find themselves in.

# Expatriate Issues

## Isolation and Intimacy

The "constriction" of life that occurs when you deploy may initially be enjoyable. However, close proximity and the difficulties involved in such work may lead to problems within the group. An unexpected intensity of emotions may be forged by proximity, shared adversity, hardships and experiences (both good and bad). This may lead to the formation of intimate relationships, which may or may not survive the return to base. On the other hand, such work may lead to difficulties in interpersonal relationships becoming worse by the inevitable occurrence of gossip which may be corrosive, divisive and damaging. Wherever possible do not be drawn into speculation and gossip; learn to keep quiet.

## Psychological

Many individuals feel homesick. Some get anxious or miserable, especially if things are going badly, which may in turn alter their use of alcohol or drugs. The events you have seen or become involved with may affect the way that you react in future situations, and how you relate to people within theatre and following your return home. It is important to be aware that your co-workers may have, or may develop, frank mental illness or drink- or drug-related problems, and that some of them may have personalities which make them extremely difficult to get on with.

## Alcohol

Be careful in your use of alcohol. Alcohol is often available easily and cheaply in expatriate communities. It is a social lubricant and serves to ease emotional upsets and help you to unwind, but it can lead to its own problems. Whilst its use at the end of a busy and difficult day is perfectly acceptable, if it becomes the preferred way of dealing with emotional difficulties it is less helpful. For example, following exposure to unpleasant events you may re-experience thoughts or images of the event in the daytime or in dreams. Alcohol is often used to help sleep or the anxiety engendered by such phenomena, but it can only add to the problem in time.

## After-work Issues

It is natural to wonder what is happening at home, and there may come a time when you question what you are achieving in-country. Such thoughts may become ruminations and lead to anxiety, worry and distress, especially if there are problems in-country, poor communications with home, isolation and boredom. It is therefore important to take time away from the work. Organise group support wherever possible and try to ensure that relationships do not become either abusive or difficult.

Isolation may lead to increased loneliness, heightened vulnerabilities and emotional distress, especially if you witness, or are involved in, dreadful and unpleasant events.

## Home Comforts and Support from Home

When things are particularly difficult, it is good to able to draw on moral, practical, financial and even spiritual help from home. Unless you are a masochist or a stoic it is important to have some home comforts, as they help to relieve feelings of isolation.

Access to a reliable postal service is highly desirable, if not essential! Letters not only form a diary for the future but also a tangible record for friends and family to read and re-read. Unlike telephone calls, letters also allow a more measured exploration of emotions and difficulties, in addition to which, people like to receive letters. In theatre, you will become rapidly demoralised if no one writes to you – so make sure you write to them! Whilst at times it is very useful, telephone communication can be quite problematic and it is often advisable to work out what you want to say before you make the call.

## Own Support Network In-country

Maintain a sense of proportion from your knowledge of the overall aims and performance of your NGO and your role and position within the effort. Acknowledge the highs and lows and the events that have had a psychological and emotional impact and meaning within the group and how you and the group has, or has not, dealt with them. Aim to draw support from those sharing the same situation.

# Repatriation, Reunion and Readjustment – Post-deployment

Repatriation is about readjustment to your previous life and the accommodation of change in both yourself and those who remained behind. In general, the more problematic the deployment, the more problematic the readjustment.

Just as you had expectations when you deployed in-country, you will have expectations of your return which may vary in their level of reality. Seldom, however, will your plans for return work out exactly as you planned.

Wherever possible, it is advisable to prepare realistically for repatriation. Whilst in-country, start to wind down and review the deployment as a group, exploring good and bad events, how the experience will benefit you, what you would do differently next time, and what you would tell other people going to the same area. Do not underestimate your achievements. Write a report and keep a copy.

In preparing for return and reunion it is important to think what those at home will expect and what you will tell them. Consider how you will deal with the feeling that "no one understands" what you achieved, experienced, saw and felt.

Following repatriation, the recent "constriction" of your existence will become obvious to you. There is often an initial period of euphoria when all goes well, followed by a desire to be in the company of those with whom you shared the experience. There will be jokes, language and events which only they can understand; it is important to recognise this and ensure that where possible you meet up again. (Of course the obverse may happen – you may wish never to see these people again!)

On return you will be asked about your experiences and initially this may be a very positive thing, but eventually people will expect you to stop talking and listen to the events in their life in your absence. If you have had particularly unpleasant experiences you are in a dilemma.

Generally, traumatic events will upset you when you think about them, and this will naturally lead you to avoid talking about them. Whilst this is understandable, it may not be the best thing in the long run. But what do you actually tell people if you do not want to upset or even traumatise them? If you have witnessed dreadful and unpleasant events you may become angry and irritable, which only adds to your difficulties and problems in relationships. There may be a feeling that "you weren't there, so you won't or don't understand", and whilst this is an obvious statement of fact it is unhelpful.

It is important to find someone who can listen. People often say that they would not wish to tell their partner things which are unpleasant for fear of upsetting them, but what would you want to know if your partner had deployed somewhere? Whatever you do, do talk and/or write about it. Some people may be envious of your experience, others deeply interested, but you may find that you do not want to talk about it and you have moved on psychologically speaking. Either way, in most cases, things resolve with the passage of time and by talking.

The return to work can be quite difficult, with a loss of excitement and arousal, a dissatisfaction with the mundane nature of the job, the lack of stimulation, petty bureaucracies and envy from those who did not go. It is possible that you may become unsettled and even move on.

## When to Seek Help?

If you have had a problematic time, do not forget that it is counterproductive to bottle things up – seek help if:

- you want help;
- someone you respect or care about suggests that you've "changed";
- *the following phenomena are severe or are not settling (or are getting worse) after 6–12 weeks and are interfering with your life:*
  - intrusive thoughts, images, smells triggered by people, places, media etc.,
  - avoiding such "triggers",
  - avoiding friends and social situations – becoming socially "withdrawn",
  - relationship problems, especially if related to irritability and anger,
  - disturbed sleep, poor concentration,
  - becoming over anxious, always "on edge",
  - becoming depressed and miserable,
  - drinking too much, misusing drugs,
  - acting "out of character" and impulsively.

## Where to Seek Help?

1. Those who shared the experience – where appropriate.
2. Family and friends – where appropriate/available.
3. Through your NGO – who should have access to, or be able to direct you to, psychological support.
4. Through your family doctor (general practitioner).
5. Private psychiatric and psychological professionals.
6. A traumatic stress service such as those run at University College Hospital, London, and the Maudsley Hospital, London.
7. If you have been tortured you can contact the Medical Council for the Victims of Torture, 96–98 Grafton Road, London NW5 3EJ.

# Stress

Stress may be defined by the following equation:

$$Event\ (stressor) + Meaning\ (to\ you) = Stress\ reaction$$

where the key to the development and resolution of a stress reaction is the meaning of the event to you. Meaning is derived from your background, life experiences, coping strategies and abilities, and the psycho-social environment before, during and after the event. Cultural aspects are also important.

There are only a finite number of symptoms of stress reactions, all of which everyone has experienced at some stage. Lists are difficult to remember, and an easy way of

| Physical | Psychological |
|---|---|
| Racing heart, difficulty breathing, nausea | Agitation and irritability |
| Dry mouth | Fearfulness and worry |
| Palpitations | Increasing obsessiveness and rigidity of thinking |
| Tightness in chest | |
| Sweating | Mood swings |
| Indigestion | Jumbled and racing thoughts |
| Nausea and vomiting | Loss of sense of humour |
| Altered bowel habit | Little joy in life |
| Teeth grinding | Worrying unduly |
| Easily distracted | |
| **Social/behavioural** | Thinking |
| Intolerance, irritability and argumentativeness | Self-doubt |
| Emotional and social withdrawal, isolating self | Boredom and loss of direction |
| Emotionally demanding, "using" others | |

recognising stress reaction is by an individual's change in personality or character as revealed by their behaviour.

## Acute Stress Reactions

Psychological reactions, which occur during overwhelming critical incidents, may range from blind panic, fear or agitation through to withdrawal or stupor. These symptoms may be seen in a minority of individuals, and the worse the event, the more likely they are to occur. They settle rapidly when the stimulus is removed.

## Post-traumatic Mental Illness (PTMI), Post-traumatic Stress Reaction (PTSR) and Disorder (PTSD)

Most individuals cope well under even extreme adversity. Whilst all will be changed by their experiences, it is wrong to assume that most individuals will be "traumatised" by traumatic life events. Personal "growth" is not uncommon following adverse life experiences, but some individuals may develop problems.

It is commonly assumed that the only mental reaction to such exposure is post-traumatic stress disorder (PTSD). This is erroneous, as *any* mental reaction or illness may occur – *PTSD is only one.*

## Genesis of PTSR

Traumatic stress reactions are the product of a complex interaction between the individual, the traumatic event, the environment during and after exposure and the culture from which the individual and group hail and to which they return.

### *Factors Involved in the Genesis of Post-Traumatic Stress Reactions*

## Normality and Ubiquity

Post-traumatic stress reactions are normal. Indeed anyone who has had the break-up of a meaningful relationship has had the symptoms of a PTSR. You re-experience

| The individual | The trauma |
|---|---|
| Previous psychiatric illness | Predictability and controllability |
| Child sexual abuse | Type and frequency of trauma |
| Previous, current and unresolved medical and personal problems | Involvement – direct or indirect |
| | Experienced alone or in a group |
| Poor coping skills | Helplessness and loss of control engendered |
| | Existential meaning of event |
| **The environment** | |
| *Before the event* | |
| Cultural beliefs | |
| Psycho-social support | |
| Current life events | |
| Pre-deployment training | |
| *During the event* | |
| Support/response to incident | |
| *After the event* | |
| Human kindness and support – extending over time | |
| Normalisation vs. medicalisation of reaction | |
| Appropriate involvement of hierarchy | |
| Media attention | |

thoughts and images of your loved one which may be triggered by events, places or people. You may avoid going to places which remind you of the relationship. It may be more difficult to get off to sleep and you may become more emotional or angry. Some individuals turn to drink and some "suffer" more than others. PTSR seem to be universal and most people cope extremely well with adversity; only a few go on to develop a post-traumatic mental illness.

## Recognition of PTSR

PTSRs reveal themselves to others through changes in behaviour and personality. These may be subtle, and individuals are often able to continue at work. The better you know your fellow team members, the easier it will be to spot the early signs of problematic PTSR. Your "reaction" to such changes in character are important clues in identifying those with problems.

The three pillars of the PTSR are re-experiencing, avoidance and arousal phenomena. They vary in intensity between individuals, but are basically the same for mild, moderate and severe post-traumatic stress reactions and disorders.

1. Re-experiencing phenomena.
2. Avoidance phenomena.
3. Arousal phenomena.
4. Associated behaviour.

See the box overleaf

## Post-incident Support

### Early

In the early days after an incident, human kindness and support should be offered. Individuals should be listened to with empathic interest. An environment should be created in which they can talk *if they wish to*, both at the time and afterwards. *Do not "force" individuals to talk*, but try to get a picture of what happened to them. Team leaders should lead by example and get involved appropriately. It is advisable to normalise the situation by keeping survivors at work or by ensuring the earliest possible return to work. Reinforce any teaching received as to the normality of the reaction. Endeavour to analyse what happened with sensitivity and involving the individual(s) in order to learn "lessons" and then enshrine them in protocols and training.

### Later

As time passes, other people's interest in those involved will wane in a similar way to grief. Despite this, the individuals concerned may still be suffering, and the main clue to this is a *change in personality*. If you notice this in others (or in yourself) do not be afraid to ask the individual if they are all right and offer access to psychological help when and where appropriate.

Traumatic incidents can alter our schemata for ourselves and our world view. They challenge our belief systems, but in most cases the initial psychological symptoms and distress settle within 6–12 weeks.

1. **Re-experiencing**
   - Recurrent, unwanted, intrusive thoughts, images, sounds, smells
   - Triggered by places, people, events leading to distress and physical arousal
   - Nightmares and "daymares" – "as if" phenomena or flashbacks

2. **Avoidance**
   - Avoiding thoughts and things associated with the event – even amnesia
   - Feeling cut off, emotionally isolated from others with a reduction in the normal range of feelings
   - Loss of interest in things previously enjoyed
   - A different view of the future – shortened life span

3. **Arousal**
   - "Jumpy", "on edge" – unable to relax
   - Irritability and aggression
   - Difficulty sleeping
   - Poor concentration
   - Forgetfulness
   - Physical responses to reminders of the event

4. **Associated Behaviours**
   - Risk taking activities and impulsivity
   - Increased accidental deaths – road accidents
   - Substance abuse, especially drinking
   - Depression
   - Relationship problems
   - Survivor guilt

If individuals fail to accommodate to the changes wrought by trauma, they are likely to involute to a greater or lesser degree, and guilt over sins of omission or commission is not uncommon.

Encourage talk to prevent "avoidance" whilst allowing due cognisance to the individuals' normal coping mechanisms. Aim to provide the "right" environment for the individual to feel able to talk and avoid coercion. It is important to give the individual a feeling that they are supported and that others are "there" for them.

Wherever possible, encourage the group to "look after its own".

## Preventive Measures

### Before Deployment

- Selection should be by high-quality, experienced staff.

- Pre-deployment training should be realistic in order to build group cohesion.
- Sort your problems out; unresolved problems play on your mind and will be there on your return adding to the difficulties of readjustment, especially after a stressful deployment.
- Expectation versus reality: obtain as much information as possible, but beware of the media.

### During Deployment

- Make sure you are well informed about the mission and your role.
- Be aware of difficulties inherent in the work and specific to theatre.
- Make sure there is work to do.
- Make sure there is time for recreation (and a few little luxuries) if possible.
- Make sure there will be smooth communication with home, i.e. mail, phones etc.
- Make sure that home issues are dealt with professionally, and by the NGO where appropriate.
- Make sure that there is access to reasonable medical, dental and psychological care where possible.
- Discuss any difficulties encountered in your work by your actions or omissions.

Whilst post-trauma mental illness is uncommon, there is little evidence that it can be prevented as its genesis is multifactorial. The earlier that help is offered to those suffering, the better the chance of success.

## Post-traumatic Stress Reactions and Grief

It may be helpful to conceptualise PTSR in terms of a normal human response to unpleasant life events such as grief. It may also be managed in a similar way.

- Both are a ubiquitous human experience.
- Both have an idiosyncratic meaning for each individual despite similar symptoms for all.
- Both "settle" in most instances in 6–12 weeks.
- Both are helped best by those who shared the experience – family, friends, colleagues.
- Some individuals go on to develop mental illness.
- All are changed by exposure to death and trauma.
- Both require an acceptance of reality for resolution.
- Psychological defence mechanisms are at play in both situations and require acknowledgement.
- In both there is a "time to talk" which must be dictated by the individual concerned.
- Some individuals require professional help to overcome their difficulties.
- Anger is common to both, although it is generally less obvious in grief.
- In both, psychological "work" is required to accept, assimilate and accommodate to new realities.

## Stress Management

Given the fact that human reactions to stress are so varied and multifactorial in their genesis, it is surprising yet true that most cope much better than an onlooker would anticipate. It is easy to overestimate potential psychiatric difficulties. It is equally easy to forget the long-term psychological cost paid by some people who volunteer to help other people in the world who are less fortunate than themselves.

Look after yourself. Seek help and advice if you need it, and accept that change is the only constancy since it is both inevitable and irrevocable.

## Coping Mechanisms

## Cumulative Nature of Stress

Exposure to gruelling work schedules, witnessing human misery and being exposed to traumatic and unpleasant events will take its toll if you do not care for yourself.

**Adaptive**
- Sit and ponder the situation constructively
- Express emotions with friends
- Get appropriately angry
- Talk to as many close friends as is reasonable
- Look for the good in the experience, and what you can learn
- Get help – practical and supportive

**Temporary**
- Keep busy, throw yourself into something
- Do something where you don't use your mind, e.g. physical activities
- Bottle things up, then "explode"
- Irritability and irascibility
- Distract yourself by treating yourself to something

**Maladaptive**
- Trying not to think
- Social withdrawal
- Denying reality
- Hiding emotions
- Constant worry
- Losing sleep
- Drinking or smoking too much

**Dealing with stress – accept reality**
- Acknowledge what stresses you
- Keep a balance between work and leisure
- Find a safe confidant
- Keep a network of friends and acquaintances
- Look after yourself
- Ask for help if you need it
- Avoid excessive alcohol and smoking etc.
- Take regular exercise
- Eat a balanced diet – always eat meals as they break up the day and relieve strain
- Maintain or develop outside interests
- Holidays exist for your mental health
- Be flexible – the only certainty is change
- Let the past go
- Assess situations objectively and accurately
- Listen to others

Learn to recognise when and what stresses you and seek help. You are not super-human. Make sure you take breaks and holidays to recharge your batteries. Work at relationships and maintain strong friendships and family ties wherever possible. Listen to others who care about you and accept appropriate offers of help. Do not do "back to back" tours of duty. If you burn yourself out you will become useless to those you may wish to help. Beware of thinking you are indispensable – you are not.

## "Addiction" to Aid Work

You may find that humanitarian aid work is the "only" work for you. The only work that makes you feel worthwhile, challenged and validated. There are people who need your expertise, so look after yourself, and keep yourself physically and mentally fit to continue. However, don't forget to be truthful to yourself when you ask yourself: *Why am I doing this (again)?*

# Conclusion

Take care of yourself.

# Planning, Related Issues and Clinical Care

# 13. Pre-Hospital Planning

Cara Macnab and Peter F. Mahoney

| Objectives | • To remind delegates/volunteers of the need to consider self-care as well as care of displaced people.<br>• To illustrate the differing working environments.<br>• To emphasise the need for pre-planning. |
| --- | --- |

## Introduction

The biggest threats to humanitarian workers in the field are from injury and illness. People deploying from a developed society are used to being able to call for and receive help easily when they are in difficulties.

Considering the Emergency Medical Services (EMS) response to an incident this implies that:

1. somebody has recognised that help is needed and call for it;
2. the means to call for help (radio or telephone) is on hand;
3. a dispatch centre receives this call and can send out a response vehicle carrying appropriately trained crews with the necessary equipment;
4. the crew can gain access to the casualty and deliver appropriate care on the scene and in transit;
5. the casualty can be taken to an appropriate receiving medical location.

In many overseas deployments the EMS facilities will be limited or non-existent. Humanitarian workers need to consider:

1. how they will get help for themselves or colleagues if they are ill or injured;
2. if they are providing such care to a population (either of expatriate workers or local people), how such care will be accessed and delivered;
3. if there is a local system in place, how will they interact with it?

The aim of this chapter is to give some guidelines and structure for the planning process for this type of eventuality. A number of these factors have been discussed in Sect. 1 in the chapters on medicine in remote areas.

# Possible Situations

There are four main situations to consider and these are outlines below. The use of the word "safe" implies that active conflict or deliberate targeting of individuals or organisations is not taking place. Real-life scenarios will include elements from one or more of these situations, but they are used here as a starting point.

## Safe Environment, Well Resourced

In this situation the infrastructure is intact (communications, roads, clinics and hospitals), personnel with appropriate skills are available, routes are secure, evacuation distances are relatively short, and the hospitals and clinics are competent.

The main considerations in this situation are how care is accessed and how it is paid for.

## Safe Environment, Under Resourced

Any of the system components outlined above may be deficient. Considerations include what needs to be done to improve the standard of care, whether better care can be accessed by contracting with private medical providers, and what additional equipment and training is needed by the deployed personnel.

## Austere Environment

This implies remote working conditions with long delays in accessing care. Supply and re-supply of medical materials may be erratic. Evacuations are likely to be over long distances. The main considerations are radio and other communications to call for help, specialist vehicles and helicopters to reach and evacuate the casualties, and the ability of the casualties' colleagues to treat them in situ for the required period of time.

## Conflict Environment.

The medical and EMS infrastructure may be damaged or inaccessible owing to road blocks or front lines between warring factions. Curfews may limit the times that vehicles can access casualties. Supply and re-supply of medical materials (drugs, oxygen, dressings) are likely to be sporadic. There will be casualties caused by fighting and munitions as well as accidents and illness.

Under these circumstances detailed assessments are needed as to what can realistically be achieved.

# Assessment

## The Population at Risk

The group needing care may be the organisation's own people (non-governmental organisation (NGO) or military), personnel from other NGOs, the local population or a combination of these.

For "own" personnel, planning needs to consider their pre-deployment health and what special needs exist. If deployed personnel have conditions such as asthma, angina or diabetes (and are considered fit for the mission), then these conditions need to be covered in the planning. If this is not possible, ask should they be deployed? Be aware that whatever the original plan, personnel from other organisations will seek help and they may or may not have undergone medical screening prior to deployment.

In areas where malaria and other diseases are prevalent consider supplying appropriate initial-treatment drug packs to personnel if access to care is likely to be delayed.

For "local" populations, the planning depends on whether this is developing or improving a service as a long-term health project, or whether it is part of an emergency intervention. In both circumstances, a "needs assessment" must be done covering the population demographics, illnesses, medical conditions and nutrition. Local input as to the needs of the community and the design of the system is very desirable. Under emergency conditions such as forced population movement or military intervention this is unlikely to be practical.

The personnel operating the pre-hospital system need to understand what care is available at the local hospital and clinics. On two recent deployments, one of the authors worked at a field hospital. NGO and military personnel would bring in local patients suffering from cancers and other chronic illnesses, despite being told that the hospital was not able to help them. The hospital was left with the problem of getting these (disappointed) people home again.

## Personnel

The personnel include doctors, nurses, paramedics, medics, communications staff, drivers and pilots. The level of care provided at the scene, during evacuation and in hospital will depend on the training and skills of these individuals. Remember that different countries have different standards of training. It may be that an agency will only want to bring in its own people, or may identify a particular area of weakness that needs assistance. In Kosovo in 1999, the training of local surgeons and anaesthetists was assessed as being very good; the problem was the lack of pre-hospital care. In some areas, NGO and military ambulances were able to bridge this gap in the system.

## Infrastructure

This can be assessed by considering the process of moving the casualty from the incident to the hospital.

Communications are dealt with in the following chapter. In the EMS context, consider what links exist from the scene to the dispatch centre, from the dispatch centre to the ground vehicles and aircraft, and from these to the receiving facility.

*Equipment.* In a well-resourced NGO or army there will be a vehicle fleet manager tasked to ensure that vehicles and aircraft are serviceable. In smaller NGOs (or when dealing with local services), check the general condition of vehicles to see if they are maintained or not. See what medical equipment (if any) is carried and whether it functions (and see if the crews can use it). If in doubt, research alternatives.

*Roads and routes.* Look at likely routes from potential incident sites to hospitals or clinics. Consider if they are passable using the vehicles you have seen (or whether 4–wheel-drive vehicles are needed) or if there are road blocks, check points or threats from mines and other munitions. It may be that the obvious choice of hospital or clinic is denied for security or logistic reasons and alternatives need to be found.

### Destination

- Can the hospital or clinic provide the care needed?
- Ask who is running it (State, military, armed faction, international governmental organisation (IGO), NGO)?
- What casualties will they accept (some military facilities will only take military personnel and send civilian casualties on to the nearest civilian NGO/IGO facility)?
- Are the hygiene standards (including sterilisation of equipment and screening of blood donations) acceptable to your organisation and personnel?
- Is the service free or not?
- Are the people you intend to bring to this facility at special risk due to their religious or political beliefs or ethnic origin?
- The "destination" may be across an international border. Additional factors to consider are customs clearance (for drugs and equipment) and immigration formalities for the patient and accompanying staff.

# Conclusions

Humanitarian workers on deployment are at risk of disease and injury. There are likely to be difficulties in accessing appropriate care. By considering the process of care from the incident through to the hospital, these problems can be anticipated and solutions developed, ideally before the first incident occurs.

## Further Reading

Kuehl A. Prehospital systems and medical oversight. 2nd ed. Mosby Year Book, 1994. St. Louis: Mosby, 1994. ISBN 0 8016 6580 9.

International Committee of the Red Cross (ICRC). Hospitals for war wounded: a practical guide. Geneva: ICRC, 1998. ISBN 2 88145 094 6.

# 14. Aviation Medicine Aspects

Campbell MacFarlane

- To introduce the aid worker to aviation medicine.
- To describe safety aspects.
- To describe medical care and life support during air transportation.

## Introduction

Medical aid personnel working in conflicts, catastrophes, and remote areas may be required to interface with aviation in a variety of ways. Firstly, they may be inserted, deployed and recovered by air, secondly they may be shuttled from location to location in their operational area by air, or be involved in medical reconnaissance or search and rescue utilising aircraft. Thirdly, they may be required to assist in the safe landing of medical evacuation aircraft, prepare patients for aero-medical evacuation, load them into aircraft, and occasionally act as flight medical attendants, accompanying and supporting patients in flight, and ensuring appropriate handover and disposal on arrival.

Some guidelines for such activities are provided below.

## Fitness to Fly

The team members must be fit to fly themselves. As this is not their primary role, and their aviation involvement may be intermittent and infrequent, the stringent medical fitness requirements as applied to aircrew or full-time medical flight staff are not applicable, but team members should have an appropriate level of general fitness and basically be "fit to fly". This implies attention to the following points.

1. Ability to equalise pressures in the middle ear (clear ears). This can be affected by various factors, the most common being upper respiratory tract infection.
2. Ability of the sinuses to adjust to pressure and volume changes. This can be affected by sinusitis.
3. Dental fitness. Gas-containing areas in infected teeth can produce severe pain (aerodontalgia).

4. Lung bullae or known tendency to spontaneous pneumothorax. This can cause massive pneumothorax at altitude.
5. Epileptic tendency. This can be exacerbated by rotor or propellor flicker.
6. Conditions which can be exacerbated by relative hypoxia at altitude, e.g. chronic lung disease, severe anaemia.
7. Gross obesity or hiatus hernia. Severe discomfort or even respiratory embarrassment can be caused by expanding gases in the gastrointestinal tract.
8. Colour blindness. This can affect the interpretation of ground-to-air signals.
9. Hearing. Must be adequate for normal aircraft communication systems.
10. Psychological aspects. Fear of flying, claustrophobia, panic attacks, stress from unfamiliarity with aviation factors, e.g. noise, vibration, turbulence, are real-life events and can be incapacitating.
11. Diseases requiring specific and regular medication, e.g. diabetes mellitus. Aviation activities may result in rapid moves, loss of meals, stress and loss of sleep. Medication may be left behind, packed in inaccessible hold baggage, or be difficult to administer in severe turbulence. Time schedules can be severely altered, with significant delays.

Those likely to be involved in aviation activities and their commanders should take note of the above *prior* to deployment.

## Preparation of Landing Areas

Helicopters are frequently utilised in catastrophes and remote areas, and medical aid workers may be required to select, mark and operate helicopter landing areas at short notice. In selecting such areas, the rough size of the helicopters in use should be known (Fig. 14.1).

Formal helipads are usually dealt with by appropriate personnel, but in the case of emergency helipads the following details should be borne in mind [1].

1. The area on which the helicopter lands should normally be a circle of at least 10 m diameter (ideally 10–20 m).
2. There should be no obstructions in the approach and take off areas (at least 25 m in those directions).
3. Obstructions to be noted include:
   high trees,
   chimneys,
   spires,
   pylons,
   power lines (these are of particular importance since they may not readily be seen from the cockpit, and have caused many aircraft accidents).
4. Beware loose objects in the landing area which can be displaced into rotors or engine intakes. Markers on the landing area should not be made of paper, cardboard, etc. for the same reasons. Loose clothing, blankets and the like should be removed from the area.

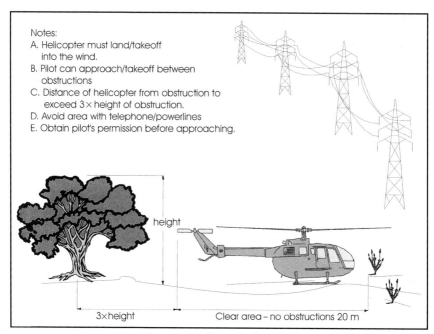

Notes:
A. Helicopter must land/takeoff into the wind.
B. Pilot can approach/takeoff between obstructions
C. Distance of helicopter from obstruction to exceed 3× height of obstruction.
D. Avoid area with telephone/powerlines
E. Obtain pilot's permission before approaching.

height

3×height

Clear area – no obstructions 20 m

**Fig. 14.1.** Helicopter landing area.

5. Landing and take-off areas should be dust-free if possible (often not possible). Dust can obscure pilot and bystander vision and can affect engines and rotors. Sand is even more hazardous. Grass and tarmac are better surfaces.
6. The maximum slope of the landing and take-off area should be 5°.
7. The distance of the helicopter from any unavoidable obstruction should be three times the height of that obstruction.
8. The optimum approach angle is 7° (helicopters can land and take off vertically if necessary, but this is affected by ambient heat, altitude, visibility and aircraft load). The approach path should have a slope not greater than 1 in 8 and should be at least 30 m wide and free from obstructions.
9. Where possible, the approach/take-off paths should be into prevailing winds. Helicopters are very sensitive to cross-winds, and in hot/high conditions with a heavy load may have to take a run into the wind to gain altitude.
10. A portable windsock is useful, but must be sited so as not to be an obstruction.
11. A fire extinguisher should be close by.
12. If time permits a large white H can be put down in the centre of the landing area, but it must not be constructed of material which can blow into critical aircraft parts. Paint or whitewash can also be used.
13. Where possible, a description of the helipad, surrounding topography and potential hazards should be transmitted to the pilot, preferably before take-off. Further identification of the area should be agreed, e.g. emergency vehicle

position, coloured smoke grenades (also give wind direction). Smoke should not be released too early, as the wind may disperse it before it is spotted by the pilot. Similarly, if it is released too late it can obscure the landing area. Wind direction can also be indicated using flags, sheets, etc., but these must be secured.

14. Flares can be used to identify the location, but can cause bush fires. They should not be fired when the helicopter is within 400 m and should never be fired directly at the aircraft.

15. Marshalling the aircraft and guiding the landing by means of arm movements to the pilot are best left to experienced personnel who understand what is going on. Increasingly, Medevac pilots ignore such signals as they have a great many other factors to consider, and they tend not to trust people whom they do not know.

16. Emergency landing areas for helicopters are not usually used at night, as the pilot is unable to see hazards, particularly wires, but this is sometimes necessary. Military pilots may use night-vision goggles or aircraft systems. (The use of night-vision goggles will restrict the use of light by people on the ground.) In more permanent landing areas with which crews are familiar, night use is possible. This will require illumination, either portable lights or using vehicle headlamps. White stroboscopic lights are also useful, as are lit portable windsocks. Do *not* shine lights directly at aircraft. Medical aid workers would not normally be involved in fixed-wing landing strip selection and operation, but might be required to assist.

## Aircraft Safety

Safety around aircraft is paramount, especially with regard to rotary wing aircraft, and is everyone's responsibility (Fig. 14.2). The aircraft commander is in charge.

While rotors are turning it is important to protect the eyes from flying particles. The patient lying on a litter requires similar protection. Medical personnel frequently underestimate the force of rotor down-blast, and it should be remembered that the aircraft must displace its own weight.

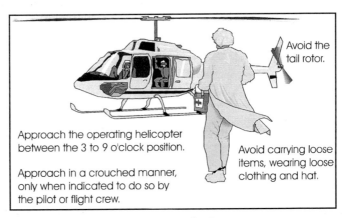

Avoid the tail rotor.

Approach the operating helicopter between the 3 to 9 o'clock position.

Approach in a crouched manner, only when indicated to do so by the pilot or flight crew.

Avoid carrying loose items, wearing loose clothing and hat.

**Fig. 14.2.** Aircraft safety.

This, plus the noise and unfamiliarity with the situation on the part of the medical personnel, can be frightening, disorientating or at least intimidating to the novice.

Personnel must be strictly controlled so that they are not a danger to themselves or others, the aircraft, or the patient.

Clothing must be secured. Headgear in particular must be secured, e.g. a safety helmet. If this cannot be effected it is better to remove headgear and store it safely. There must be nothing loose that can affect rotors or engine intakes.

Personnel must take up position safely on the perimeter of the landing area. No one approaches the aircraft until so directed by the aircraft commander or medical crew, usually by means of a thumb's up sign or by torch light at night. Once directed, the correct approach is from the front of the area in the view of the pilot. Once it is clear how the aircraft is going to land, personnel should take up position on the perimeter, usually kneeling, within the safe area, i.e. within the area from 3 to 9 o'clock in front of the aircraft, and await instructions. (The safe position varies from aircraft to aircraft. The Chinook, for example, may have it at the rear.)

Personnel should stay low when approaching the helicopter, as wind gusts can change the height of the rotor blades.

It is the responsibility of the flight crew to control doors and hatches. Any equipment being carried, e.g. stretchers or ladders, must not be angled upwards. With engines running, speech is precluded and signals between personnel must be visual or by touch. If the aircraft has landed on a slope, personnel should not approach or clear the area in an uphill direction, as the rotor blades are then closer to the ground [2].

Caution must not be abandoned when the aircraft engines shut down, as the rotor blades dip even lower as they slow to a stop.

Of particular danger is the tail rotor, which can be nearly invisible at speed. Personnel must never approach the rotor or attempt to reach the other side of the aircraft via the tail. Fatalities are not infrequent. Particular care must be taken when rear-loading through clam-shell doors. In preparing the patient, all equipment, blankets and straps must be secure, and it is important that medical equipment is not blown away or displaced by down-blast. If the patient is conscious then explain what is going to happen, as this can be a very frightening experience for a helpless patient.

With regard to fixed-wing aircraft, this is usually a safer and more controlled environment, but again personnel must stay well clear of propellors and jet engine intakes.

# Aviation Physiology

This is a complex subject, but the medical aid worker can get by with an understanding of a few basic principles:

## Boyle's Law

When the temperature remains constant, the volume of a given mass of gas varies inversely to its pressure. This means that with altitude, as the pressure decreases, the volume of a gas expands. The reverse occurs on descent. This is of great significance to patients, medical attendants and certain equipment.

## With Altitude, the Atmospheric Oxygen Content Decreases

Relative hypoxia commences above 8,000 ft. (by convention, in aviation, altitude is still expressed in feet), and in an unpressurised aircraft, oxygen supplementation for all on board is necessary at 10–12,000 ft. Depending on their pathology, patients may need to commence oxygen before then. In the event of such altitudes being antcipated in an unpressurised aircraft, it is vital to ensure that adequate oxygen supplies are on board for flight crew, medical crew and patients.

## With Altitude There Is a Drop in Temperature

This drop is roughly 2°C per thousand feet and aircraft heating systems can be temperamental.

It is also important to realise that cabin air can be very dry, which is of significance to the patient's mucous membranes, and may necessitate the humidification of delivered oxygen. It is also a predisposing factor for dehydration over a long period.

The above phenomena apply particularly to unpressurised aircraft, but it is important to understand that even in large, pressurised passenger jets, flying at 30–40,000 ft. the cabin altitude is equivalent to around 8,000 ft., not sea level, and that these phenomena still apply to a certain extent. Thus, a border-line hypoxic patient can slowly become hypoxic due to the slight oxygen reduction at that altitude. As a simple example of the effects of Boyle's law, it can be noted that when a large passenger jet takes off and its cabin altitude is adjusted to around 8,000 ft., the air in the middle ear expands. The extra volume is normally expelled spontaneously through the eustachian tube (unless there is inflammation in the nasopharynx).

On descent, however, the air in the middle ear now contracts. In order to equalise air pressure on both sides of the tympanic membrane, air must now go up the eustachian tube into the middle ear. The construction of the eustachian valve is such that flow in this direction is less easy in most people. In some cases this occurs spontaneously and the ear "pops", but many people have to assist the process by yawning, swallowing or holding the nose to perform a Valsalva manoeuvre in order to push air into the middle ear so that the pressure can equalise. It is easy to understand that air force fast jet pilots who may have to perform rapid manoeuvres at varying altitudes are considered unfit to fly when they have a cold, as oedema at the eustachian valve could result in severe damage to the tympanic membrane and incapacitating pain. In passenger aircraft, babies not infrequently experience discomfort on descent and cry vigorously. This usually has the desired effect of equalising the pressure in the ears. These effects are naturally much greater in unpressurised aircraft. In certain sophisticated Medevac aircraft the cabin altitude can be adjusted to sea level if required. Normal passenger jets do not like to do this as it creates a greater pressure gradient between the inside of the cabin and the ambient atmosphere.

The normal operating heights for helicopters is such that the above phenomena are not usually of great significance, but should a helicopter be taking a patient from a coastal area to a mountainous region, even though the aircraft has only been 2,000 ft. above the ground, the overall ascent to the destination may be such that altitude effects can be present.

## Assessment and Preparation of Patients

This is probably the most important aspect of aero-medical practice. The patient must be fully assessed medically, anticipating any potential in-flight problems, and a decision made on fitness to fly. Depending on the situation, it may be better to fly specialised personnel or resources to the patient. In a disaster situation there may be no choice but to fly, and as much as possible must be done to limit complications.

In acute trauma there may only be a short time to do this when helicopters are employed as the primary response to a scene, but in fixed-wing flights over long distances, considerable attention needs to be directed to assessment and preparation.

A full medical assessment of the patient needs to be done, in conjunction with the staff of the facility requesting aero-medical evacuation (if such a facility exists or if the staff is not the medical aid worker him or herself). History, examination, investigations, treatment, medication, progress and present status need to be taken into account, documentation completed, and necessary medication obtained. Administrative matters such as passports, permission to enter the other country in the case of international flights, the agreement and appropriateness of the receiving institution, vaccinations and health requirements, accompanying relatives, funding, etc. must be dealt with, and the flight crew can be of great assistance here. In acute trauma situations it is vital that airway, breathing and circulation be fully dealt with.

## Airway

It is vital that a patient's airway be maintained in flight. If there is any doubt about it, it is better to deal with it, e.g. by intubation, beforehand. This is particularly true of head-injury patients, whose level of consciousness can fluctuate. They do, in any case, have a tendency to vomit. If one adds to this the expansion of stomach gases and a possible element of motion sickness, the possibility of airway obstruction by inhalation of vomit is high.

In case of in-flight vomiting, it is often better to transport non-intubated patients on their side rather than strapped firmly on their back. In non-intubated head-injury cases the possibility of vomiting remains, and it may be advisable to pass a nasogastric tube, aspirating air and stomach contents as necessary and allowing egress of expanding gases. In transferring a patient with a wired jaw by air, the wires should be cut and replaced temporarily with elastic bands. In-flight vomiting in a wired-jaw patient can be a serious emergency, with the possibility of inhalation and airway obstruction.

## Breathing

A major in-flight problem can be expansion of air in a pneumothorax. This can be massive and rapidly fatal. Any pneumothorax of whatever size being transported by air needs a drain in place, and this must be checked and seen to be functioning. Spares must be available in the event of blockage or displacement. In a situation in which there is a possibility of a pneumothorax developing, e.g. multiple fractured ribs, but none can be detected, it is safer to insert a drain prophylactically prior to flight. The argument that if a pneumothorax develops in flight one can quickly insert a drain may be true, but in the aircraft environment it may be difficult to detect a pneumothorax until it is dangerously advanced, and turbulence or thunderstorm activity may preclude any procedures or even assessment of the patient.

It is important to assess the requirement for ventilation carefully, as a patient who can manage on the ground may not be able to cope at altitude. The pulse oximeter is a particularly useful instrument in aviation medicine and will give a quick idea of how a patient is progressing. With regard to oxygen requirement, this is not usually a problem in a short helicopter flight, but in a long fixed-wing flight it is important to ensure that there is enough oxygen on board to cope with patient demand for the whole flight. As an aid to the calculation of oxygen requirement at altitude, the following altitude oxygen requirement equation is useful [3]:

$$\frac{FIO_2 \times BP_1}{BP_2} = FIO_2 \text{ required}$$

where $FIO_2$ is the fraction of inspired oxygen that the patient is currently receiving, $BP_1$ is the current barometric pressure and $BP_2$ is the barometric pressure at altitude. Thus the patient's oxygen requirement at any cabin altitude can be calculated.

It is necessary to couple this with probable oxygen usage. This is dependent on the various mask and cannula delivery systems, and usage varies considerably with the type of equipment and the flow rate. For example a simple mask with a per cent $FIO_2$ of 40 uses 5–6 l/min. A partial non-rebreathing mask at 90% uses 9–10 l/min.

The patient's oxygen requirements when ventilated may be easier to estimate (because $FIO_2$, respiratory rate and tidal volume are set). If the ventilator itself is driven by gas and the gas is oxygen, this also needs to be accounted for.

A useful equation with regard to oxygen cylinders is

$$\text{Working time} = \frac{O_2 \text{ cylinder content (l)} \times 100}{\text{Minute volume (l)} \times O_2 \text{ concentration} + 10\%}$$

This only gives a rough guide, and allowances must be made for losses and delays.

## Circulation

Where possible, patients should be resuscitated to a haemodynamically stable situation before flight. This naturally includes control of bleeding. This may not be possible where a helicopter is functioning as a flying ambulance in a primary response situation, where a patient is being taken to a resuscitation/surgical unit, but in the case of a fixed-wing long-distance transfer it may be in the patient's best interests to delay the flight to allow surgical intervention to control bleeding. If no such facility is available, there may be no alternative but to fly. This implies full resuscitation en route and is a hazardous and stressful exercise with a possibility of in-flight death. With adequate warning, the Medevac aircraft may be able to transport extra blood with it.

Under more controlled circumstances, haemoglobin concentration should not be less than 7.5 G/dl for aero-medical evacuation [5].

In the assessment of the patient and preparation for flight the above-mentioned physiological effects of flight must be considered further.

## Other Considerations

Boyle's law applies to other areas as well as the ears and chest. If there has been a fractured skull with air inside the skull this aerocoele can expand, acting as a space-occupying lesion with potentially dire results. In such a case, a skull X-ray before flight is useful to clarify the situation, if this is possible. Such a patient is not normally considered fit to fly, but if there is no alternative the altitude of the flight must be as low as possible.

Intestinal gases in the abdomen can expand. If the patient has had an intestinal resection with anastamosis, it is better to wait 7–10 days for healing to take place and ileus to resolve, otherwise expanding intestinal gases can disrupt the anastamosis. For the same reason, neonatal intestinal obstruction patients are not normally transported by air, as expanding trapped gases can disrupt the intestinal tract.

Equipment is also subject to these effects. The air in pneumatic anti-shock garments and splints will expand during ascent, acting as dangerous tourniquets if not vented. With regard to patients in plaster of Paris, these splints should be split before take-off. With the lower pressure at altitude limbs tend to swell, and the air spaces in the plaster do so also, possibly resulting in vascular compromise. The split should be right down to the skin, as encircling bandages can still act as a tourniquet, especially if there is blood in the dressings, which hardens in the dry air.

It is important to realise that air in the bulb of an endotracheal tube will expand on ascent, possibly causing increased pressure on the trachea mucosa. This air can be vented, but the usual aero-medical practice is to fill the bulb with water, which is not affected by altitude. Catheter balloons should also be filled with water. The flow rates of intravenous (IV) fluids can also be affected by altitude/pressure variations and may need to be adjusted during different phases of the flight. It should be noted that the above altitude/pressure effects reverse on descent, and that counter adjustments need to be made to compensate. If a pressurised aircraft's cabin pressure can be adjusted to ground or sea level, these effects will not occur.

## Cold

Patients must be protected against hypothermia at altitude. In addition, the dry atmosphere can predispose the patient to dehydration. Additional oral or IV fluids may be necessary to deal with this. Mucous membranes may need to be moistened and humidification of inspired gases instituted. On long flights, the patient's contact lenses should be removed.

## Loading of Patients

Loading of patients is performed in conjunction with the flight crew, i.e. it is a team effort. This is an opportunity to discuss routes, timings, weather and altitude. Requests for low-altitude flight, sea-level compression, flight time and destination airport can also be dealt with.

Prior to movement, it is important that all IV lines, catheters, drains, etc. are re-checked for effective function, and secured against movement and snags. Any final adjustments or re-siting is then done. Unnecessary lines are removed and dressings checked. As much as possible should be done on the ground, since space and access may be limited on the aircraft.

Generally, procedures can be done in flight, but there is always the possibility of severe turbulence, which would prevent any such activity. Swinging traction weights are not appropriate on aircraft and can be dangerous. Fixed traction should be substituted.

Last-minute assessments such as auscultation and pulse checking are done, as this may be impossible in flight. All straps and lines are secured. Occasionally, patient loading devices are available, but not usually. In executive jet type aircraft, which are commonly used for Medevac duties (but may not be medically dedicated full-time and therefore not permanently fitted for patients), loading can be tricky and many hands are needed. There is usually a steep set of stairs, and commonly a narrow door, which makes the manipulation of a litter difficult. For example, it may be necessary to allow air into a vacuum mattress (used for spinal immobilisation and protection) to give enough flexibility for it to bend, and then re-vacuum it once inside. It is at this point that IV lines and catheter bags can snag and be displaced.

Underwater seal systems for chest drains are not appropriate for aircraft, especially if the litter has to be placed on the cabin floor. These should be replaced with Heimlich one-way valves, with urine bags attached to deal with drainage, or with field drainage sets. Spares must be available, as these valves can frequently clog with blood. Commercial field drainage kits containing bags with non-return valves are better if they can be obtained.

Once the patient is in the plane, everything must be secured against the motion of the flight and turbulence. This includes medical equipment.

The commonest cause of injury to flight medical crew is being struck by inadequately secured medical equipment during turbulence.

Classically, head-injury patients are transported head forward so that the acceleration forces during take-off do not predispose to head congestion.

The patient and the equipment are checked again, necessary in-flight medication is obtained, and checks are made that the necessary case notes, charts, documentation, X-rays and test results are present. Depending on the length of the flight and aircraft facilities, attention is directed to the toilet needs of the crew and the provision of food and drink. Because all the concentration has been on the patient the latter is sometimes forgotten, with severe physical and psychological results. It is probably best to task the flight crew with this responsibility.

When the flight medical crew are ready and safely strapped in, engine start-up may commence. In the case of a helicopter primary response mission, things have to be done quickly but safely. In a "hot load" situation, with rotors turning, safety is a high priority, especially when rear-loading. Personnel assisting in loading but not accompanying the patient must observe the rules on leaving the aircraft and depart through the safe area, crouching and in sight of the pilot.

## In-flight Activities

During take-off, it is important to ensure that the patient remains secure. Reassurance should be given to a conscious patient who is unfamiliar with flying. This should be done during movement to the runway. During the ascent to cruising height, attention is directed to the physiological effects mentioned above, and any necessary adjustments are made.

During the flight, routine observations are made and recorded. Auscultation and pulse assessment may be impossible, especially in a helicopter, and reliance is placed on observation and electronic monitoring. ECG, end tidal $CO_2$ measurement, pulse and blood pressure are measured in this way and the pulse oximeter is very useful in assessing cardio-respiratory effectiveness. Difficulty in ventilating and a deterioration in the measured parameters may be the only way of detecting the early development of a pneumothorax in flight.

IV fluids and medication are given and recorded, as is any drainage as well as urine output. During the flight, it is appropriate to radio ahead and give an up-date on progress, confirm the diagnosis, indicate the expected time of arrival and confirm that there will be transport to meet the aircraft. If customs and immigration produces are necessary, it is useful to warn the relevant officials in advance. In-flight emergencies are dealt with as best they can be under the circumstances, bearing in mind the inherent disadvantages. If necessary, in-flight advice and supervision can be obtained by radio if such a system has been established.

An in-flight assessment of patients in helicopters is even more difficult owing to the noise and vibration levels and there is little room to perform any procedures. In the event of an in-flight emergency, it may be necessary to request the pilot to land immediately a safe area is seen, in order that this can be dealt with.

## De-planing and Hand-over

Once the engines have shut down, the patient is reassessed and documentation is updated. The unloading procedure can be as tricky as the loading and care must be taken by the medical flight crew (who may be quite tired) that once again IV lines, drains, etc. remain intact. After any necessary customs and immigration formalities, the patient is transferred to an ambulance, or from a fixed-wing aircraft to a helicopter. Ideally, the medical flight crew should accompany the patient to their final destination, giving a full hand-over, including in-flight progress, and delivering all documentation.

Once this has occurred the crew can recover equipment, arrange for cleaning or replacement, and organise the replenishment of disposables, fluids and drugs. Drug accounting must be scrupulous. A full mission report should be written as soon as possible after the flight, while events are still fresh in the memory.

In the case of a helicopter primary response, it may be necessary to unload the patient with the rotors still turning. This "hot unload" can be dangerous and should be done by the medical and flight crews only. Hospital staff should not be allowed to approach the area, since they can be a danger to themselves and everyone else if they are untrained, irresponsible or excited by the event. The crew should carry the patient safely to the perimeter, where the litter can be placed on a hospital trolley. In less urgent cases it is better to wait until the aircraft has shut down completely, remembering the danger of drooping rotor blades when they are slowing down. Trolley and staff can then approach the aircraft. In acute resuscitation situations it is often useful for the medical flight crew to be part of the resuscitation team at the receiving institution, depending on the staff and facilities, and also bearing in mind the possible immediate re-tasking of aircraft and crew for another emergency.

# Conclusions

The above guidelines should be helpful to medical aid workers who may have to interface with aircraft and aircrew. Ideally, the problems of moving casualties by air should be thought through, rehearsed and practised before it has to be done "for real".

# References

1. Boyd ST. Air ambulance manual. Durban: Natal Provincial Administration, 1989; 18.1–18.5.
2. Stoy WA and the Center for Emergency Medicine. Mosby's first responder textbook. St. Louis: Mosby Lifeline, 1997; 279.
3. Sharp GR. The earth's atmosphere. In: Aviation medicine 1. London: Trimed Books, 178; 1–14.
4. Nehrenz GM. Aeromedical physiology. 1987; unpublished manuscript.
5. Harding RM, Mills FJ. Aviation medicine: articles published by the British Medical Journal. London: British Medical Journal, 1983; 20.

# Further Reading

McNeil EL. Airborne care of the ill and injured. New York: Springer, 1983.
Ernsting J, King P, editors. Aviation medicine. London: Butterworths, 1988.
Rayman RB. Clinical aviation medicine. Philadelphia: Lea & Febiger, 1989.

# 15. Communications Technology and Range

John F. Navein, Simon J. O'Neill and
Craig H. Llewellyn

**EDITORS' NOTE** – This chapter and the following one are lengthy and detailed. This is our intention, as we believe that most medical persons are unfamiliar with this important area. Aid personnel frequently depend for their lives and safety on their ability to communicate effectively.

| Objectives | • To introduce the topic to the non-expert. |
| | • To describe communications systems and devices. |
| | • To advise on the choice and use of appropriate technology. |

## Introduction

Good communications are a fundamental requirement of everyday life. Whether they are at the basic level of the telephone, newspaper or radio broadcasts, or more sophisticated media such as video teleconferencing and the internet, people are becoming ever more reliant upon them to live their lives. In an emergency or disaster situation, uncertainties increase and with them the need to communicate also increases, sometimes dramatically. At the same time though, the communications infrastructure required to support that need often becomes overloaded or destroyed altogether.

Disaster medicine has been defined as the application of various health disciplines to the prevention, immediate response and rehabilitation of health problems arising from disasters, in cooperation with other disciplines involved in comprehensive disaster management [1]. Good communications are essential to enable cooperation between disciplines to occur, and are crucial tools for effective and comprehensive disaster management. The first part of this chapter will look at the practical aspects of communicating in remote or austere environments, and list the various modalities available along with their relative merits. The second part will look at the application of those technologies to conflict and disaster medicine. It will take a problem-orientated approach to communications in each of the three phases of an emergency or disaster [2] and suggest ways in which the rapidly growing capabilities of technology could be used to re-engineer the way we practice.

The re-engineering of healthcare delivery by telemedicine is one such concept. Telemedicine has been described as the use of communications and information technology to provide health care remotely [3]. Within that definition there is a broad spectrum of applications, some of which are applicable in the disaster situation, although many others are not. We will discuss the pros and cons of telemedicine, provide guidelines by which to judge the applicability of emerging technologies in the context of conflict and disaster medicine, and suggest some principles to guide planning for developing technological solutions to operational problems.

## Communications Technology for the Layman

Communication is defined as the ability for two or more parties to exchange information either directly or remotely, with or without the use of accessories or equipment. Within this definition, communication can either occur face-to-face through the senses of sight, sound, touch and smell, or through the medium of remote access equipment to exchange information at a distance. Generally this uses sound only, although increasingly sight is also used. Since the invention of the telephone, humans have become adept at communicating using sound alone. We *feel* the other person's emotions and even sense their honesty without the need to look them in the eyes. However, the old adage that a picture paints a thousand words still holds true, and indeed some data elements would be very difficult, if not impossible, to communicate without the addition of a visual element.

How would you describe the Mona Lisa for example? Perhaps you would say "….an attractive young woman in her mid-twenties, posing against a rural background with a wry smile on her face…." Immediately each of us would conjure up a different picture in our minds due to a variance in interpretation of the description given, whereas a picture, even a low-resolution or black and white picture, would leave us with much less room for confusion.

There is a natural tendency to want the best tool for a given job, the highest levels of quality, total reliability and all at the lowest price. In the real world there has to be some degree of compromise, and in the world of conflict and catastrophe medicine a key question is what capability do you really need to achieve a given goal. In addition, the very best technical capability may well be totally inappropriate to both the task in hand and the environment in which that capability would be destined to operate.

In this section we will describe the range of communications technologies available and the pros and cons of each, so that planners and practitioners of conflict and catastrophe medicine can get the biggest and most appropriate bang for an ever-limited buck. We will cover the following areas:

- choosing the right technology – an overview;
- fixed-wire links;
- wireless systems;
- satellite networks;
- the future.

# Choosing the Right Technology

There is no doubt that the key to good communications is choosing the most appropriate technology for the job. The spectrum ranges from two tin cans and a piece of string through to satellite-based video teleconferencing. Each achieves its goal, but neither is applicable to the austere environment of the conflict and catastrophe situation. Between the two is a range of technologies of expanding capabilities and reducing costs, each of which is the right solution in one situation but may well be wrong in another. Some factors to consider are listed below.

## Functionality

People buy technology for a variety of reasons. We tend to buy a car based on the right look, the right colour and the right image, but when we buy say a washing machine, we are more interested in wash temperatures, the spin-speed and the economy of the system. Communications equipment should be the washing machine and not the car. Remember that it is merely the medium to deliver your working solution and the capabilities of each of the communications media are fundamentally different from one another. If you get it wrong, it could be analogous to transporting the Manchester United supporters club to an away match on bicycles. Functionality should determine choice, not what is the latest or looks the best.

## A Word About Bandwidth

Bandwidth is a key concept when discussing communications and how the capability of a given communications technology relates to its functionality. Bandwidth is defined as the communications capacity of a transmission line or a specific path through a network. A useful analogy is to regard bandwidth as the size of your communications pipe. For example, a kitchen sink requires a 1.5-inch pipe to handle the flow of water, whereas a mains pipe may be several feet in diameter. These sizes could be described as the bandwidth of the connecting pipes. Obviously, a narrow point anywhere along the network will be rate-limiting and will define the capacity of the whole
Communications technology can be either digital or analogue. Digital equipment transmits information as the ones and zeros of computer language, and each one or zero is called a "bit" of information. Analogue equipment, on the other hand, transmits energy in sine waves of amplitude versus time (Fig. 15.1). The capacity of a digital system to transmit information is its bandwidth and is expressed as the data transport rate, measured in bits of information transmitted per second (bit/s). Do not get confused with bytes, which are eight times bigger than a bit (i.e. 1 byte = 8 bits). The traditional plain old telephone systems (POTS) we are used to in our homes generally use analogue circuits where the bandwidth is expressed in hertz (Hz). For the sake of simplicity in this chapter we will use digital units throughout.
To take the hose-pipe analogy further, you can increase the flow of information by increasing the pressure through the pipe, or rather by compressing it. Compression of data is either "lossy" or "lossless" depending on whether the data lose quality

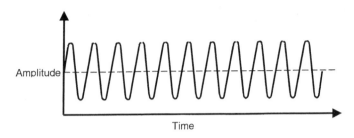

**Fig. 15.1.** Analogue sine wave.

**Table 15.1.** Capability of a system for different bandwidths

| Bandwidth | Capability | Typical medium | Time to transmit A4 page |
|-----------|-----------|----------------|--------------------------|
| 2.4 kbps | Voice, fax, data | Mini-M Satphone | 1.5 min |
| 9.6 kbps | Voice, fax, data | Inmarsat B Std | 30 s |
| 33.4 kbps | Voice, fax, data | Standard phone | 8 s |
| 64 kbps | Voice, data, VTC | ISDN / HSD B Sat | 3.5 s |
| 128 kbps | Voice, data, VTC (good) | 2 x ISDN / HSD B | 2 s |
| 1.34+ Mbps | Broadcast-quality video | Fibre-optic / VSAT | 0.2 s |

along the way, but if we assume there has been no compression, then a rough idea of capability for a given bandwidth is given in Table 15.1.

From Table 15.1, it is clear that bandwidth and time are on opposite sides of the same equation. If you increase the bandwidth you increase the capability but also reduce the time it takes to transmit a given amount of data. Less time, then generally less cost. For instance, a high-speed data link across a satellite link transmits 64 kbits of data every second but it costs about four times as much per second as a low-speed data link transmitting one-seventh the amount of data. A message that is bigger may be cheaper in the long run, but be aware that the economics of sending small volumes of data on high-capacity links may not add up, and needs to include the costs of links themselves and the cost of the equipment.

## Synchronicity[1]

Communications can be either synchronous or asynchronous. This is an important distinction. Synchronous communications are when both parties are communicating

---

[1]This definition refers to synchronicity in its message sense rather than its communications sense. The relative communications definitions are *synchronous*, i.e. transmission in which data bits are sent at a fixed rate with the transmitter and receiver synchronised. Synchronised transmission eliminates the need for start and stop bits, whereas *asynchronous* transmission is when time intervals between characters may be of unequal length, and the transmission is controlled by the addition of start and stop bits at the beginning and end of each character.

in real time, e.g. when people talk to each other either face to face or on the telephone. Letters and e-mail (generally speaking) are asynchronous forms of communication. Asynchronous communication is far easier to manage as it does not mean that the two people need to be in a given place at a given time, an important practical point when the link is poor or when they are in different time zones. On the other hand, synchronous communication can allow a far faster development of an idea or faster decision making through discussion in real time, but it takes far longer on-line, which again may be an important factor when it to comes to cost. A standard e-mail message will take less than a minute across a low-bandwidth satellite phone at around US$2.50, whereas a standard phone call of say 10 min will cost US$25.00. It can add up very quickly. Note that e-mail can be synchronous, and hence asynchronous clinical e-mail is called "store and forward" to differentiate it from the real-time alternative.

## Wire Versus Wireless

The answer to the question of wire versus wireless varies considerably according to circumstance. Normal wire-based telephone networks are notoriously unreliable in areas afflicted by conflict or catastrophe, but they are also one of the first utilities to be repaired. They are also sometimes subject to eavesdropping. On the other hand, an area with a telephone network, especially if it is linked into a local internet service provider, can provide the basis for a very reliable, cheap and comprehensive range of capabilities.

Satellite phones (at least Inmarsat) are independent of a local infrastructure, whereas a global system for mobile (GSM) phone coverage is very unlikely in an area where the telephone network is not working. Where telephones are available, GSM can be more convenient and more reliable than the traditional telephone network as the infrastructure is generally much more modern.

## GSM Versus Satellites

An important difference between GSM phones and satellite phones is that GSM is under the control of the country that you are in when you make or receive calls. The way the billing works means that the local mobile phone company (and therefore the local economy) gets a share of the revenue. Satellite communications are under the control of international companies, and the billing generally excludes a contribution to the economy you are in. The practical consequence of that is that many governments are not at all keen on satellite phones and may confiscate them on entry. This is potentially a serious problem, and the situation in a given area changes frequently with time. Therefore, if you are planning to go to a country that you do not have recent practical experience of, contact your supplier or the network operator before deciding which system and manufacturer to choose.

An important practical consideration is that satellite phones, although they work virtually anywhere in the world, have a low building penetration. This means that they do not work indoors and will not work without a direct line of sight from the aerial to the satellite. GSM phones, on the other hand, work well indoors but suffer from poor geographical coverage. We cover this important factor in more detail under the relevant section.

## The Box Itself

Communications equipment is getting smaller, faster and better all the time. The weight and volume (wt/cube) of the equipment are obviously important, and for larger pieces you should check simple things such as whether it has wheels, whether it is rugged, whether it will run off dual-voltage mains, batteries and a car lighter socket, or will only operate with special batteries with a limited life. Also make sure that it is easy to use, although most systems are very good in this regard nowadays.

Does it look like a phone? One of the solutions to the problem of getting satellite telephones through customs is to choose a Thrane and Thrane handset. This can be split up into a number of different components, none of which remotely resembles a satellite phone.

## Cost

Working out costs can be tricky, and we would recommend that you form a close relationship with an independent communications company and take advice.[2] The main elements of cost are the capital cost of the equipment, the bandwidth/time equation discussed above and the per-minute tariffs. Drive a hard bargain and shop around for the best rates, and if your usage is a lot higher than you anticipated then re-negotiate. Re-negotiate annually anyway. The competition is intense and costs are coming down all the time. GSM networks are also expanding rapidly and there are GSM mobile networks in some of the most unlikely places. GSM is often cheaper than satellite, and increasing coverage may take in an area where you are operating making a changeover sensible. However, you must remember to include in the equation that GSM operators usually charge you for the cost of incoming calls when roaming on your GSM phone, which may be the international element of the whole call. Incoming calls on a satellite phone should be free.

Beware the pricing structure. On some systems (e.g. Inmarsat) you will get charged a fixed rate regardless of the destination or time of day, whereas in others (GSM and Iridium) the price will vary considerably depending upon where the call is to. Some you'll win, some you'll lose. So, if you are not sure then ask, but remember that your decision will almost certainly be a compromise to match your needs with the available tariffs, so be prepared to review your options as your requirements change.

Finally, be aware that the costs can vary dramatically depending on which way you are calling. This is particularly the case when calling into an area from a First World landline. There is fierce competition in the overseas market, especially with the emergence of "resellers" who buy bulk bandwidth from the major carriers and resell it at a

[2]Simon O'Neill, the technical author of this chapter, is happy to advise on the question of relative costs or any other technical aspect of communications, and can be contacted on simon@icomms.com

discount. Hotels often charge a big mark-up for calls out, but not for calls in. Check out the differences, in and out, for the areas in which you are working and adjust your communications plans and procedures accordingly.

## Fixed Wire Links

Fixed-wire links, as already discussed, can be divided into either analogue or digital. Simple digital circuits and the more common analogue systems both generally operate across ordinary copper wires. Although these are often laid up in groups of say 8 pairs or 16 pairs, each is usually limited as to the kbits/s it can transmit, for example ISDN at 64 kbits/s. The more advanced modern fibre-optic cables usually have very high data transport capacities, or bandwidth, well into the Mbit/s (megabits or a million bits of information per second).

## Analogue

A conventional analogue telephone line operates at the digital equivalent of around 9.6 kbps. This is fine for telephone conversations and transmissions from a fax (fac-simile) machine which produces a paper copy of the document at the other end. Analogue transmission is a mode in which data are represented by a continually varying electrical signal It has a signal throughput capacity of 3 kHz. Although the early telephone equipment restricted the data flow to a digital equivalent of around 9.6 kbps, modern technology now enables multichannel ISDN to operate over a simple pair of copper wires. It is also possible, however, to transmit digital data from a computer-driven device across an analogue network by passing the data through a modem. This converts the digital signal transmitted from the PC into an analogue signal recognisable by the analogue network. Fax machines do not require modems to operate across standard telephone systems as the necessary conversions are carried out internally. Standard modems and fax machines sample the input signal about 6,000 times per second, leading to a digital capacity over a conventional telephone in the region of 33 kbit/s. This is ample for most domestic applications including e-mail, as well as for the live transmission of basic vital signs used in telemedicine. At 33 kbps, a 1 MB file will take around 10 min to transmit. Video tele-conferencing (VTC) is possible at this bandwidth, and can even be done across the internet if both ends have the same software. This can provide a very cheap (the cost of a local call at both ends) and imaginative method of communication, but the quality is currently not good and it is often referred to as "talking heads" VTC.

## Broadband

Broadband is the definition given to the higher-magnitude bandwidth obtainable using different adaptations such as digital asynchronous transfer modes (ATM) of communication, which offer the means of greatly improving the bandwidth of copper conductors. Various different concepts have been trialed throughout Europe to bring broadband services to the doorstep of the end-user at a reasonable price.

These have included the use of the domestic electricity supply network and national rail networks to transmit data, and have, by and large, been successful. It is likely, therefore, that these and other utility providers will develop their own national infrastructures to become telecom carriers in the near future.

## Digital

We have established that analogue communications have their limitations and the more advanced user may need additional bandwidth. This can be achieved by the installation (where available) of an ISDN (integrated services digital network) line. Telephone exchanges use "all solid-state switching" and offer a digital connection from end to end, so that broadband services can be achieved as well between continents as they can across national networks. A few years ago, ISDN was rare and expensive, but it has since spread to many countries, at least in the capital cities, and that trend is likely to continue (Fig. 15.2).

A note of caution is that many countries are encouraging de-regulation of their telecoms industries. Whilst this should ultimately mean better quality services, it can lead to difficulties with inter-carrier connectivity. For example if you are using Carrier A which does not have an ISDN gateway to Carrier B, you will be unable to exchange data via ISDN to Carrier B subscribers. Many companies also use their ISDN lines for voice and fax as well as data, so be aware that whilst the voice element will almost certainly work every time, fax and data may experience difficulties to certain destinations. This problem is certainly improving with time as carriers get their own house in order and develop links and agreements with each other. In the meantime, if you are experiencing problems, check with your carrier before assuming that any problem you have with connectivity is the result of your faulty equipment.

ISDN is a circuit-switched network or dial-on-demand service where connections are established on a call-by-call basis. Typically, you would expect to pay a rental for the line and the cost of any calls made, just as with the conventional telephone system. Most PTTs (posts, telephone and telegraph – although the acronym is now more widely used to mean the national telephone network) offer two data rates across ISDN: basic rate (BRI) and primary rate (B-ISDN or broadband). The basic rate service, also referred to as 2B+D, consists of two user channels each carrying 64 kbit/s and a third smaller channel carrying 16 kbit/s known as the D channel and

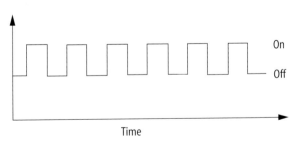

**Fig. 15.2.** Digital signal.

used for network signaling purposes. For applications requiring greater bandwidth, the two user channels can be combined to give a combined speed of 128 kbits/s (ISDN2). You should note, however, that many carriers do not offer a discount for multiple line usage and therefore this option would simply be double the cost of a single link.

The primary-rate service comprises 30 user channels (often referred to as a "pipe", or 30B+D) A combined data rate of 1920 kbits/s is available to the user, and in its full capacity offers greatly improved and even broadcast quality video transmission, but the cost is significantly higher, although there are generally more options for the billing of these high-capacity lines.

An alternative is to pay a rental or lease fee for the line with no additional charges for the traffic across them. This is known as a "nailed up line", and is ideal for a point-to-point connection such as one organisation office to another, or from a hospital to a health centre. Once installed, any calls made across the link are effectively toll-free, and so the more it is used, the better value it becomes. The leased-line option limits the user to the two end points where the line is installed, and without the addition of a licensed "breakout" capability, calls cannot be made to numbers outside of the local area network (or LAN). Those who use the dial-on-demand ISDN can dial any other subscriber with ISDN an line, and many schemes are evolving which will enable the ISDN user to use standard analogue equipment as well across the same link, and consequently connect with any other telephone in the world. However, this does require a digital–analogue converter, which may be in the handset or alternatively can take the form of a small box fixed to the wall beside your ISDN port. The economics and choice of which ISDN link to use depends directly on the traffic across it (Fig. 15.3).

In Fig. 15.3, the solid lines represent the difference between the cost of a leased line and that of a dial-up circuit such as normal phone usage. It is not to scale, and merely indicates how the curves relate to each other. Therefore, it is not an accurate representation as the relative actual costs will vary considerably from region to region and

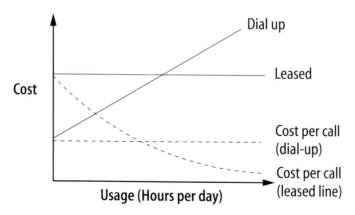

**Fig. 15.3.** Cost differences between a leased line and a dial-up circuit.

even from carrier to carrier. The dotted lines show the effect on the cost of an individual call assuming that the destination is constant and traffic volume is the sole variable.

ISDN will, almost certainly, not be appropriate for connectivity in the field. It is fairly sophisticated technology which requires an intact infrastructure to support it. We have considered it at some length, however, because it is now relatively cheap and may be the right solution for the central organisation for inter-agency communications, and even increasingly for communications from an agency to the capital city of an area affected by a catastrophe. Also, in some circumstances in the post-conflict situation, ISDN may become available fairly early as part of an infrastructure regeneration programme. As well as being able to pass more data more quickly, and enable a number of telephone extensions to be used across one link simultaneously, ISDN2, at 128 kbits/s, delivers enough bandwidth for good quality VTC.

## Teleconferencing

Teleconferencing is a very cheap and efficient way of doing business. It enables any number of people to share in the same telephone call and to hold a virtual meeting. In its simplest form it entails using an extension or desktop conference phone, but most teleconferencing utilises a multi-point bridge whereby any number of callers can call into the bridge on the same number and teleconference. Teleconferencing tends to feel uncomfortable if it is between people who have not met, and in line with traditional conferences needs a good chair person and a degree of discipline. Most major telecoms companies offer this service, and many also offer translation or transcription as an optional extra. Although there is a slight premium over normal calls, the host can elect to cover the whole cost, ask participants to pay a local call charge and cover the difference, or ask them to pay for the whole cost themselves. Teleconferencing provides considerable savings in travel time and costs and will work with calls from abroad or from mobiles.

## The Internet

The internet started in 1969 when the US Department of Defense got together with a few academics and industrialists to develop a new way to send messages. The aim was to develop their own private network to pass around nuclear secrets. All went well, and the first e-mail message, which included the famous @ sign, was sent in 1972. ARPAnet, as it was then called, continued to develop steadily but it wasn't until 1993, when Marc Andreeson came up with a way to make web browsing pictorial and easy, that the web as we know it today became a reality

The internet is rather like the road network but for information. It is a collection of public and private networks that are linked together using a set of protocols called TCP/IP (transmission control protocols/internet protocols). The web is the internet with pictures. Its that bit of the internet that exchanges multimedia information, pictures, sound and video (using hypertext transport protocol or http).

The internet and the world wide web (WWW) will transform our lives over the years to come, and specifically will transform our capability to prepare for and manage humanitarian and emergency projects. Cyber cafes, where anyone can gain access to the internet, are spreading world-wide. They will enable anyone to gain access to vast amounts of data for educational research or planning purposes, or to share and develop ideas (for good and bad) with others sharing the same interests elsewhere. Real-time news is available through newspapers and news corporation sites, and it is possible to use the web as a modality for telephone calls and talking heads VTCs, all for the price of a local phone call.

There are concerns about security on the internet, especially if you are using local internet service providers, but for practical purposes the web is a safe and reliable means of communication; it was, after all, designed to pass around nuclear secrets and it certainly beats telephones and the mail on both counts.

## Wireless Systems

The expert's definition of what constitutes a wireless system is ill-defined, and ranges from personal mobile radios, through cordless phones in the home, to mobile phones and beyond. The simplest way to describe a wireless system is one that does not rely on a wired link between its users. It therefore includes all the above examples, but to date the most successful is undoubtedly the global system for mobile telecommunications, or GSM.

## GSM

Many of us already use GSM telephones. In Northern Europe and Scandinavia, we enjoy the most mature GSM networks in the world. The handsets are now commonplace in most walks of life and across all generations. Currently, GSM operates at low bandwidth with data transmissions for e-mail and web surfing possible at up to 9.6 kbit/s. The available bandwidth will expand with time, but note that not all currently available handsets are data-compatible. From the telemedicine perspective, ECGs and photographs have both been successfully transmitted across the GSM network [4].

GSM is a terrestrial-based digital system which is a second generation of the earlier TACS and ETACS analogue cellular services. Adopted by more than 250 network operators worldwide, the digital infrastructure allows subscribers to operate in many different locations, including internationally, using the same handset and phone same number. The networks tend to be concentrated in areas of high population density, and coverage varies greatly from country to country and even from city to city. It is currently predicted that GSM coverage will never exceed 15% of the world's land mass, or 60% of the population. Furthermore, the regional nature of the system creates a complex billing structure that makes call cost analysis difficult and somewhat arbitrary.

Ironically its global growth has been fueled by the evolution of portable satellite systems which worried many developing countries in which they were destined to be used. Satellite phones do not necessarily provide a revenue stream in the country of use, and are often deemed to be a violation of sovereignty. GSM solves this because the transmitters are land-based and therefore under local control, and many countries have chosen to make the substantial investment necessary to build a GSM network in order to retain control and ensure that they earn revenue from visiting subscribers as well as their own domestic market.

The GSM network in a given area will operate on one of three different bands (900 kHz, 1,800 kHz, 1,900 kHz), and whereas there is usually a single bandwidth for a given country, some (e.g. Russia) countries have a number of operators who operate on different bandwidths. Most mobile phone handsets are single band and will only operate on networks in areas using the same band as their service provider. Increasingly though, newer handsets are dual band, and top-of-the-range phones are tri-band and will work anywhere in the world where there is a network. Where you can communicate using your domestic mobile phone therefore depends on the handset you have, which service provider you are signed up with, and which overseas networks they have reciprocal arrangements with.

When you are abroad and out of your native network you are deemed to be "roaming". This works with little or no input from the user and often provides a choice of host network providers. But beware of call costs. When you roam, you, as the subscriber, are responsible for all your outgoing calls, which are charged at the local cellular rate PLUS the international call charge to your destination. In addition, you will also be charged for the international leg of any INCOMING calls. This presents most of us with a new billing concept that is easily forgotten at the time of a call, but which comes flooding back when the bill arrives! The advantage, however, is that anyone at home can call your mobile number as normal and get through to you wherever you are at the cost to them of a normal national mobile call. Many tariffs require you to call your service provider before you leave to ask them to switch on roaming for the country you are going to. Many also require that you switch it off when you come home so that the billing system knows when to revert to the domestic tariff. You should also check costs for both incoming and outgoing calls before you go.

GSM has excellent building penetration, which means that it can be used easily in cities and on the move, and is a great advantage over satellite systems. The mobiles are also very easy to use and familiar, especially if you take your own phone away with you when you travel. GSM also tends to cheaper in many places than satellite. These are substantial advantages over satellite, and the differential is likely to get wider as the GSM networks expand and costs fall. However, coverage is patchy and often very poor, especially during the active phases of conflict or catastrophes. Check before you go.

As has already been mentioned, GSM is terrestrial-based and requires a sophisticated and intact infrastructure in the area where the phones will be expected to work. GSM will therefore not be suitable for most conflicts or during the acute phase of a disaster, although they may have a place in the pre- and post-disaster phases in some countries, and in the management of the acute phase of an isolated catastrophe in an otherwise functioning locality.

## The Emergency Override

The UK mobile phone networks operate a system called ACCOLC. This stands for ACCess Over Load Control and is a way of ensuring that the Emergency Services and other priority personnel such as Local Authorities and Coastguards can have priority access to the network during an emergency.

Invariably a local disaster will attract a great number of media operators who also require telephone lines to their offices in order to keep the world up to date with developments. Journalists' standard practice when there is the opportunity for a scoop is to establish a link with their office and then keep the line open in order to guarantee that it is there whenever they need it. As there are a finite number of lines in any given area, this type of practice could easily flood the network and prevent the emergency services from getting any access to the system.

There is a procedure for gaining access to the ACCOLC system, and applications need to be approved by the Home Office. They decide who is eligible for the service in order to control numbers. Similarly, ACCOLC is not in automatic operation all the time. It has to be invoked by an authorised police officer or local authority representative.

# Satellite Networks

Satellite communications offer substantial advantages over GSM, and low-bandwidth satellite telephones (satphones) are now cheap enough to buy and use and to be considered the technology of choice in many situations. Building penetration is poor, but coverage is more or less worldwide regardless of the infrastructure on the ground. Broader bandwidth systems offer greater bandwidth than GSM up to ISDN speeds of 64 kbit/s and beyond. The potential functionality of a satellite-based system is therefore currently much greater than GSM

Although their main application is in support of conflicts and catastrophes overseas where other forms of communication are not available, satellite communications may be appropriate in First World catastrophe situations too. They are independent of the GSM and radio networks and rarely get overloaded. They also operate effectively in GSM black-spots where GSM coverage is patchy or absent altogether.

## The Origins

In 1945, the author of *2001: A Space Odyssey*, Arthur C. Clarke, produced a feasible theory on how communications satellites could act like a mirror by bouncing the signal from one place to another on the planet's surface within seconds. With that, the idea was born, and the first Sputnik satellite was launched in 1957. Since then over four thousand satellites have been launched, and in the next 2 years another 280 are expected to be launched for communications alone!

Traditional satellites orbit at an altitude of some 35,000 km above a specific point on the equator. In this position they will orbit the earth once every 24 h and therefore appear to remain stationary in the sky when observed from the earth. This is known as a geosynchronous or geostationary earth orbit (GEO), and the footprint of each satellite is over a fixed region of the world's surface. The satellites reflect the signal down to a land Earth station operated by the major telecoms companies (BT's is at Goonhillie in Cornwall) and from there into the terrestrial network. Inmarsat satellites operate in this manner.

The footprints of geostationary satellites often overlap, and so in many parts of the world it is possible to access two satellites. This can be important in an emergency situation when multiple users are accessing the same satellite at the same time. Very occasionally a satellite will get overloaded, and by simply turning around and accessing the next satellite you can regain connectivity.

The new hand-held systems will operate via low earth orbit (LEO) satellites which will be on the edge of space at an altitude somewhere between 640 and 1,600 km. At this height they have an orbital period of around an hour and therefore move very quickly relative to the ground. Visibility is limited to a few minutes at a time, so LEO systems operate a "hands-off facility" whereby calls are handed on to the next satellite in the orbit to provide an uninterrupted service. Hands-off technology is proving challenging at the moment.

Medium Earth orbit (MEO) systems orbiting between 6,400 and 19,200 km are also under development. They will operate in much the same way as LEO systems but require fewer satellites to cover the same area, and each one will have a greater duration of visibility to a given point during each orbit.

One of the great misconceptions about mobile satellite telephone calls is that the subscriber is responsible for all or part of the cost of an incoming call. Most reputable operators will not charge for either incoming calls, or unsuccessful calls such as unobtainable or busy. Many also operate on a purely call-by-call tariff basis with no connection fees or monthly subscriptions to pay, which tends to suit most organisations dealing in conflict and catastrophes. Most will deploy a satellite terminal on a given project and use it extensively for a limited period of time only. The terminal will then sit dormant on a shelf until the next project or assignment. Monthly fees are therefore inappropriate. On the other hand, if the organisation will be using a terminal full-time, then a monthly fee may be attractive if accompanied by a reduced call fee. As with GSM, ask an independent adviser and shop around for the best deal

It is possible to transmit broadcast-quality pictures by connecting several satellite systems together (multiplexing) or by forfeiting the real-time element and using a store-and-forward solution. Store and forward allows the images (or data) to be captured and stored in a compressed file to be transmitted at a later time, for example the video footage pictures of Richard Branson aboard his Global Challenger balloon flight in 1998. Although they were considered as "live" pictures, most of them were compressed and transmitted store-and-forward via a 64-kbps Inmarsat satellite to a chase plane at fixed times of the day before being decompressed, edited and distributed to the world's media.

Using a similar principle, high-resolution images can be transmitted across a Mini-M satphone using a compressed transmission protocol, whilst still maintaining a real-time link, thus enabling "live" text messaging between the two parties. They can discuss the contents of the image(s) and even annotate it for more detailed reference, and all at 2.4 kbits/s and from anywhere in the world.

## Inmarsat

Inmarsat was formerly a governmental agency with some 88 member countries until its privatisation in April 1999. It is the original global satellite service operator. Now on their third-generation satellites, they operate four geosynchronous earth orbiting satellites giving coverage of virtually the entire surface of the planet. (Owing to the curvature of the earth, their footprints do not quite extend to the poles.)

## Mini-M

Mini-M has brought satellite communications within reach of most global travelers. The combination of a light portable terminal at an affordable price, with worldwide coverage and reduced airtime rates, has pushed the connection figures beyond 50,000 terminals worldwide over the last 2 years.

The Mini-M, is a self-contained unit about the same size as a laptop computer. Mini-Ms require no more technical expertise to operate than a standard telephone, weigh less than 2 kg and cost around US$2,750. There are now only two manufacturers, Thrane and Thrane and Nera, both of whom offer the same functions and the choice is merely one of ergonomics.

Mini-M, being Inmarsat-based, will work virtually anywhere on the surface of the Earth and can provide voice, fax and data calls to any other phone, fixed or mobile. The service is dial-on-demand, which means you pay for what you use in 1-s increments at a rate which should be under US$2.50 per minute. In many parts of the world, this is cheaper than a hotel phone. Call charges do not vary with time of day or destination, provided the call is to a fixed-line phone and not to another mobile.

A Mini-M can also easily be connected to a laptop computer for e-mail and data traffic, but the maximum data rate of 2.4 kbit/s is desperately slow if you are used to moving large files and documents around on normal phone lines.

## Inmarsat B

Inmarsat B portable systems come in a number of different shapes and sizes from a number of different manufacturers around the world. In its basic form, data are transmitted at 9.6 kbits/s, and there is the option to expand this to high-speed data (HSD) at 64 kbits/s. Although referred to as a portable system, the Inmarsat B is really a transportable system, with a basic volumetric size equivalent to a tea chest or large packing case. However, it will give you "ISDN in the sky", with greater bandwidth being possible by multiplexing units together. Inmarsat Bs have been used successfully to provide telemedicine services using video-teleconferencing for remote communities in austere environments [5]. The systems cost around US$20,000 each with an HSD capability, and HSD airtime should be less than US$10 per minute, which may work out cheaper than a Mini-M in some situations (see section on bandwidth). The main problem with Inmarsat B systems has always been one of true portability, and it is this factor that led to the development of its successor, the M4.

## M4

M4s were launched in the final quarter of 1999 and the service became available via a limited number of land Earth stations. A full service will be available in 2000. M4 provides a considerably enhanced capability over the Inmarsat B and is considerably smaller and cheaper too. The minimum communication standard is to provide data at 64 kbit/s on a terminal about the same size as the Mini-M, to give subscribers full and portable access to the internet, connection to their local or wide area network, transmission in real time and store-and-forward video, and the capacity to send pictures and broadcast-quality voice on a plug-and-play platform. Again the ergonomics vary dramatically between manufacturers.

Inmarsat are also introducing the Inmarsat packet data service (IPDS). IPDS will offer a full-time data connection to the network which will only be charged when it is used, and then it will be charged per transmitted Mbit of data rather than by the minute. This will provide true flexibility, choice and cost savings, particularly for those wishing to have regular access to e-mail or data. Users will effectively be able to leave the system in a stand-by mode watching the network, and pay only for the data transfer when it arrives.

In summary, the M4 is the size of a standard laptop computer, boasts full ISDN compatibility (64 kbps), and is truly portable with an all-up weight of around 4 kg. The costs of the equipment will vary a little from country to country and depending on specification, but should be less than US$9,000 with airtime around US$8.00 per minute. Therefore, it only replaces the Inmarsat B. If all you need is voice and low-end data transmission, then the Mini-M remains the better option.

It is possible to split the 64-kbps ISDN link to give $8 \times 8$ k voice channels by attaching a satellite-ready reverse multiplexer to the unit. A reverse multiplexer connects directly into the M4 terminal and provides RJ45 outlet ports to allow up to eight additional handsets to be connected. Each time a call is made, however, the entire channel will be operating at 64 kbps, with the associated increased call cost of US$8 per minute rather than US$2.50 for a Mini-M. If it is likely that several handsets will be often be used simultaneously, a split M$ may prove an economically sound option.

## Iridium

Iridium are the first hand-held satphone operators, operating 66 LEO satellites in a birdcage pattern around the Earth. Because these satellites orbit every hour or so, it is necessary for the system to perform some quite complex inter-spacial hand-offs to pass your call from one satellite as it sets over your horizon to the next as it comes into view. It is rather like a mobile phone network on the ground which will hand your call off from one base station to another as you drive past, the only difference being that with Iridium you are effectively standing still whilst the network revolves around you (Fig. 15.4).

Iridium terminals are hand-held and a little bulky compared with GSM mobile phones, but the true comparison should be with the laptop-sized Mini-Ms rather

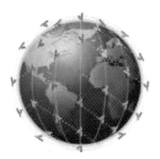

**Fig. 15.4.**  Typical iridium spot-beam map.

than the terrestrial GSM phones. As with Inmarsat there is little building penetration and so they cannot be used indoors or between tall buildings. Most terminals have the option of a remote external antenna which can be fixed up to 80 m away to give greater accessibility to internal or restricted spaces.

## Radio

This section must also include the many private mobile radio (PMR) networks which are in operation. The most common are those used by the emergency services. Although expensive to install and generally restricted in their regional coverage, there are no call charges and so the operational costs are limited to maintenance and servicing. Currently there are plans to produce a national radio network for the ambulance services of England. This will provide a backbone network down the length of the country with individual wireless local area networks (WLAN) integrated into it, to enable different services to share information on their own private network. The next progression will be to produce a truly integrated system that encompasses satellite, GSM and PMR in order to offer guaranteed delivery of patient data to the destination hospital whilst en-route, and regardless of environment.

*The provisioning of integrated access to broadband multimedia services either from wired or wireless networks is the goal of the next generation of both private and public networks.*

The current microelectronics revolution is making it possible for smaller and smaller handsets to perform a number of stand-alone and/or integrated functions such as fax, e-mail, VTC and good old voice telephony. The next generation of terminals may also offer us the ability to access home shopping, banking, entertainment, and in fact a whole variety of PC-based user-interactive services through one handset. The user does not need to know which transmission medium they are currently operating under, but merely that they will have a guaranteed line regardless of global whereabouts and environment.

**Table 5.2.** Summary of communication options

| | Cost of kit | Cost per min London–Lagos | Bandwidth[a] (kbits/s) | Capability[b] | Time (s) to transmit 1 page of A4 | Needs intact local infrastructure | Building penetration | Geographical coverage |
|---|---|---|---|---|---|---|---|---|
| POTS | V. low | $0.50 | 9.6 | V,Dd | 8 | Y | N/A | ++++ |
| GSM | $100 | $1.00 | 9.6 | V,D | 30 | Y | Y | + |
| Radioc p/s VHF | V. high | Free | 9.6 | V | N/A | N | N | +++ |
| Inmarsat Mini-M | $1700 | $2.50 | 2.4 | V,D | 90 | N | N | ++++ |
| Inmarsat M4 | $9K | $2,50 | 64/26 | MV,D,VTC | 3.5 | N | N | ++++ |
| Inmarsat B | $25K | $3.60 | 9.6/64 | V,MV,D,VTC | 3.5 | N | N | ++++ |
| Iridium | $1,200 | $2.40 | 4.8 | V | N/A | N | N | ++++ |

[a] Or equivalent for analogue services.
[b] V, voice; MV, multiple phone lines; D, data; VTC, video teleconferencing.
[c] Public service radio domestically or VHF for overseas links.
[d] Data with the addition of a modem.

# Summary

Table 15.2 summarises the relative merits of the various options available for communicating around the world.

## The Future

It is interesting to try and predict the future in an industry where the technology is out of date virtually as soon as it hits the marketplace. We remember hearing a quote in which IBM bosses stated that the world market for PCs world be lucky to exceed a million, and there are now more than 35 million in the UK alone! It was also an IBM executive who, only 20 years ago, famously predicted that "one day a computer will weigh less than a ton".

In telecommunications, however, it is clear that the future will be greater bandwidth, over as few wire links as possible, and available to everyone at a realistic price.

A wire link is prohibitively expensive. Once installed, it is a costly item to move around and so the emergence of close-proximity wireless communicators is a welcome development. There is a project known as "blue tooth" which does exactly this. Already many of the big names in telecommunications and computing have pledged themselves to blue tooth in order to create a wireless office solution in the coming years. This means that users will be able to walk into an office with their laptop, sit down anywhere and then access all the usual features of a local area network The printer, the fax machine, other PCs and the telephone would all "see" them when they register and be sitting waiting for instructions from them and any other registered users. Currently, the technology is working from a radio transmission perspective rather than some of the line-of-sight solutions that are available today.

The idea is that you will have one telephone handset that you keep with you all the time, with your own telephone number. When you are in the office it connects via the office system, when you leave the office it will use a terrestrial or satellite network depending on where you are in the world, then when you get home it automatically logs you on to your home system. People calling you do not need to know where you are, they just dial your number regardless and they will always get through to you. Extend that concept now to your PC, the internet and e-mail and you are well on the way to understanding how and why blue tooth will be important to us all in the not too distant future.

Interestingly, though, it does not matter how technology progresses, our fundamental demands on the system remain the same. We require a reliable and resilient medium, which may need to be global as well as local and mobile, have 24–h readiness and be flexible and adaptable, and of course all at the right price. Add to that a full convergence of all available networks and there will be no need to worry about who the carrier is at any given time. In fact an ideal that seems some way off at the moment is that the carrier, network and technology may all change whilst a call is in progress. In the same way that a GSM network passes your call from one terrestrial base station to another, your call could be passed from one network to another, perhaps even across the boundaries of different technologies presenting true convergence.

The futuristic vision above may not find favour with many readers of this chapter, but it is worthy of note that many of these capabilities will be independent of a terrestrial infrastructure. In short, they could well make the whole business of providing support to a conflict or catastrophe situation considerably more reliable by providing one of the cornerstones of good management, i.e. good communications.

# References

1. 1. Gunn JW Humanitarian, non-combatant role for the military. Prehosp Dis Med 1994;9:546–8.
2. Llewellyn CH The role of telemedicine in disaster medicine. J Med Sci 1995;19:29–34.
3. Lilley R, Navein J. A telemedicine toolkit. Oxford: Radcliffe Medical Press, November 1999.
4. Freedman S Direct transmission of electrocardiograms to a mobile phone for the management of a patient with acute myocardial infarction. J Telemed Telecare 1999;5:67–9.
5. Navein J, Ellis J Telemedicine in support of peacekeeping operation overseas – an audit. Telemed J 1997;3:207–14.

# 16. Spectrum of Capability and Applied Communications

John F. Navein and Simon J. O'Neill

**Objectives**

- To discuss the range of capability using communications modalities.
- To discuss the principles of using communications technology in hostile environments.
- To discuss problems and solutions.

## Introduction

The range of communications modalities described in the preceding chapter give a range of capabilities around which providers can build support for an operation. As with the enabling technology, they can be divided into low-bandwidth and high-bandwidth capabilities.

## Low Bandwidth

### Paper

Paper-based communication in the form of books, newspapers and posters remains one of the mainstays of communications. It is cheap and easy to produce and can easily be archived as a permanent record. On the other hand, paper-based information is difficult and slow to transmit, difficult to update and time-consuming to collate into any form of useful database. Most people, however, are more comfortable accessing information by reading from a piece of paper than they are reading from a screen.

### Broadcast

Simple one-way communications by broadcast, either by radio or TV, is the other main way that most people gather information, and even the Pentagon is known to rely on CNN for much of its real-time information-gathering during a crisis. Although broadcasting is useful as an information-gathering tool, it is also a very effective way of projecting information to affected populations in time of crisis, radio being less powerful but also less fragile and more ubiquitous than television. Important questions surrounding the manipulation of the press and information vs. propaganda need to be considered when using broadcast mediums to inform, but such questions are outside the scope of this chapter.

## Simple Voice Communications

Voice is the most basic form of communication and probably the most important. It is real-time and interactive, and most interactions between people can be done in person, by telephone or radio. Voice does have disadvantages, however, in that it requires two people to be together or at either end of a link at the same time for it to work, and there is generally no "hard copy" for the record. Voice is also sometimes inadequate, and as a medium it fails to get enough information over accurately or quickly enough. It is difficult to describe the scene of a catastrophe or the clinical situation in a hospital accurately and succinctly by voice alone. Also, visual cues such as body language are not transmitted, which can lead to misunderstandings between people who do not know each other well. By and large, though, voice works and is cheap, reliable and low-tech.

Teleconferencing (see previous chapter) is a very useful capability which is, in our view, under-utilised. Teleconferencing allows people in multiple sites to hold virtual meetings with considerable savings in time and money over the traditional face-to-face meetings. More importantly perhaps, teleconferencing allows virtual meetings to occur when real meetings otherwise may not, and those that do occur will be timed more appropriately to the job in hand.

## E-mail

E-mail has transformed communications. Although it has been used by the military and research establishments since 1973, it is only in the last 4 or 5 years that it has become a mainstream method of communication. You can access your e-mail wherever and whenever you want, and can reply at your convenience wherever you are. E-mail is generally asynchronous in that it does not require the sender and the recipient to be on-line at the same time (although real-time e-mail is possible), which can be a distinct advantage over the telephone.

E-mail also makes it easy to copy messages to a large number of people at the click of a mouse. E-mail etiquette is much simpler than the traditional written form, so that the reply to a message may be a single word. Less time, no paper and much quicker than mail. However, its ease can also be its problem. Because it is so easy for people to copy messages, they tend to do it without really thinking about what they are doing and whether there is a real need for all those people to know. This has the potential for information overload amongst the recipients. It tends to create an "ad hocracy" out of a hierarchy as the normal communications channels are short cut by "information" copies up the chain. Also, the ease of sending e-mail messages and the short reply time means that disagreements and misunderstandings can easily get out of hand as the calming influences of time (mail) or having to deal directly with people (telephone) are avoided.

## Store and Forward

Store and forward is a telemedicine term for clinical e-mail with attachments. In this context, store and forward attachments can include documents, digital photographs, X-rays or video clips. Clinically, store and forward can be used for up to 80% of telemedicine consultations, and takes less specialist time and resources than traditional practice. Because distance ceases to be a consideration, store and forward consultations can go to the next available or the most appropriate specialist rather than the most local. In time, store and forward will lead to a substantial change in the way medicine is practiced, but in the setting of conflict or a catastrophe it provides the vehicle for importing a whole range of expertise into the situation which would not otherwise be available. The same principal also holds for other disciplines such as engineering, The same communications system which sends clinical details and a photograph of a patient to an expert can also be used to send the engineering equivalent information and a photograph of, say, a damaged bridge.

Administratively, digital photographs can be used in lieu of lengthy descriptions, and the technology now exists whereby a picture can be transmitted and discussed in real time by voice concurrently (see above). White-boarding, where the correspondents highlight features on the picture rather like sports commentators highlight an action, can be a useful adjunct.

## The Internet

The internet as we know it became available to personal computer users only in 1993 when the first web browser, known as Mosaic, was released. This allowed users to search the internet using a user-friendly graphical interface. Its growth since then has been awesome. It is doubling its traffic volume every 4–5 months, and it is estimated that there will be 163 million users by the year 2000, a mere 7 years after the launch of Mosaic. Penetration of the market is low outside North America, Europe and the Asia Pacific Region, as shown in Fig. 16.1. Internet access in these areas will always lag well behind the developed world, but it is still growing rapidly and each new user constitutes a new source and recipient of information which was not there before.

The internet can also be used to communicate as well as to gather information. With the help of a cheap software package such as NetMeeting® (IBM), it is possible to talk across the net to anyone else on the net who has the same package at local call rates. Conference calls and video teleconferencing is also possible, although the quality is poor at present. Some web sites include chat sites where people from around the world with an interest in a particular topic can exchange ideas and develop new concepts, usually by e-mail, although conferencing is becoming more common despite the scheduling problems that it brings. It may well transform the scientific process over the next few years from one of peer-reviewed articles and text

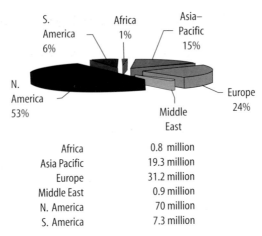

| | |
|---|---|
| Africa | 0.8 million |
| Asia Pacific | 19.3 million |
| Europe | 31.2 million |
| Middle East | 0.9 million |
| N. America | 70 million |
| S. America | 7.3 million |

**Fig. 16.1.** Internet users as of 1998. Africa 0.8 million; Asia–Pacific 19.3 million; Europe 31.2 million; Middle East 0.9 million; North America 70 million; South America 7.3 million.

books such as this to one where ideas are posted on the web and developed by discussion until a consensus is reached [1].

## High Bandwidth

Video teleconferencing (VTC) adds a two-way, real-time video image which can be worthwhile in certain circumstances. Although VTC is possible at low bandwidth across the web the quality is poor, and clinically useful VTC needs to be at 64 kbps as a bare minimum. VTC is difficult between people who do not know each other, but is a good tool for enhancing communications between those who do and within organisations. The addition of video to a link is reassuring to people at the distal end and can provide a valuable "situation awareness" tool for reporting purposes.

VTC is increasingly being used by organisations with dispersed structures as a routine means of holding virtual meetings, obviating the need for the participants to travel. As with voice-only teleconferencing (see above), up to 32 different sites can call into a multi-point bridge on a single number. Input can be via wire, GSM or satellite links. Costs can be high, but so can the costs in time and money of moving up to 32 people to the same place for a meeting. Nevertheless, the question should always be asked as to whether the additional modality of a video link is worth the extra cost as against a voice-only link. As well as holding virtual meetings, VTC is also being used for telemedicine, distance learning and a variety of administrative functions such as career interviews.

# Applied Communications in the Conflicts and Catastrophes

In this section we focus on the application of communication technology in the three phases of a conflict, catastrophe or disaster.

## The Pre-disaster Phase

Communications are an important consideration during the pre-disaster phase in two distinct ways. First, good communications are a key enabler in pre-disaster planning and dissemination of the results of that planning, and second, the communications plan itself is a key component of those plans.

### Using Communications to Write the Plan

#### The Internet

The internet is revolutionising communications and our ability to plan and prepare for disasters. The internet, and access to it, is rapidly spreading across the world to provide a cheap, fast and open method of exchanging and disseminating information. There are internet cafes and internet service providers in most major towns, making previously isolated expertise and communities part of a network from which they can learn and to which they can add.

The utility of the internet is two-fold. Firstly it provides access to vast amounts of information, and secondly it provides the means to communicate either by e-mail or by voice and basic VTC.

#### Information Sources

Information sources can be divided into base-line archive information which does not really change very much with time, and rapidly changing emerging stories surrounding acute events. The internet is useful for both.

Although most disasters and conflicts are predictable and predicted, many of those responding to them, especially those from outside the affected community, may have little available information by which to plan. Most academic institutions, commercial and voluntary organizations, and government departments in the developed world have web sites open to the internet which are valuable sources of archive data and can be used as regularly up-dated information sources. For example, the Center for Disease Control in Atlanta Georgia (www.cdc.gov) posts detailed medical threat assessments for all countries of the world, whilst foreign ministries give advise (often conflicting) regarding the security situation in hot spots. The latest medical information and access to MedLine is available through a number of web sites, including the National Library of Medicine (www.nlm.gov), and journals such as the *British Medical Journal* (www.bmj.co.uk) are published electronically. Weather forecasts are available via the CNN web site (www.cnn.com), and researchers can find more detailed information about individual countries by specific country searches.

Internet users must always question the reliability of this base-line general information. The quality of information found on the web is dependent upon its source web site and the time since it was last up-dated. You will need to make an assessment of whether the source site is reputable and whether the information on it is either out of date or time-sensitive. With reference to purely medical data there are a number of quality search filters which can help. They have established some measure of quality, and they surf the net for medical-orientated sites, establish which fit the criteria and filter out the rest. Two such sites are Omni (http://www.omni.ac.uk) and Health on the Net (http://www.hon.ch/). Although it is easy to be critical about exactly how accurate and current web-based data is, it is a considerable improvement over what planners had available even 3 or 4 years ago and the quality will continue to improve with time.

The major problem with the internet is information overload. There is so much information available that it is difficult to find the information you need from a reliable source. Web search engines help with this by enabling the user to define the search parameters and to cut down the number of options on offer. They also include "bookmarks" which the user can use to mark a useful site for future reference. A well-prepared web browser with appropriate bookmarks in place to identify proven reliable sites will enable planners to generate a comprehensive initial assessment of a location very quickly.

Disaster plans themselves will also become accessible on the web. The electronic format makes modification easy and dissemination cheap, but depending upon the type and extent of the expected disaster, a paper version needs to be available should communication links go down.

### The Communications Plan

Adequate planning and preparation is essential in all aspects of conflict and catastrophe medicine, none more so than with the communications plan. Maintaining a currently viable communications plan is not easy because of the rapidly changing technical capabilities and cost structures available. A rule of thumb is that technical capability is doubling and costs are halving every 2–3 years, and the deployment of LEO systems will only compound the problem. Given the pace of change, it is not helpful for this textbook to define what the communications solution for a given situation should be because the solution, and certainly the cost, will have changed by the time it is needed.

Although on-going change is a problem for planners looking to the future, it is also an opportunity as long as certain rules are observed We will describe those rules and the underlying principles, and cover the factors which need to be considered when developing a plan.

### Underlying Principles

There are two underlying principles and one set of rules which should underpin any communications plan. The underlying principles are (a) that the plan must be based on a user requirement, and (b) to recognise that communications is a specialist

| A communications solution must be appropriate for the situation in which it is expected to operate. Specifically it should be : | |
| --- | --- |
| Required | It should be designed around a user requirement i.e. those who will use the system should define what they will need it to do and the technical solution should answer that requirement. |
| Reasonable cost | Communications costs can be high, both in terms of equipment and call charge and the capability it provides must justify the cost. Sometimes, however, high bandwidth equipment may provide better value over low bandwidth because it transfers higher volume of data per minute and, beyond a certain break even point, will be cheaper. |
| Robust | The equipment and its supporting network must be robust yet light and portable. |
| Reliable | Network overload can be a particular problem, especially across mobile phone networks |
| Really easy | To use with no requirement for technical support in country. |
| Resource constrained | Equipment and networks must be appropriate to a resource constrained environment. Equipment should be able to operate from multiple power sources including batteries and generators, be weather proof and not rely on local infrastructure if that is likely to be destroyed or overloaded. |
| Routine | Communications systems should be used routinely, preferably as a part of daily work practises but a least on regular exersices if they are to be expected to work in the event of a disaster. |
| Reviewed | The capabilities and costs of communications solutions are changing at an increasing rate and therefore plans should be regularly reviewed. |

**Fig. 16.2.**   The rule of the eight Rs.

area which should be planned by a specialist. The rule governing a communications solution in austere environments is the rule of the eight Rs (Fig. 16.2).

A communications solution must be appropriate for the situation in which it is expected to operate. Specifically it should satisfy eight conditions.

Required It should be designed around a user requirement, i.e. those who will use the system should define what they will need it to do and the technical solution should answer that requirement

Reasonable cost Communications costs can be high, both in terms of equipment and call charges, and the capability it provides must justify the cost. Sometimes, however, high-bandwidth equipment may provide better value over low band-width because it transfers a higher volume of data per minute and, beyond a certain break-even point, will be cheaper

Robust The equipment and its supporting network must be robust yet light and portable

Reliable Network overload can be a particular problem, especially across mobile phone networks

Really easy The equipment should be easy to use with no requirement for tech-nical support in-country

Resource-constrained Equipment and networks must be appropriate to a resource-constrained environment. The equipment should be able to operate from multiple power sources, including batteries and generators, be weather-proof and not rely on a local infrastructure if that is likely to be destroyed or overloaded

Routine Communications systems should be used routinely, preferably as a part of daily work practices, but at least on regular exercises if they are to be expected to work in the event of a disaster

Reviewed The capabilities and costs of communications solutions are changing at an increasing rate and therefore plans should be regularly reviewed

### Establishing the User Requirement

The user requirement is the fundamental foundation for the application of any tech-nology. It is the process by which the users at all levels define what it is that they wish technology to do, and what attributes it will need to have to be useful to them where they will use it. The user requirement is best worked out as a team using standard brain-storming methodology.

The product of this exercise should be a prioritised list of capabilities on the one side and constraints on the other. Examples of capabilities might be that two (or three or four) people at given locations need to be able to communicate freely with each other, or that there is also a requirement for the movement of data between those given locations. The constraints will include the rule of the eight Rs, but addi-tional constraints might be that communication needs to be real-time, it might need to be simultaneous across a number of sites, perhaps include a visual element and be at a defined level of security. The data transfer service may need a turn-around time of say 24 h, and again may have a security element to it. It is important to note that there is no mention at all about technology; no mention of satellites, radios, band-width or anything else technical. In fact the user requirement could be met in some circumstances by face-to-face meetings, couriers and the mail.

From the user requirement comes the technical solution, which should be based purely upon that requirement. Any temptation to add capability just because it is possible should be resisted unless it does not impact on the eight Rs, especially if the result would be that the solution becomes less robust or less reasonably priced.

### Communications Is a Specialist Area

Communications in an austere environment is a specialist area and therefore a specialist should be tasked with converting the user requirement into a technical solution. In addition to the technical expertise needed to decide which is the most appropriate solution to a given user requirement, there also a need for logistical expertise to get the equipment across borders, especially in regions where there is armed conflict and where satellite equipment (which is outside of the control of the incumbent regime) can be very attractive. Call tariffs for satellite phones can be very complicated (LEOs) or very simple (Inmarsat), and can differ by a factor of five or six. Even within one technology, the cost of calls can differ by a factor of 20% depending upon which service provider you chose.

Larger organisations can afford to have their own communications staff and this is the preferred solution where possible. Individuals or smaller agencies cannot and need not justify such expense and should develop a relationship with one of the companies who specialise in providing communications in their particular circumstances. The choice should be a company which acts as an agent for a wide range of technologies and therefore has no vested interest in a particular solution. Some will offer discounts and may even offer a leasing service or short-term rental so that customers do not need to buy capital equipment which may soon become obsolete. After-sales service is important and problematic. No companies currently offer in-country servicing should your equipment break down, and it is wise to build some redundancy into your plans to allow for this (as defined by the user requirement). Most companies will offer a return to base (RTB) warranty and will dispatch a replacement as soon as a unit breaks down. It is wise to get any agreement in writing, but most specialist providers are very aware of the environment in which agencies work and will do their best to help. However, if the service you receive is not up to scratch there are plenty of other providers in the market.

## The Acute Phase

The first serious attempt to use information and communication technology to support a community in the aftermath of a catastrophe was in 1991 when NASA established a link between Yerevan in Armenia and four US medical centres [2] in the aftermath of the major earthquake there in 1988. Since then progress has been slow but steady as people have worked to establish the appropriateness of evolving technology in the disaster setting.

### Information Sources

#### The Internet

Major news agencies have very active and regularly up-dated web sites which are particularly useful for breaking news. Some have direct audio and even video links into their news programmes across the web. A "surf" around various international news agencies, many of which are multilingual, can provide an interesting perspective on how other communities see a particular situation. The protagonists on both sides of armed conflicts often have their own web sites which provide useful insight into their view of the world. Although much less common in the developing world at present, the internet has started to spread there too and will continue to do so. Web sites are generally easy to navigate around and usually include the date when they were last up-dated, thus giving the user some idea of the information's currency. Most sites are linked to other web sites of interest by hypertext links. These are in highlighted text or as an address within one site which immediately links through the allied site at the click of mouse.

The great lesson of history is that we forget the lessons of history, and the development of the internet offers us the opportunity to record and exchange lessons learnt across organisations by posting them on the web. It is a feature of the response to conflicts and disaster that most of those responding have never done it before. Over the days, weeks or months that they work, they build up considerable experience, which is sometimes recorded on paper and very occasionally archived. It is rare for it to be published or for anyone else to benefit from it. Ready access to electronic reports via accredited and user-friendly web sites will be of immense help to planners, and mean that valuable experience is available to others without going through the rigours of publishing in the peer-reviewed literature.

Prospectively, development agencies [3] and NGOs should consider developing programs which put rugged IT and communications capability into existing infrastructures in disaster-prone and politically unstable areas, after suitable training programs and other support systems have been developed so that they are available when needed. It is interesting to consider whether the presence of a reliable communications infrastructure is a stabilising or de-stabilising influence. Perhaps freely available communications across an ethnic divide, for instance, may become a tool to prevent the downward spiral into violence.

### The User Requirement of Communications in the Early Acute Phase

The major requirement of a communications system in the early acute phase of a disaster is to communicate the extent and nature of the problem (disaster assessment) and to coordinate the initial response to it. There is therefore a requirement for communications both within the affected area and with/between those parties outside the area who are trying to respond to it. Local authorities have responsibility for the coordination of a response but may have lost the ability to do so effectively. They must be included within the decision-making process as soon as possible and therefore need to be included within the communications loop.

### Initial Disaster Needs Assessment

A wide range of information needs to flow into and out of the disaster zone to multiple agencies around the world. Accurate determinations of the extent of the disaster and exactly where it is are required. It is also necessary to discover what resources are available locally and the condition of transport and other infrastructures. Outside expertise (national and perhaps international) needs to be directed towards working out priorities and solutions. Traditionally that expertise has travelled to the disaster area, has often been ill-prepared for the conditions found there, and has consequently placed an additional burden on an already stretched community. Assessment teams need to be self-sufficient, particularly in communications, so that they can keep up to date with the evolving situation and easily relate their assessment of the situation on the ground to those who need to know.

### Catastrophes Where a Robust Infrastructure Remains Intact

Following a catastrophe (such as a rail or plane crash) where the local communications infrastructure is robust and largely intact, the routine communications system of the agencies involved, perhaps with additional channels being made available, is the solution of choice. In most cases this will involve a combination of public service radio networks and GSM phones. As previously noted, satellite telephones may be a useful adjunct in some cases where there is a GSM black spot or system-overload. Many GSM operators have mobile booster systems which they normally use to reinforce their networks during major events and which they will make available to cover a catastrophe, especially if they have been included in the pre-disaster planning.

National and local news organisations also provide a useful source of information, although the content needs to be treated with some caution. Major news organisations often have early access to key individuals who are managing the scene, but also need to meet deadlines to provide the latest up-date. As with all sources in the early acute phase, reliable information may simply not be available in all the confusion. Agencies responding from outside the region should remember that the national news for the affected area may be available live on the internet

### Regions Where the Communications Infrastructure Is Poor or Destroyed

Currently, Inmarsat satellite communication is the communication medium of choice. They operate almost totally independently of the local infrastructure and work effectively worldwide at a reasonable cost. In the unusual event of the satellite becoming saturated there is generally an alternative regional satellite available in most parts of the world.

Mini-Ms are light and will work from a range of power sources, including car batteries and internal batteries, as a short-term solution. They can be made far more versatile by adding a basic laptop (with word processing and e-mail packages) and a digital camera. Mini-Ms provide cheap voice communications and a very low-bandwidth (2.4 kbps) data transfer, which is fine for e-mail and faxes but is very slow for larger files such as photographs. Remember, though, that a Mini-M attached to a computer with the right compression software can become a very useful data transfer tool with white-boarding and simultaneous voice transmission, and is ideal for discussing photographs and diagrams.

The Inmarsat B is obsolescent, and is soon to be replaced by the cheaper and much smaller M4. The M4 is the solution of choice for sending large amounts of data or if you need to run a number of telephone lines simultaneously. Mini-Ms also enable a reasonable quality of video teleconferencing, including the transmission of video clips. You can transmit compressed video footage if you link a Mini-M to a laptop with the right software, and this makes store and forward video a reality as a method of reporting an assessment at a reasonable cost. It is our belief that this could transform the art of disaster assessment and begin to put a degree of science into it.

M4 call charges are three to four times as expensive as those of the Mini-M, but they can transmit 25 to 30 times as much data per minute (or much more with compression). Therefore, if you just want a single-voice channel and the occasional small-scale data transfer, the M4 is not for you, but if your user requirement is for a more ambitious capability then it probably is.

The Inmarsat B does still have a niche in the capability spectrum. The B is bulky and uses a lot of power relative to the other two, but some models have the advantage of having the option of using both low bandwidth at 9.4 kbps at $2.50 per minute and ISDN-level bandwidth at $9. It is therefore appropriate for both single-voice calls and higher bandwidth data transfer.

VHF radio may also have a role in this situation, particularly for larger organisations which have already invested in the equipment and have the in-house expertise to set up and run a radio network.

## The Future?

The current system of disaster assessment does not work well. Multiple teams, some ill-prepared for the environment to which they travel, descend upon a disaster area only to become a further burden on an already stretched community. Communications technology offers a re-engineered solution to address this problem, and is starting to be actively considered by some members of the United Nations Disaster Assessment and Coordinating Committee (UNDACC) and other agencies.

The re-engineered solution is to establish standing, field-trained, assessment teams who can quickly be inserted into a conflict or disaster area at the earliest opportunity in the evolution of the situation. The team will be self-sufficient in food and shelter etc., and will undertake an assessment using video, still photographs and a pre-prepared electronic questionnaire. Once the initial assessment has been completed, the team will transmit its assessment openly to all interested parties, be they responding agencies or potential donors, and post it on the internet. Such teams will reduce the footprint of the assessment effort considerably at a time when the local infrastructure is least able to cope, whilst improving the quality and timeliness of the information available to planners.

The team would deploy with a high-bandwidth capability to enable video footage to be transmitted, and to allow VTC meetings to take place between key personnel from within the locality of the disaster and those coordinating the relief effort from outside. It will establish direct links between donors and recipients to ensure that the planned response meets the real needs of the affected community. Mutual suspicion may be allayed by the opportunity to "meet" across the link, and the inevitable logistical and political problems will be resolved more easily and quickly. It will also reduce the need for outside politicians to visit the disaster area.

The addition of a specialist may be appropriate in given situations, especially following the outbreak of disease where the nature and extent of the outbreak is unclear. A specialist in tropical medicine or public health with electronic access to their resources back home should be able to resolve many of the problems much more quickly than is currently the case, and then leave the on-going surveillance to appropriately trained local staff while retaining a direct communications link over time. This would also support the principle of self-reliance in the local community.

In the longer term, the team will stay in-country for some time to provide continuity and on-going up-dates as the situation evolves. Outside planners will be able to direct the team to specific questions which need to be addressed, and to verify the arrival and distribution of aid in order to close the audit loop, again making all information available to all agencies.

We recognise that this concept has a number of disadvantages associated with its implementation, particularly the cultural change which would have to occur for agencies to trust an outsider to provide them with the information they need in an accurate and timely manner, but the concept has been proven in theory [4] and interest in it is growing.

## Coordination of the Disaster Response

It is very likely that the communications tools which are appropriate for the co-ordination of the acute phase of a conflict or catastrophe will be the same as those needed for the initial assessment, particularly those used at the scene. However, as the response matures and services begin to be restored or new ones introduced then fixed-wire systems will often become available. A regular review of the communications plan is therefore wise, and as additional options become available they should each be measured against your user requirement and a change made if appropriate.

Redundancy should be considered depending on circumstances. If, for example, you had been using a wireless system on a modern service contract (i.e. no monthly fees), then you should retain your wireless system as a fall-back until you are satisfied that the replacement meets your requirements, is reliable and provides better value for money. Conflicts and catastrophes are notoriously unpredictable and a fall-back is wise, especially if it is free.

### Routine Reporting

The need to establish a reporting routine will vary depending both on the situation and the structure and management style of the organisation responding to it. In general, a routine reporting policy is good. People need to know what is going on at the scene in order to provide efficient support and the logistics to deliver it; at least some people need to know some things. The team at the scene is invariably too busy to provide all the information that their organisation would like, when they would like to receive it. Therefore, part of the communications plan must be to prepare, by consensus, a standard reporting format which provides only that information that is required to do the job and at a frequency which is appropriate. This is the minimum data requirement. Ideally, a mechanism should also be in place for its review with time. In general, people on the ground will do their best to provide information if they feel it is worth while, and hence this should be an exercise in consensus and persuasion rather than dictat. Short daily reporting with a two-way transfer of useful information works best. The timing should be at the convenience of those in the field.

The coordination of the response to a conflict or catastrophe overseas remains the responsibility of the local authorities and they are often ill-equipped to deal with the task. They need to be able to communicate with their own resources in order to launch and manage a local response, whilst at the same time coordinate across a wide range of national and international agencies and organizations who are keen to support them. The early insertion of an effective communications capability (with technical support) to enable that coordination to occur will generally prove very valuable. The capability should have three nodes, the disaster area itself, the local national ministry responsible for coordinating a response and a link into the international communications network. The choice of system will depend upon the particular situation, but will probably be a combination of routine telephones and satellite/GSM.

### Projection of Expertise

Disasters, by definition, require the assistance of outside resources and expertise, at least in the early stages. Questions of public health, engineering, communicable diseases, nutrition and many others will need to be answered by those on the ground who may not have the knowledge or experience to answer them or the means or time to learn. The traditional method of solving this problem has been to import the expertise into the area for a "specialist visit", even though this may bring many of the problems outlined above. However, much of this help can be given satisfactorily by the movement of information rather than the movement of experts, especially if the organisation and technology delivering that expertise is trusted by both parties. An information transfer system which permits ready access to international libraries and databases may reduce the need for such expertise by providing the local specialists with the information to make their own decisions. Alternatively, the transmission of appropriate pictorial or written information to an appropriate expert, or even video teleconferencing, may achieve the goal satisfactorily.

### High Level Communication

There is often a requirement for officials at the highest levels to communicate. Discussions at ministerial level may be required to reduce the bureaucratic barriers to the delivery of aid. These discussions do not often occur at present. Easy, open communication between desk officers reduces the need for higher-level intervention, and easy open communications at higher levels, should it become necessary, also reduces the risk of misunderstanding and the need for high-level travel.

### Audit

An audit is becoming more important as the response to conflicts and catastrophes becomes more mature and professional, and donors require more accountability for money spent. A tracking system or method of recording that aid has arrived where it was supposed to, and that it had the desired effect, is required but not often available. This sort of information closes the loop logistically, but also provides the basis for a reliable evaluation of a given aid effort. A range of options is available from bar-coding linked to the satellite network, and tracking of vehicles using the geographical positioning system (GPS), to more simple reporting procedures with data transfer of delivery notes or photographs by e-mail or fax. The solution should fit the user's requirements.

### Communications to Support the Team

Teams deployed into an area of conflict or catastrophe work under stress and are often away from home for many months. Regular communication with home is an important tool to reduce the impact of both. Daily calls home can be very expensive and the post is often slow and unreliable. E-mail, with photographs as attachments, allows daily contact with home cheaply as a supplement to less frequent phone calls. Internet phone calls are also cheap where available, and a modest investment in the right software at both ends may be a high-value, low-cost solution.

## Post-disaster Rehabilitation Phase

The post-disaster rehabilitation phase is the period between the time a community ceases to be overwhelmed by the effects of the disaster and the time when it returns to normality. It starts days or weeks after the disaster strikes and may go on for years. It is often the time when most effort goes in to the pre-disaster planning phase for the next one, as lessons are learnt and memories are fresh in the minds of the community. It is also the time when a community is still in need of support for their efforts, and when the external resources available to provide such support often begin to fall off as media and public attention shift elsewhere. On the other hand, this can be an important time because communities are often at their most amenable to the consideration of a permanent change from pre-disaster practices, to their ultimate long-term benefit.

Good communications and telemedicine can be the infrastructure upon which a new health care system can be built, focusing on para-professional personnel in remote areas and linking them to various higher levels of consultation and care. This can re-focus the health care system on primary care and create new categories of health care personnel, thus providing new employment opportunities.

An example of this occurred in the later stages of the siege of Sarajevo, when the destruction of the medical infrastructure and the emigration of a large proportion of health care workers coincided with the introduction of new ideas from outside. These new ideas were born out of necessity and the influx of aid workers from around the world to create a fertile period for change that would not have been possible had the war in Bosnia not occurred. The post-conflict phase is also the time when many well-intentioned promises are made at farewells which soon begin to slide down the priority list because focus and funding move elsewhere. The user requirement at this stage is to enable those promises to be kept whilst reducing the need to maintain a strong physical presence in an area, which may be financially unsustainable. Supporting a reduced in-country team with a virtual presence from outside is relatively cheap to do and easy to deliver; it is also a good way to begin to taper-off support as self-reliance grows.

## On-going Expert Assistance

On-going redevelopment through education and development programmes are the mainstay at this stage in a conflict or catastrophe. The imaginative use of communications can greatly enhance the value of programmes designed to meet these needs. Expert visits are an expensive but important element of such programmes, and to some extent communications technology can be used to replace or augment them.

An important proviso to put in here is that distance learning or virtual "meetings or visits" do not work well if the people at either end of the link do not know each other. There is some element of the human psyche which means that people have to meet and touch before they can communicate easily in any important way. Therefore, teleconferencing, e-mail, distance learning and especially VTC meetings between people can only support a wider programme and need to be based on established personal relationships to work well.

Currently, much of the value of expert visits is lost through lack of follow-up and reinforcement. An on-going link with ready communication between visits can greatly enhance the value of the programme by reinforcing the original messages and establishing a progressive programme between visits in addition to intense work during them. The communications solutions you chose will depend upon what you wish to achieve, but e-mail will be a minimum.

## Distance Learning and Twinning

The medical infrastructure, and particularly the medical talent, of a country is sometimes weakened following a catastrophe and is always weakened following conflict. Many experienced doctors and nurses will be killed during the fighting, and many of the remainder will migrate and may establish thriving careers elsewhere. A new generation will need to be trained to take their place, and distance learning programmes linked with specialist visits, as mentioned above, are a good and cost-effective way of doing that. It is even conceivable that some of those who migrated would wish to help out in this way. Such help may be important, but it needs to be relevant. Current distance learning packages tend to be generic and designed around Western medical practice, which may not be relevant either in content or in culture.

Twinning is an arrangement whereby medical communities in post-conflict regions are twinned with specific institutions overseas. The links are normally multiple, with each one focusing on a specific speciality. This is the ideal arrangement to combine the concepts of specialist or exchange visits and distance learning schemes because it creates an integrated package which is aimed specifically at the particular circumstances operating in the affected area. Quite sophisticated communications links may be appropriate to support mature and well-funded schemes, which may include commercial satellite links, which are otherwise outside the scope of this chapter. A well-planned broad-bandwidth link may also make commercial sense in the post-conflict environment because there will probably be the opportunity to share costs or subcontract time or capabilities to other organisations. This will defray costs and may even lead to a profit.

## Training Can Go Both Ways

The Uniformed Services University of the Health Sciences has undertaken a number of tele-training projects overseas using Inmarsat B-based VTC links. It quickly became apparent that the links were also valuable to the university since they exposed staff and students to conditions and problems they would not normally come across. This is an important principle, both because of the opportunities that it opens up and also because reverse-teaching programmes are a powerful way to improve the morale of a medical community trying to recover from a prolonged period of hardship.

## The Internet

Establishing internet connections can be a valuable and cost-effective stand-alone way of supporting post-conflict recovery. E-mail and links to specialist chat nets and web sites reduce the sense of isolation felt by many clinicians working in post-conflict settings. Access to MedLine is also very valuable in countries without medical library facilities, and some sites will provide electronic copies of articles by e-mail. The ability to share experiences is important to people during this phase, and establishing a home page on the web may help. A web site provides a medium to describe what happened and to pass on lessons learnt to those who will follow. Internet access may well be all that is required, since it will give practitioners the tools they need to help themselves [5].

## Technology and Returning Refugees

The technology exists to assist with the difficult question of the management of returning refugees and to assist in the reunification of families. As a minimum we should be trialling the use of appropriate telecommunications and IT applications in the early response to refugees and displaced persons. These could be used at the point of registration and the initial medical encounter for counting, documentation, the issue of new identity documents, and the initiation of new medical records. This can be done in the field with laptops, e.g. using hand-held devices such as the Palm Pilot transmitting to the laptop by IR digital cameras to produce images for photo-identification cards and embedding critical medical information on the card.

## Telemedicine and its Role in Conflicts and Catastrophes

Telemedicine is defined as the use of information and communications technology to provide medical care remotely. The definition includes a broad range of technologies from the POTS (the plain old telephone system), through store and forward to VTC, with a broad range of concepts and capabilities to match them. Although still in its infancy, telemedicine is gradually coming of age and may have some applications in conflict and catastrophes.

Telemedicine is not a single entity, but rather a range of "telespecialities" each with its own technical solution. Some specialities such as dermatology or radiology are well defined, others less so. The introduction of technology into a process does not of itself bring benefits, it is the resultant re-engineering of the underlying process which effects useful change.

It is tempting to use telemedicine to project expertise from an intact and thriving community into one struck by conflict or disaster, but care is needed. Carers working in a warm well-resourced functioning hospital have little concept of how to provide care in the austere and resource-constrained environment of a disaster. The medical priorities are very different, and those working at the scene need to rely on their own training and local resources rather than those from outside. Those providing care via telemedicine need to be experienced and know what is available and appropriate where the care is to be delivered.

There is a feeling that telemedicine may be inappropriate in the conflict and disaster setting. However, a number of applications are emerging which could lead to a significant and beneficial change over current practice.

Surgical hospitals covering many conflicts are often a long way from the fighting and located at the end of a long, arduous and dangerous evacuation chain. Many casualties who make the journey do not need surgical intervention, and could well be managed closer to home by non-surgical care [6] without going through the added trauma of a long evacuation. A re-engineered and preferable model of care might be to provide the resources to give good non-surgical care at the head of the evacuation chain, and to establish a telemedicine link to the surgical hospital at the end so that the surgical team can give advice when it is needed on who should and who should not be evacuated to them. Such a link would require an experienced war nurse equipped with a voice link only at the head of the chain, perhaps with the capability to transmit the occasional photograph. Such a system would have the added benefit of advising the surgical hospital what casualties to expect so that they could plan their surgical lists accordingly.

Many agencies provide support to a conflict or catastrophe by evacuating medical cases away from the area for care elsewhere, a process which is called Medevac. Very often these decisions can become politically charged, and the in-country staff are put under considerable pressure to approve cases which are not necessarily appropriate. In addition, many patients are moved inappropriately because those making the decision in-country do not necessarily have sufficient expertise in that particular condition to know what questions to ask, and therefore insufficient information reaches the receiving specialist centre to enable them to make the right decisions. Store and forward telemedicine would considerably improve decision making in this contentious area by enabling all relevant clinical records, including test results and X-rays, to be scanned and sent to the receiving specialist centre for an opinion, and an answer could be received same day. In some cases, a VTC link enabling the receiving specialist to speak to the patient direct and examine them by proxy (through an experienced clinician who would be with the patient) would be a further refinement.

Not only would this improve the decision making about who to move and who not to move, but it would also remove the pressure on the in-country team to make a clinically inappropriate or politically driven decision.

# The Principles of Using Technology in a Conflict or Catastrophe

This chapter has covered the range of communications technologies that are available to people responding to a conflict and catastrophe situation and the capabilities that they release. We went on to discuss some process re-engineering opportunities that modern technologies can provide. It is important not to get over-enthusiastic about technology, especially in an austere or resource-constrained environment, and to retain a position of healthy scepticism. The right technology will revolutionise the way we do business; the wrong technology will be an expensive and frustrating mistake. Planning based on user requirements makes all the difference.

The principles listed below will guide those considering a technological solution to a particular problem.

## Principle 1. Technology Must Be Targeted on a Problem

Technology should be the solution to a problem, rather than being a solution looking for a problem to solve. The basic problem in applying communications technology to a conflict or catastrophe situation is obvious, but the cost and complexity of the various solutions to the same problem can vary considerably. The user's requirements are the key to getting the balance right. Focus on getting the user's requirements right, dividing them into "must haves" and "nice to haves", and accept that the solution may either be very simple, such as the post, or else may simply be to improve management rather than investing in technology. If technology is the answer, there will probably be a number of options open to you.

## Principle 2. The Solution Must Be Appropriate

Having decided on the range of options available, you next need to make sure that they are appropriate for what you want to do. The various options need to be assessed against the rule of the eight Rs. As with the user's requirements, it is very important for this assessment to be made by the users, or at least by people with experience of working in the environment in which the equipment will be used.

## Principle 3. Technology Should Not Be Layered on Top of the Existing System

Technology can be used either to automate the current system or facilitate fundamental changes in the way you do business. If you are introducing a new technology or a new capability, then as a general rule it will not achieve its full potential unless it is associated with some degree of re-engineering of the underlying processes, e.g.

using store and forward telemedicine to streamline Medevac by moving information not patients.

## Principle 4. You Must Follow the Rules of Good Business Practice

Before proceeding to procurement, you will need to measure your solution against a clinical and business case. The clinical and business case is not just a financial judgement, it measures the changes and technology that you wish to introduce against the vision, value and philosophy of your organisation and against the user's requirements which you defined at the beginning. Cash will be one variable, but it is likely that efficiency, service and quality will be as important if not more so. Decide what factors are important to you, weight them relative to each other and then measure them before making a realistic assessment of what they will measure afterwards. The difference is the clinical and business case for (or against) change.

## Principle 5. Stay in Your Own Lane

Many projects fail because the wrong person with the wrong skills and experience makes the wrong decisions. Most of the key decisions about the introduction of technology need to be made by the users. In telemedicine, clinicians at both ends need to define what they want the technology to do. Management changes are decided by management, and technical advice should come from people with technical expertise in providing communications in the sort of environment you will be working in. This principle may appear obvious, but it is our experience that it is often forgotten.

## Principle 6. Training and Evaluation

People must be trained if they are to be expected to use new or unfamiliar technology. The training is best undertaken in the environment in which it is to be used, so-called "situational training". Similarly, a system of evaluation needs to be put in place to provide an early insight into evolving problems, and to provide a quality feedback which can be used to make improvements in the future.

# Conclusions

Good communications are crucial to the effective response to, and management of, conflicts and catastrophes. Planning is the key to delivering a solution which will meet your needs.

The authors are happy to answer any specific questions from readers and can be reached via e-mail

# Glossary

| Term | Definition |
|------|-----------|
| ATM | Asynchronous transfer mode: a Dell-based data transfer technique in which demand determines packet allocation. ATM offers fast packet technology and real-time, demand-led switching for efficient network resources. |
| B-ISDN | Broadband ISDN offering 30◊64 kbps channels plus two network control channels. It has a total user rate of 1920 kbps and is often referred to as a 2-Meg link. |
| BRI ISDN | Basic rate interface allowing 2◊64 kbps and 1◊16 kbps channels to be carried over a single pair of copper wires. Through the use of bonding techniques, the 64 kbps channels can be aggregated to create more bandwidth. |
| Broadband | A term describing any network that can multiplex several independent network carrier frequencies on to a single cable, thereby producing a high data transfer capability. |
| CODEC | (COder/DECoder): a device that converts analogue signals into a form suitable for transmission on a digital circuit. The signal is decoded back into analogue form at the receiving end of the link. |
| Ethernet | A LAN and data-link protocol based on a packet frame. Usually operating at 10 Mbps, multiple devices can share access to the link. |
| GEO | Geo-stationary Earth orbit: a satellite orbiting the Earth at some 35,000 km and apparently stationary in the sky to an observer on Earth. |
| GSM | Global system for mobile telecommunications (originally it was the French Group Speciale Mobile, but was changed as it became the global standard}. |
| Inmarsat | Now a private company offering global satellite services via a number of LESO. (Inmarsat was formerly a multinational co-operative with some 88 member countries until it was privatised in April 1999). |
| Internet | A group of networks that are interconnected so that they appear to be one continuous network. |
| Iridium | New-generation satellite operator: the first to launch hand-held satellite telephones (November 1998) with true global coverage using LEO satellites. |
| ISDN | Integrated digital services network: a switched digital network capable of handling an amalgam of digital voice, data and image transmission. |

| | |
|---|---|
| LAN | Local area network: a communication system that links computers into a network. |
| LEO | Low Earth orbit satellite, typically transitting the world at an altitude of about 800 km, just at the edge of space. |
| LESO | Land Earth station operator: usually operated by the national PTT, and responsible for landing satellite traffic from space and distributing it to its destination. |
| Packet | A collection of bits, including the address, data and control information, that are switched and transmitted together. The terms frame and packet are often used synonymously. |
| PMR | Private mobile radio such as that operated by the Ambulance Service. |
| PSTN | Public switched telephone network: the ordinary telephone network for switched access to local and long-distance services. |
| Store-and-forward | Clinical e-mail with attachments, not in real time. |
| VTC | Video teleconferencing link: often referred to as video conferencing, this is the capacity for a group of operators to be interlinked so as to share real-time conversation and video. |

# References

1. Smith R. What is publication? BMJ 1999;318:142.
2. Rayman RB. Telemedicine: military applications. Aviat Space Env Med 1992;135–7.
3. Ferguson EW et al. Telemedicine for national and international disaster response. J Med Syst 1995;19(2):121–3.
4. Navein J, Hagmann J. Telemedicine and the remote assessment of disasters. Prehospital and Disaster Medicine, 9WCEDM, 10/S1, May 1995.
5. Groves T. SatelLife: getting relevant information to the developed world. BMJ 1996;313:1606–9.
6. Hayward J. Hospitals for war wounded. Geneva: International Committee of the Red Cross, 1998.

# 17. Acute Medical Problems

Claire Walford, S. Nazeer, A. McGuinness,
Jim Ryan and A.J. Thomas

**Objectives**
- To heighten awareness.
- To indicate the range of conditions which might be encountered.
- To highlight particular risks to locals and expatriate carers.
- To discuss general principles of prevention and mitigation.
- To discuss the broad principles of recognition and management of important conditions.
- To describe on-going health care.

## Introduction

The authors of this chapter include emergency physicians, primary care physicians and a surgeon. All have experience of the complex problems faced by health professionals in attempting to provide acute medical care in the face of adversity following natural and man-made disasters and in other austere settings. In this context, it is impossible to draw a line between public health medicine and acute medical care. Thirst, starvation, diarrhoea and communicable disease are all illnesses requiring management and are the lot of the acute care health professional as well as the public and community health professional. Inevitably this has lead to some overlap with other chapters and sections in this manual. We see this as reinforcement, not repetition, and perhaps it also shows an additional viewpoint. This chapter attempts to deal with a vast array of medical problems in a wide variety of conflict settings. It is not intended for the experienced senior physician, seasoned by numerous deployments. The authors recognise that readers of this manual are more likely to include elective students in medicine and professions allied to medicine, junior doctors, nurses and a range of other health professionals. The age and experience of this diverse group will also vary greatly. Therefore, the chapter does not attempt to be an exhaustive treatise on medical therapeutics. Such specialist texts already exist and are listed in the suggested reading section at the end of this chapter, and in the Resources section.

A variety of other impacting issues may confound and disrupt the delivery of care and need to be considered when reading this chapter. These include:

- the nature of the disaster, i.e. natural or man-made;
- climate, i.e. hot/cold, winter/summer;
- environment, i.e. urban or rural;
- infrastructure, i.e. intact/compromised/destroyed;
- political situation;
- transport and communications.

## Medical Problems – Scope

Bearing in mind the sheer scale of potential medical problems, a structure or framework is demanded. The following main headings are used:

- water supply, food and sanitation;
- shelter;
- mass gatherings;
- climate, hot and cold;
- pre-existing disease;
- envenomation;
- miscellaneous.

## Water Supply, Food and Sanitation

In developed societies, the provision of clean water, sufficient food and energy sources are taken for granted. In a conflict setting, water and food are closely associated with health problems – access may be a matter of life and death. Sanitation, which includes waste disposal and vector control, also has an important impact on health.

A delicate balance exists between the affected population with its needs for water, food and energy, and the environment and its problems such as the pollution of drinking water by human waste and the over-use and possible exhaustion of food and energy sources.

An imbalance between population needs and environmental capacity resulting in outbreaks of disease is a frequent finding in the aftermath of a conflict or catastrophe, and the restoration of that balance is one of the most urgent tasks faced by aid workers.

### Water

#### Water Needs – Quantity

There is now general agreement on the minimum standards required in terms of quantity and quality. Water needs refer not just to drinking water, but must also encompass overall needs.

In determining water needs a number of variables need to be considered, making it difficult to describe absolute quantities for any given conflict or catastrophe.

The absolute minimum physiological quantity of water needed for survival is widely agreed to be 3 litres/person/day in a temperate climate. If hygiene needs are added, this figure rises to 15 litres/person/day. This minimum figure will rise in a conflict or

> **Water needs**
> - Drinking water
> - Food preparation
> - Personal hygiene
> - Laundering

> **Water needs – variables**
> - Climate/geography/ambient temperatures
> - Cultural aspects
> - Impact of illness
> - On-site medical facilities
> - Technical factors

catastrophe setting – aid organisations now regard 20 litres/person/day as the minimum standard if there is to be a positive impact upon the health of a population.

There are needs in addition to the minimum standard described above. These are listed in the box below.

There are clearly many variables, but the following indicators give a feel for the sort of quantities that may be required:

> **Additional water needs**
>
> - Public toilets (hand-washing and cleaning)
> - Laundries
> - Hospitals
> - Malnutrition centre
> - Perineal cleansing
> - Health centres
> - Cholera and diarrhoea centres
> - Animal needs (livestock)

Cholera centre – up to 60 litres/patient/day;

Malnutrition centres – up to 30 litres/patient/day;

Livestock needs – up to 30 litres/large animal/day.

### Water Needs – Quality

Water must be palatable and of adequate quality to be drunk and used for personal purposes without causing significant risk to health from short-term use due to water-borne diseases, or to chemical or radiological contamination. The phrase potable water is widely used and is defined as *water which contains no substances posing a danger to health when consumed or used for any domestic use.*

The concept of palatable water needs to be clarified. Water that is over-chlorinated will not be consumed. Further, the degree of sterilisation should be a balance between needs, availability and the risk of excess infection. The local water supply in many areas subject to conflict or catastrophe will be contaminated in any event to a greater or lesser extent. The aim is to prevent excess infections, particularly in areas of mass gathering.

Water which must be treated includes:

- all drinking water for home use;
- piped water for large populations (one water stand per 250 people);
- water exposed to chemical or radiation contamination.

The means of treating water are listed below.

- Tank storage: allowing sedimentation (less chemical for sterilisation required).
- Transparent reservoir: exposure to UV rays from sunlight eliminates most pathogens.
- Filtration: slow filtering through sand and porous membranes.
- Chemical: the use of aluminium salts facilitates sedimentation. Free halogens act as disinfectant. The effective dosage of free halogen is 0.5 mg/l acting over a period of 30 min.
- Boiling: seldom used because of energy availability constraints.

### Water Needs – Storage

Storage and treatment are closely linked. Storage is in itself a form of water treatment. Each family should have two water collection vessels of 10–20 l. These should preferably have covers, or at least narrow necks.

## Sanitation

The disposal of human waste is of equal priority to the provision of water when faced with mass gatherings. The reasons are obvious. One gram of human faecal matter may contain:

Viruses    – poliomyelitis $10^6$
           – hepatitis A $10^6$
           – rotavirus $10^6$

Bacteria   – *Vibrio cholera* $10^6$
           – *Salmonella* $10^6$
           – *E. coli* $10^8$

Parasites  – amobae $10^4$
           – *Giardia* $10^5$
           – ancylostomes 800 eggs
           – ascarids 10,000 eggs
           – schistosomes 40 eggs
           – Shigella $10^6$

Human faeces are very variable in pathogenecity, for example children's stools are more infectious than adults. This also holds true for the sick, with cholera for example, and for healthy carriers of a variety of pathogens.

Contamination can occur for many reasons.

- Inadequate hygiene after defaecation leading to faecal/oral transmission.
- Transmission from person to person by dirty hands.
- Faecal contamination of water destined for consumption or domestic use.
- Contamination of food in a variety of ways, for example washing fruit or vegetables in contaminated water. Insect vectors may also do this; the ubiquitous fly is the best example.

Minimum standards are now agreed by most aid agencies. These include:

- a sufficient number of toilets; there should be 1 toilet per 20 people;
- toilets no more than 50 m distance from dwellings or 1-min walk;
- safe, comfortable toilets which are accessible day and night;
- hand-washing facilities close by;
- good vector control;
- appropriate attention to gender issues related to society, age and reproduction.

## Disposal of Waste

The general principles of waste disposal are control at source and proper disposal. *Note that in the very early stages of a conflict or catastrophe it may be necessary to create a defaecation area until a more permanent solution is found.* The permanent method of choice in the field is either a dry pit latrine or a pit system incorporating ventilation. These systems are best erected by expert engineers.

Solid waste disposal extends to include the dead and perhaps body parts. Management of the dead should respect traditional beliefs and customs, but must take into account health risks which may have to over-ride tradition – for example cremation rather than burial in epidemics.

Finally, waste other than human waste must be safely collected and disposed of. This includes:

- market and commercial waste;
- industrial waste;
- domestic waste;
- medical waste;
- "sharps" and hazardous waste.

## Food and Nutrition

The enormous logistic requirements of a food programme for refugees and internally displaced people (IDPs) is beyond the skills and resources of individuals and most small non-governmental organisations (NGOs). The distribution and control of provisions are best left to large international aid agencies which have the necessary resources to acquire, transport, prepare and distribute food aid. However, you may be involved in assisting a food programme, and therefore a knowledge of the principles is mandatory. Some useful guidelines are listed below.

- There is rarely sufficient food in the refugee/IDP location and importation from abroad is the norm.
- A means of food preparation is needed, as are cooking and feeding utensils.
- Food appropriate to the population should be used; Western food, and in particular military field rations, are usually inappropriate.
- As a guide, the minimum daily need is 2000 calories.
- Calories are best provided as a combination of cereals, pulses and oil.
- Ration cards assist in fair distribution.
- Feeding centres for the malnourished and medical centres have higher calorific needs and specialist supplements will be needed.
- A survey to identify malnutrition in children should be part of the initial assessment survey (rapid health assessment) – see below.
- Malnutrition/nutrition surveys must be repeated at regular intervals.

The basic principles underpinning access to food are:

- assessment of nutritional needs;
- availability of food resources;
- recognition of the balance between needs and resources;
- recognition of the impact of natural or manmade disasters on supply and distribution.

The minimum standard to be achieved must include a general ration for everyone of the correct quality and quantity, and may include additional complementary or supplementary rations.

Quantifying food needs in conflict and catastrophes has caused much controversy. A generally agreed view states that "nutritional needs represent the average quantity of nutrients a person needs every day to remain in good physical and mental health, taking account of his or her physiological condition, sex, weight, age, environment and physical activity."

For mass gatherings, for example, it is possible to estimate an average nutritional requirement for the group. The methodology is as follows. Start by accepting an average individual's needs as 2,100 kcal and 50–60 g protein. This figure will vary for any specific individual because of age, gender and degree of physical activity. Other impacting factors include pregnancy and lactation. To calculate the overall need more accurately, it is necessary to know the rough percentage in each category.

In addition to protein and calorific needs, consideration must be given to the prevention of vitamin and trace-element deficiencies. In particular, food programmes should aim to eliminate or prevent illnesses such as beri beri, scurvy, pellagra, congenital malformations (folic acid in pregnancy) and anaemia, in particular in children, the elderly and pregnant women.

Other matters to be considered in providing food and nutrition in conflict and catastrophe settings should include:

- transport, storage and distribution;
- food provided should not cause food-borne disease;
- local diet and taste should be taken into account;
- pre-existing malnutrition will affect the quality and quantity of food required.

There are specialists NGOs with particular expertise in food and nutrition and in managing malnutrition. They should be involved at an early stage. In particular, readers should note the expertise of Oxfam, Save the Children, WHO and the World Food Programme.

## Shelter and Energy Provision

Displaced people are vulnerable to the elements and will often congregate in areas with no natural shelter. Early provision of shelter reduces the risk of communicable disease, assists security, reduces exposure to extremes of weather and also provides a degree of privacy.

Ingenuity may be required, at least for a time. The use of natural ground features and local vegetation may be all that is immediately available. With the arrival of aid agencies, more appropriate shelter may be provided by:

- heavy duty plastic sheeting (the cheapest);
- imported tents;
- huts/shelters built from local resources, e.g. wood, clay and wattle;
- existing buildings repaired or re-roofed with plastic sheeting.

Longer-term shelter needs careful planning and facilitates food distribution, administration and control, and provision of sanitation.

Ideally, each family group should be provided with a minimum of 3 m$^2$ per person – an ideal rarely met.

In addition to shelter, some form of energy provision is required for food preparation, to permit effective personal hygiene and to provide heat in cold climates (remember, nights may be extremely cold even in warm climates).

## Mass Gathering

Mass gathering under normal circumstances is associated with large groups of people gathering for sporting occasions or music festivals. The problems faced by medical attendants are those associated with the disease and illness profile of an otherwise healthy group. There may be anxieties concerning trauma and mass casualties, but communicable disease is rarely an issue. Mass gathering due to the displacement of individuals or groups following war or conflict is a different matter. This section is therefore concerned with conditions associated with catastrophe and conflict. These are typically related to overcrowding, poor sanitation, deficient nutrition, adverse environments and lack of shelter. Many conditions are not specific to war or disaster, and are encountered under normal circumstances but become epidemic under conditions of mass gathering. There is also a non-specific group of conditions – acute diarrhoeal diseases are an obvious example. Others conditions are specific to certain geographic regions and climates, and while endemic under normal circumstances, become a problem both in terms of numbers and severity in a mass gathering scenario: vector-associated conditions such as malaria or yellow fever are examples.

There are multiple classifications of the important conditions. Thus classification can be by pathogenic agent, as is conventional in most medical texts, or by means of transmission, which is more appropriate in conflict and mass-gathering settings. In this chapter, conditions are classified according to *means of transmission*. Although a fairly exhaustive list is produced below, the discussion will only be broadened for the more important conditions which are likely to be encountered.

## Communicable Diseases Associated with Mass Gatherings – Grouped by Means of Transmission

1. Vector transmission
   - Malaria
   - Yellow fever
   - Typhus and related conditions
   - Plague
   - Human African trypanosomiasis
   - Schistosomiasis
   - Onchocerciasis

2. Faecal contamination
   - Acute watery diarrhoea (*Vibrio cholera* and related organisms)
   - Acute bloody diarrhoea (bacillary dysentery)
   - Chronic diarrhoea
   - Amoebiasis and giardiasis

- Enteric fevers (typhoid and related fevers)
- Viral hepatitis
- Ascariasis
- Hookworm disease

3. Air/droplet transmission
    - Measles
    - Acute respiratory infections
    - Tuberculosis
    - Meningitis

4. Sexually transmitted
    - AIDS
    - Syphilis
    - Gonorrhoea

5. Direct (contact) transmission
    - Scabies
    - Impetigo
    - Conjunctivitis
    - Trachoma
    - Fungal skin infections

Volunteer's requirements in terms of depth of knowledge of the above conditions will vary depending on training, qualifications and assigned role. All of these conditions are covered in depth in various texts which are listed at the end of this chapter and in the Resources section. However, many of these conditions are of such importance that they merit further discussion here. In discussing selected conditions, it is wise to remember that risks apply not only to the local community, but also to volunteers, in whom the risks may be greater because of lack of prior exposure.

## Vector Transmission

### Malaria

Malaria is a vector-borne disease. The vector is the female anopheline mosquito. Disease results when an infected mosquito bites a human and injects the malaria parasite into the victim's bloodstream. Four varieties of parasite give rise to disease in man:

- *Plasmodium vivax*;
- *Plasmodium falciparum*;
- *Plasmodium ovale*;
- *Plasmodium malariae*.

All present with fever accompanied by headache, nausea and muscular pains. These paroxysms commence with chills and then shaking, followed by a febrile phase and ending with drenching sweats, lasting in all about 10 h. The periodicity of paroxysms varies with parasite type. In *vivax* and *ovale* malaria, episodes occur every 48 h. In *malariae* malarias, episodes occur every 72 h. *Falciparum* malaria has no definite periodicity and fevers may be continuous. *Falciparum* is also the most dangerous type with the risk of complications and death. Established *falciparum* malaria is a life-threatening emergency demanding immediate management. Chemotherapy will depend on local expert advice.

Malaria is a major health problem affecting refugee and displaced populations in times of catastrophe and conflict. The disease is prevalent in tropical and subtropical regions of the world. It is endemic throughout South and South–East Asia, Africa, parts of the Middle East, and South and Central America. Epidemics may start in endemic areas with the arrival of a displaced and vulnerable community. The disease poses risks to refugees, IDPs and aid volunteers alike.

The best option is prevention, which for the aid volunteer implies chemoprophylaxis prior to deployment and the use of repellents and nets. This is further discussed in the chapter on medical electives abroad. The regimen used will depend on the area of deployment, prevalent parasites and the level of resistance. **Expert advice must be sought**. Mass prophylaxis for vulnerable communities is more contentious. Programmes are expensive, difficult to implement and monitor, and may result in adverse drug side-effects and the emergence of resistant parasites. The decision to provide chemoprophylaxis for a particularly high-risk group (for example pregnant women at risk from drug-resistant *falciparum* malaria) should be made at a high level by aid officials well versed in managing the condition.

Whatever your role you should understand the principles underpinning prevention. Pre-deployment prophylaxis has been discussed. The other measures are:

- avoidance of proximity to water sources;
- application of larvicides to vital water sources;
- periodic residual insecticide spraying – check local guidelines;
- use of impregnated mosquito nets over sleeping accommodation;
- wearing long-sleeved trousers and shirts at dusk and dawn.

The management of established malaria will depend on parasite species, severity of illness, risk factors (children, pregnancy or the presence of P *falciparum* are some examples), local drug resistance and available resources. There is no standard treatment for malaria. Growing resistance and adverse drug reactions complicate matters. Expert advice must be obtained before deployment.

### Yellow Fever

This disease and a wide variety of related conditions are caused by arboviruses (arthropod-borne viruses). Yellow fever is fully preventable by vaccination, which should be mandatory for expatriates travelling to at-risk areas. Related diseases include Marburg disease, Lassa fever, Ebola disease, Rift Valley fever and Dengue fever.

You must check if any of these diseases are prevalent in your deployment area. If so, take expert advice.

Epidemic yellow fever occurs when the *Aedes aegypti* mosquito with an urban breeding cycle transmits the virus to humans. The disease is characterised by fever, jaundice and a bleeding diathesis which may cause fatal haemorrhage.

Confirmation of the disease requires serological testing. Management is by case isolation and symptomatic treatment of symptoms since no specific therapy is available (Lassa fever excepted). Prevention requires good vector control and immunisation if that is feasible.

## Typhus and Related Conditions

These conditions are important vector-borne diseases. They include a range of diseases caused by the Rickettsial group of microorganisms. Disease is transmitted by lice, ticks, mites and fleas. Displaced populations associated with overcrowding and poor personal and community hygiene are particularly at risk. The diseases are under-diagnosed and under-reported.

Louse-borne typhus is the most important as it may occur as an explosive epidemic in vulnerable communities. Severity varies, with case fatality rates from 10 to 50%. The main reservoir of the disease is the convalescent typhus patient.

The classical features of this disease group are:

- an incubation period of 3–14 days;
- sudden onset of malaise, myalgia, headache, fever and chills;
- vomiting with diarrhoea or constipation;
- a maculopapular rash which may become confluent;
- photophobia;
- generalised lymphadenopathy and splenomegaly common;
- circulatory collapse and death in severe cases.

Diagnosis in early cases must be confirmed by serological techniques. Thereafter, a clinical diagnosis may be made. Treatment is with antibiotics. Rickettsiae are very sensitive to tetracyclines and chloramphenicol (7-day course of tetracycline or chloramphenicol).

Prevention is by vector control and improving sanitation and personal living conditions. In at-risk settings a surveillance programme aimed at monitoring lice infestation is recommended.

## Plague

In plague, the infecting organism is *Yersinia pestis*, which primarily affects wild rodents and their fleas. Plague is transmitted to humans through flea bites. There are three clinical varieties.

- Bubonic – marked by fever, and painful lymphadenopathy (bubos) which may suppurate. Bubonic plague is the most common form, with a case fatality rate in the region of 50%.

- Pneumonic – marked by extensive pneumonitis and mediastinitis, either alone or with bubonic disease. This variant is highly contagious and lethal, with a case mortality approaching 100% if untreated.
- Septicaemic – usually a progression from the varities above. This is rapidly fatal if untreated.

Diagnosis and early treatment is vital. Serology and culture of the organism is needed initially to confirm the diagnosis; thereafter, clinical diagnosis is acceptable. Blood culture and gram stain identification may be used in a resource-constrained environment.

Treatment demands isolation of pneumonic plague victims and administration of either a tetracycline or chloramphenicol. In the presence of an epidemic, all expatriate and other aid staff should receive prophylaxis.

Preventive measures include vector control, control of rodents and education of those at risk.

### Human African Trypanosomiasis

The incidence of this disease, also known as sleeping sickness, is rising sharply as a consequence of war and conflict displacing communities into susceptible areas in sub-Saharan Africa. The disease is caused by a parasite of the *Trypansoma brucei* group. There are two clinically important species: *T. gambiense* and *T. rhodesiense*. Transmission to man is by the bite of an infected tsetse fly. The condition is lethal if untreated. The clinical picture is one of a progressive meningitis and encephalopathy leading to dementia, and it inevitably ends in death if untreated.

The condition should be suspected if a vulnerable group arrives in an infected area. Confirmation of the disease is by serological testing and the detection of the parasite in blood, lymph nodes or cerebro-spinal fluid.

Treatment should only be commenced once the diagnosis is confirmed. It relies on the administration of a range of expensive and toxic agents such as suramin, pentamidine and oral difluoro methyl ornithine (DFMO). The decision regarding choice of therapy is an expert one and advice must be sought in advance.

Preventive measures include education of the population at risk and control of the tsetse fly.

## Faecal Contamination

### Acute Watery Diarrhoea

Acute watery diarrhoea is an increasing public health problem in developing countries and among displaced communities. It is hard to overstate the importance of diarrhoea as a major cause of morbidity and death. The annual death toll from diarrhoea of all aetiologies is 4,000,000 children under the age of 5 years, with 80% being under the age of 2 years.

Poor water and sanitation, overcrowding and malnutrition are invariable pre-cipitating factors, and these circumstances are best exemplified in refugee camps and in areas where displaced people assemble. Figures quoted by the International Committee of the Red Cross (ICRC) indicate that diarrhoeal diseases account for up to 40% of all medical consultations among displaced people.

Acute watery diarrhoea is caused by a wide spectrum of organisms, with Vibrio cholera heading the list. The following organisms have all been implicated:

- *Vibrio cholera*
- *Vibrio parahaemolyticus*
- Non-typhoid *Salmonellae*
- *Escherichia coli,* enterotoxigenic (ETEC) and enteropathogenic (EPEC);
- *Clostridium perfringens*
- *Cryptosporidium parvum*
- *Rotavirus*
- Enteric adenoviruses.

NB: *Falciparum* malaria may present with acute watery diarrhoea.

*Cholera*

Cholera is a disease of poverty and malnutrition, and is a constant threat in refugee camps and among displaced communities, particularly if the community passes through or settles in a cholera endemic area.

*Clinical features.* All age groups are susceptible. Infection results from ingestion of contaminated food or water. The majority of patients have a mild, self-limiting disease or are completely asymptomatic. In symptomatic cases there is an acute onset of watery diarrhoea. The classic description is of "rice water stools" – a white diarrhoea flecked with mucus. Fever may be a presenting feature in children. Mortality is variable, and is highest in locations where hygiene is poor and no trained personnel are available to manage the outbreak. Mortality rates, or more accurately case fatality rates (CFR), in the last decade have varied between 2% and 25%. Good management should result in CFR below 2%. In fatal cases, death results from profound dehydration, metabolic acidosis and renal failure. Dehydration may be so severe as to cause uncompensated hypovolaemic shock and death within hours.

> **Case definition**
>
> "any patient developing a rapid onset of severe watery diarrhoea resulting in severe dehydration"

*Managing an outbreak.* The first aspect of management is preparation. Plans should be in hand for populations at risk and should include systems for

- early detection and agreement on case definition,
- agreed protocols for case management,
- establishment of cholera treatment units with standardised equipment,
- measures to improve personal and food hygiene,
- health education.

*Case management.* The corner-stone of management is oral rehydration with glucose-electrolyte solution, and this usually suffices in up to 80% of cases. In shocked patients, intravenous therapy is needed. One to two litres of WHO intravenous diarrhoea treatment solution or Ringer lactate solution should be infused rapidly and further boluses given according to clinical findings. In austere circumstances, the return of a strong, easily palpable radial pulse indicates a good response to therapy. The initial bolus in children can be calculated by the formula 20 ml/kg body weight. Boluses can be repeated until clinical improvement is observed. Vascular access in children may be difficult and the intra-osseous route may have to be used.

**WHO recommends a single dose of doxycyline (30 mg/kg) for adults. For children, take expert advice.**

*Prevention and control.* Vaccination, even with current inactivated vaccines, is not recommended for displaced communities. The reasons are ineffectiveness, cost and logistic difficulties. The best control/preventive measures are health education, surveillance and preparedness.

> *Afternote. While cholera is a discrete disease, it is in ways similar to other watery diarrhoeal disease and management is much the same for all.*

### Enterotoxigenic E. coli (ETEC)

This is the organism usually associated with traveller's diarrhoea. It is also a common cause of acute watery diarrhoea in children. It is rarely a cause of severe illness, and management is with oral rehydration salt solution.

### Enteropathogenic E. coli (EPEC)

A cause of watery diarrhoea in children age 6–18 years in the tropics. Treatment is as described for other causes of acute watery diarrhoea.

### Non-typhoid Salmonellae

These organisms may also result in acute watery diarrhoea in children and adults. Primary spread to man is from contaminated food – secondary spread follows the

> ## The following organisms have been implicated
>
> *Shigella dysenteriae, flexneri, boydii and sonnei,*
> Entero-invasive *E. coli* (EIEC),
> Entero-haemorrhagic *E. coli* (EHEC),
> *Etamoeba histolytica,*
> *Salmonellosis,*
> *Campylobacter jejuni,*
> *Yersinia enterocolitis*

usual faecal–oral route. A chronic carrier state can occur. The disease may progress to involve the colon, resulting in the onset of bloody diarrhoea.

### Acute Bloody Diarrhoea (Dysentery)

Acute bloody diarrhoea or dysentery differs from acute watery diarrhoea in a number of important ways. Whereas watery diarrhoea is associated with entero-toxin-induced diarrhoea, dysentery is associated with an inflammatory colitis following bacterial invasion of the colonic epithelium and, in some cases, the production of cytotoxins causing epithelial cell death. The result is bloody diarrhoea

In the context of displaced communities, Shigella dysenteriae Type 1 is the most virulent and in addition to colonic invasion produces a powerful cytotoxin. As with so many lethal communicable diseases, it flourishes in a climate of poverty, overcrowding, poor hygiene, inadequate water and malnutrition.

*Clinical features.*  The classic feature of dysentery is blood in the stool, but this may take some time to develop. The condition typically presents with fever, lassitude and onset of watery diarrhoea. Following colonic wall invasion, visible blood appears in the stool. Anorexia, vomiting and abdominal pain are common features. The disease is highly contagious and only requires a low infecting dose to cause clinical disease. Attack rates vary from 5% to over 30%, with CFRs fluctuating between 2% and 20%. Low rates are associated with good epidemic management – the higher rates are associated with inadequate treatment or none at all. All age groups are susceptible, but children and vulnerable groups are particularly at risk. The disease also has a "sting in the tail". Anorexia coupled with a protein-loss diarrhoea result in the early onset of malnutrition. In displaced communities, many will be malnourished for other reasons. Dysentery may then lead to overt protein energy malnutrition. Dysentery is thus inextricably linked to malnutrition among displaced and vulnerable populations.

*Management of an outbreak.*  The advice given for acute watery diarrhoea outbreaks also holds good for dysentery, but the case definition is different. A suggested definition is: "any case of diarrhoea with visible blood in the stools". An outbreak of epidemic proportions should be suspected if

- there is a sudden and consistent rise in the number of new cases,
- an increased number of deaths from bloody diarrhoea is reported,
- there is an increase in the proportion of cases of bloody diarrhoea compared to overall diarrhoea cases.

Bacteriological proof of an outbreak is vitally important but can be difficult due to the fragility of the organism. Multiple media may have to be used. Expert advice should be sought.

*Case management.*   If possible, cases should be managed in hospital where considerable control can be exerted. Oral rehydration therapy is used, but dehydration is usually severe. Adequate nutrition is essential and is another reason for hospital treatment if this is feasible. The use of antibiotics is fraught with difficulty – resistant strains are emerging and more and more antibiotic regimens are now useless. Expert local advice is needed before embarking on mass use of antibiotics.

*Prevention and control.*   The most effective measures are hand-washing, adequate disposal of faeces and care in food preparation.

## Amoebiasis

Amoebiasis is a protozoal disease afflicting displaced and impoverished communities. It is caused by the protozoon *Entamoeba histolytica*. Infection follows the ingestion of cysts passed in the stools of carriers and which contaminate food or water. Person to person spread also occurs.

The disease presents with nausea, colicky abdominal pain and bloody diarrhoea, which can lead to an incorrect diagnosis of *Shigella* dysentery. Conversely, cysts of *E. histolytica* may be found while investigating an outbreak but may be an incidental finding. The disease is characterised by remissions and exacerbations and may ultimately lead to bowel perforation or haemorrhage. Amoebic abscesses may form in the liver and brain. Investigation is complex and beyond the scope of this handbook. Readers are referred to the reading list for detailed information. The condition should be remembered as a cause of dysentery and it may be appropriate to treat the condition pragmatically. The condition responds well to metronidazole. Alcohol should be avoided when using this agent.

## Enteric Fever

Enteric or typhoid fever is endemic worldwide and is a particular hazard for displaced and vulnerable communities. It is caused by the following bacteria:

- *Salmonella typhi*
- *Salmonella paratyphi* A
- *Salmonella paratyphi* B

The organisms are transmitted to man by ingestion of food or water contaminated by the faeces or urine of infected patients or asymptomatic carriers. Healthy carriers contribute significantly to the spread of the disease, especially if they are employed in food preparation. Most cases are mild and never reported.

*Clinical features.*   After infection, bacteraemia occurs and is followed by colonisation of the small intestine leading to enteritis, which manifests itself as a diarrhoeal illness. Patients have fever, chills, headache, meningism and lassitude. A relative bradycardia (lower than expected pulse rate) is described. A typical rash, described as "rose spots" and affecting the trunk, appears after several days. A variety of psychiatric and neurological signs have been described but are inconsistent. This, coupled with under-reporting of mild cases, make case definition difficult.

*Management.*   Suspected cases require serological confirmation or the identification of organisms in blood or bone marrow. After the first week, organisms maybe cultured from stools and urine The presence of a leukopenia (low white cell count) is supportive. Case treatment requires antibiotics, but local expert advice on drug resistance should be obtained.

*Prevention and control.*   There are no easy solutions. As with all communicable diseases, great care must be taken regarding group and personal hygiene, storage and use of water and food preparation. Aid volunteers should be vaccinated, but this is not practical for entire displaced and at-risk communities. Personnel involved in food preparation may need screening and vaccination to prevent outbreaks under high-risk conditions.

## Viral Hepatitis

Viral hepatitis is a worldwide infection posing health risks to displaced and impoverished communities, and to expatriate volunteers. Viral hepatitis incorporates several distinct diseases.

*Hepatitis A (HAV).*   Infection is caused by ingestion of water or food contaminated by faeces containing the virus. It is usually a mild self-limiting disease. Vaccination is recommended for expatriate volunteers only. The disease is best prevented by health education aimed at safe and secure water and food supply and good sanitation.

*Hepatitis B (HBV).*   This disease has a very different epidemiology. Transmission is parenteral, sexual and foeto-maternal. There is some evidence that faecal–oral transmission is possible. Vulnerable communities are at risk. Routes of transmission may be perinatal, related to sexual activity, or from contaminated blood transfusion or needles. Aid volunteers are at risk from needle-stick incidents, unprotected sexual contact and occasionally from IV drug use. The disease is characterised by chronicity, which may lead to cirrhosis and hepatocellular carcinoma of the liver. There is no specific therapy. Vaccination is mandatory for all health care workers. Immunisation is also recommended for infants in endemic areas.

*Hepatitis C (HCV).*   This is similar to hepatitis B in many respects. It is usually transmitted by contaminated transfusion. There is no vaccine against HCV. Chronic active HCV disease can be treated with alpha-interferon.

*Hepatitis D (HDV.*   This is similar to, and transmitted with, HBV. Combined B and D infections are particularly prone to chronicity, cirrhosis and liver cancer.

*Hepatitis E (HEV).*   This is similar to HAV but poses a particular risk of fulminating hepatitis in pregnant women.

## Worm Infestations

Infestation by worms, or helminthiasis, is a worldwide problem but is of particular significance for displaced and vulnerable communities. Many are asymptomatic or show minimal signs and symptoms. The purpose here is to provide a classification and to highlight the few conditions of clinical significance to displaced communities.

*Classification*

*Roundworm disease*

- Ascariasis
- Hookworm disease
- Strongyloidiasis
- Trichinosis
- Trichuriasis

*Tapeworm disease*

- *Taenia saginata*
- *Taenia solium*
- *Echinococcus granulosus*

*Trematode flatworms and flukes*

- Schistosomiasis
- Liver fluke disease
- Lung fluke disease
- Intestinal fluke disease

*Filariasis and onchocerciasis*

- Lymphatic filariasis
- Loiasis
- Mansonella perstans
- Mansonella streptocerca
- Onchocerciasis
- Dracunculiasis

It is worth elaborating two important conditions.

*Schistosomiasis*

This disease, also called Bilharzias, is of increasing importance to displaced communities and is increasingly being reported. The disease is caused by three varieties of trematode flatworm which, depending upon the variety, cause liver, gastrointestinal or bladder disease. Spread of the disease requires a water source and an appropriate snail to act as the intermediate host to motile larvae which subsequently, as motile cercarial larvae, penetrate the skin of humans paddling in contaminated water. Volunteers as well as displaced people are at risk. Prevention is by health education and siting camps away from high-risk areas. Water can be treated to destroy the eggs and larvae. Effective treatment is now available, but expert advice should be sought locally.

*Drancunculiasis*

This condition, also known as dracontiasis, is caused by the Guinea worm (*Dracunculus medinensis*). It is exclusive to man. Infection occurs by ingestion of water containing the water flea *Cyclops* containing Guinea worm larvae. Mature female worms later migrate to skin overlying the legs and feet. Skin ulceration occurs with the tail of the worm protruding through the skin. Immersion in water results in the exposed female worm releasing larvae – thus the cycle continues.

It is a disease of refugees and displaced people in North, West and East Africa, and parts of the Middle and Far East. Ulceration and abscesses at multiple sites over the feet and lower legs cause pain and disability. Treatment is by the age-old method of removal, namely by rolling the worm on a stick taking care not to break it as it is gradually withdrawn through the skin. Prevention is best achieved by health education, boiling or filtering drinking water and using insecticide to eradicate the Guinea worm.

# Air/Droplet Transmission

## Measles

Measles is one of the great "Captains of Death" affecting refugee and displaced children. Large-scale epidemics among displaced and vulnerable communities have caused millions of childhood deaths, particularly among the youngest, weakest and most malnourished. Médecine Sans Frontière (MSF) lists measles as number two in its top ten priorities for intervention in the acute phase of a relief programme.

A mass vaccination programme for children aged 6 months to 15 years is an absolute priority during the first week (see Ch. 19). Details on surveillance, immunisation programmes, case management and prevention can be found in the selected reading list at the end of this chapter.

## Influenza

This world-wide disease is important for refugees and displaced communities because of the complications of the condition among the weak and vulnerable. Death is usually due to secondary bacterial chest infections. It is under-reported, but should be considered if there is an outbreak of fevers of unknown origin leading to severe respiratory infections in vulnerable groups. There is promise of a cheap and universal vaccine in the future.

## Pertussis (Whooping Cough)

Whooping cough is a leading cause of death in non-immunised and vulnerable populations. It tends to present after an interval in well-established camps. In at-risk populations, whooping cough can be prevented by immunisation as part of an expanded programme on immunisation (EPI) activity in the post-emergency phase.

## Tuberculosis

This disease is a major public health problem in developing countries, and among refugees and displaced people. The annual incidence of new cases of all forms of the disease is between 7 and 10 million cases. It is estimated that the tubercle bacillus infects one-third of the world's population and kills 2.5 million people every year.

Establishing and managing tuberculosis is a task for specialist NGOs, and programmes are not usually established until after the acute emergency phase has been completed.

From an expatriate health worker's point of view, there are a number of key points to remember:

- protect yourself – check your BCG status before departure;
- be aware of the association between HIV and tuberculosis;
- BCG vaccination should be part of the expanded programme of immunisations for refugees and displaced communities.

## Meningitis

Acute bacterial meningitis, caused by *Neisseria meningitidis*, is endemic in parts of the world associated with concentrations of refugees and displaced communities. The disease thrives where there is overcrowding and poor sanitation and, not surprisingly, large outbreaks and epidemics are frequent in refugee and IDP camps. Case fatality rates in untreated cases reach 70%, so surveillance and early detection and treatment are vital. Expatriate health workers in high-risk areas, or where an outbreak is anticipated, should be vaccinated. The decision to vaccinate a community is difficult and demands expert consultation. Current vaccines do not cover all serogroups, there are logistic constraints and protection is short-lived. Treatment requires expert, local advice.

## Sexually Transmitted Disease

### HIV – AIDS

Transmission of HIV and the subsequent development of AIDS is fraught with ethical, legal and moral difficulties at the best of times, but even more so when present among refugee and displaced communities. These problems are beyond the scope of this chapter. The emphasis here is protection of the expatriate and local health workers. Workers should understand the main avenues of viral transmission. These are:

- sexual intercourse;
- transfusion of contaminated blood;
- injection with contaminated needles;
- mother-to-child transmission.

Prevention of infection is achieved by adopting safe practice in each of the above areas. The management of AIDS patients is a specialised subject and readers are directed to the earlier chapter dealing with medical student electives and to the Resources section at the end of this Handbook.

# Climate – Hot and Cold

Heat- and cold-related illness is a potential hazard faced by both indigenous victims and expatriate volunteers. However, the expatriate is likely to be more at risk because of lack of acclimatisation. Illness rates even among acclimatised victims may be severe if there has been loss of shelter. The pre-existing ill, the young and the old are particularly at risk.

## Heat Injury

A number of syndromes or conditions are recognised. These range from the benign to the potentially lethal. Note that core body temperature varies in a healthy individual. The normal ranges are:

- at rest – 36.5 to 37.5°C;
- during exercise – 36.5 to 38.5°C.

The most common heat-injury conditions are described below.

## Dehydration

This may affect displaced and exposed individuals or communities who have limited or no access to drinking water. It may also affect expatriate volunteers engaged in vigorous (and unfamiliar) physical effort. The severity is related to the extent of body weight lost. The following list is a good guide:

- 2% loss – severe thirst;
- 2–5% loss – severe thirst, anorexia, headaches and altered consciousness level;
- 5–10% – all of the above, plus dyspnoea, cyanosis and neurological signs;
- 10% – the above plus visual disturbances and uncontrolled rise in core temperature (see heat exhaustion and heat stroke below).

Weight loss of 10% or greater signifies an immediate threat to life. As a general rule, losses above 5% are best treated by intravenous fluids (intra-osseous access may be necessary in babies and children younger than 6 years). The initial bolus in an otherwise healthy adult is 2 l isotonic crystalloid. In a child, the initial volume is calculated by the formula 20 ml/kg body weight. These are initial challenges and may be repeated. Urinary output is an excellent guide to clinical response. An output of greater than 30 ml/h in an adult indicates effective volume replacement.

## Sunburn

This is caused by excessive exposure to sunlight. Expatriate volunteers should ensure liberal use of UV blocking creams and should avoid prolonged exposure. Displaced people without shelter are vulnerable, with infants and small children being particularly at risk. Prolonged exposure may lead to heat stroke. Management is by protection under cover, non-adherent dressings to blistered areas, oral rehydration and simple analgesics.

## Heat Cramp

This is the mildest in a range of hyperthermic conditions. It typically occurs in a non-acclimatised individual engaging in vigorous physical activity. The characteristic muscle cramps are caused by a combination of salt and water depletion. Treatment is with oral fluids if tolerated. If vomiting is a symptom, replacement by the IV route may be required.

## Heat Faint

Also known as heat syncope, this is associated with prolonged vigorous exercise in a non-acclimatised expatriate volunteer. It is a more severe variant of heat cramp. Dehydration and widespread peripheral vasodilation are major features. Management is by resting in a shaded place and fluid replacement by oral or IV routes.

## Heat Oedema

Similar to the above conditions but with dependant oedema in addition. Associated with heavy manual labour and prolonged standing. Treatment is by rest and elevation of affected limbs, in addition to the measures outlined above.

## Heat Exhaustation

A potentially lethal condition and a more severe variant of the above. In addition to hypotension and fainting, there is an alteration in consciousness level and severe headache. This condition requires immediate management consisting of:

- cessation of all physical activity;
- removal to a cool place;
- tepid sponging and fanning;
- intravenous fluid resuscitation using an isotonic solution until clinical improvement.

## Heat Stroke

This is the most severe and immediately life-threatening hyperthermic syndrome. It usually follows a failure to recognise the onset of less severe hyperthermic conditions. It includes all of the events outlined above, plus a rapid rise in core - temperature and a failure to loose heat. At 41°C, organ failure commences. If untreated, changes become irreversible and convulsions leading to coma follow. If suspected, the central temperature must be recorded using the rectal or oesophageal route.

Prevention is better than cure. Follow the advice given below.

- Avoid hard physical labour until acclimatised.
- Wear appropriate clothing.
- Cover your head.
- Drink plenty of fluids before and during heavy manual labour.
- Use sun-screen creams liberally.

Central to effective management of heat stroke is rapid cooling. The following approach should be adopted:

- tepid bathing, but avoiding ice-cold fluid which results in vasoconstriction and thus limited heat loss;
- evaporative cooling of moistened skin by fanning; the skin must be moistened to achieve heat loss;
- administration of oral rehydration salts if tolerated;
- administration of 1–2 l electrolyte solution IV over one hour in an adult. In a child, 20–40 ml/kg body weight is used as a guide to the volume required.

Cooling should be stopped when rectal temperature falls to 38.5°C to avoid overshoot and resultant hypothermia. A benzodiazepine administered intravenously or rectally may be required to control convulsions.

In a catastrophe or conflict setting it is unlikely that advanced laboratory or critical facilities will be available, and treatment must be based on clinical observation. Rapid lowering of core temperature, rehydration with resulting improved urinary output, and good control of convulsions are the keys to survival.

*A final note. It is often the young, enthusiastic and very fit expatriate who succumbs to heat illness.*

## Cold Injury

Cold injury poses a particular problem for displaced communities in war and disasters. Even in warm climates it is often very cold after dusk. The risk factors may include any or all of the following:

- lack of shelter;
- inadequate clothing;
- presence of vulnerable groups (children and the elderly);
- pre-existing disease;
- open wounds.

### Classification

#### Local Injury

Three variants of local injury may be seen:

- frost-nip;
- frostbite;
- immersion (non-freezing) injury.

*Frost-nip* is the mildest form of injury and is characterised by pain, pallor and numbness of the affected part (fingers, toes, nose or ears). If recognised before progression to frostbite, it is easy to treat by re-warming. Frost-nip injury does appear to predispose people to subsequent injury.

*Frostbite* results from the freezing of tissues with intra-cellular ice crystal formation. The extent varies from superficial through partial skin thickness injury to deep injury involving muscle and bone (as with burns). The condition is characterised by hyperaemia, oedema and vesicle formation in superficial injury, to frank necrosis in deep injury. Urgent management is needed either to prevent necrosis and gangrene or to limit its extent. Re-warming is the key element in treatment, but should not be undertaken if re-freezing is likely. If possible, the injured part should be placed in warm circulating water at 40°C until it turns pink and re-perfuses. Treatment may be painful and require analgesia. Following re-warming, the injured parts remain vulnerable and need to be protected. Antibiotics should be used only if clinical signs of infection are evident. It may take several weeks to determine the extent of tissue loss, so early surgical intervention should be avoided. If re-freezing is likely, the frozen part should be left frozen until definitive re-warming can take place.

*Immersion injury* is the non-freezing variant of cold injury, and is usually seen in victims who have had prolonged exposure to wet conditions in temperatures just above freezing. It was endemic among soldiers during the Falkland Islands War in 1982. It typically affects the feet, but may effect hands also. Injury tends to be more superficial than with frostbite. The appearance varies from widespread superficial necrosis to an intensely painful hyperaemia. Management is by gentle re-warming in circulating warm water at 40°C and by protecting the injured part from further injury and infection.

*Systemic Injury*

The most clinically important cold-injury condition is systemic hypothermia, which may be life threatening. Accurate diagnosis requires measurement of the core body temperature using special thermometers capable of measuring low temperatures. Health care workers in war and disaster settings may not have access to such equipment and will have to use their clinical judgement.

By convention, the condition is classified as mild, moderate or severe.

- Mild – 35 to 32°C.
- Moderate – 32 to 30°C.
- Severe – below 30°C.

*Recognition.*   Awareness and a high index of suspicion are essential. Displaced communities, with many elderly, young, ill and injured among their number, are particularly vulnerable. Provision of shelter and some form of energy source for heat is vital. Key physical signs include:

- a drop in core temperature (low-reading thermometer);
- altered level of consciousness;
- cold peripheries (cold to touch);
- a grey appearance with central cyanosis (a blueness around the lips and tongue).

Alterations in vital signs such as pulse rate, respiratory rate and blood pressure are not helpful except in patients close to death.

*Management.*   The best management is prevention by provision of shelter and heat. Where the condition is suspected or proven by a core temperature reading, the following steps are recommended:

- remove from the cold environment;
- remove wet, cold clothing and cover in warm blankets or dry clothing;
- administer high-flow oxygen if available;
- cardiac monitoring if possible.

Regular re-assessment is essential. If the patient is improving, they should be protected from exposure and given hot fluids and drinks. If there is no improvement, consider the administration of warm (body temperature) intravenous fluids – ideally an isotonic electrolyte solution. The volumes administered will be determined by age and pre-existing disease. However, in a healthy adult, 2 l of warmed electrolyte solution is recommended. In a child, a dose of 20 ml/kg body weight as an initial bolus, which is then repeated, is a safe approach.

Under austere conditions, it is unlikely that anything further will be possible. Techniques such as active core re-warming and the use of anti-arrhythmic agents require a critical-care environment.

## Pre-existing Disease

A displaced community reflects society in general, and consequently pre-existing, universal illnesses may be expected to be present. Further, some of these universal conditions or illnesses are likely be more prevalent and severe because of general vulnerability. These universal conditions cover the whole spectrum of disease, but the more important are listed below.

- Upper and lower respiratory tract infections.
- Non-specific gastrointestinal tract infections, including inflammatory bowel disease.
- Peptic ulcer disease.
- Hepatobiliary disease.
- Peripheral vascular disease.
- Cardiac illnesses including angina, congestive cardiac failure and congenital heart conditions.
- Endocrine conditions, including diabetes mellitus.
- All forms of malignancies (cancer).

The difficulty in the emergency phase is that patients with these pre-existing and often chronic diseases often pose insurmountable problems for carers. The emergency phase is rightly focused on driving down overall mortality with attention to initial assessment, provision of shelter, food and water, and control of lethal communicable disease. Inexperienced volunteers are often horrified at the apparent lack of attention given to patients with pre-existing disease. Lack of means to manage such patients in the aftermath of a crisis or disaster may mean that no other approach is possible. Many will be on complex drug regimens or require sophisticated investigation and monitoring of their conditions. In other cases, in less well-developed societies, these conditions will have been neglected prior to the crisis because of the absence of any form of health care. Thus, patients will present with florid and advanced disease, not seen in developed practice outside the pages of a nineteenth century textbook of pathology. Even with the transition to development at a later stage it may be impossible to provide an adequate service for many universal conditions, particularly those on long-term treatment regimens. *A sense of realism, coupled with compassion must prevail (see also Ch. 21).*

## General Approach

This topic is covered superbly by Dr. Pierre Perrin in his *Handbook on War and Public Health* listed in the Resources section. While the initial medical management impetus is to treat life-threatening conditions related to the crisis, the establishment of a long-term health care facility is a priority.

### Establishment of a "Chain of Care"

This concept has been well described by Dr. Perrin and others. It works on the principle that a normal standard of care, provided by health professionals, is not possible. It also recognises that accessible facilities may not exist within striking distance of the crisis area. Care is provided at various levels or echelons, described as primary, secondary or tertiary. This has a distinct relationship to military levels of care in war.

#### Primary Level

Provided by non-professional carers or community health workers. These may include traditional healers utilising traditional remedies. Do not dismiss this approach since it may have as much validity as so-called Western medicine. At this level, therapies such as basic wound management, oral rehydration and psychosocial interventions should be encouraged. Primary facilities may be located in a health room or within the affected community.

#### Secondary Level

The size, complexity and staffing at this level will vary depending on circumstances. The principle here is that care is provided by a health care professional. Equipment scales for these facilities have been recommended by such organisations as MSF and the World Health Organisation (WHO) (see reading list in Resources section).

#### Tertiary Level

This is care within hospital facilities, often located some distance from the affected area. Within an affected area it is rare to find total destruction of *all* medical facilities, including hospitals. The need is to identify what remains and to liaise. Large organisations such as the ICRC have particular skills in taking over or assisting in the functioning of affected hospitals. The Leonard Cheshire Foundation, for example, have developed a "Fast Track" referral programme to match refugees and IDPs to hospitals which are still functioning. A general rule concerning tertiary level care is that it should take place within the borders of the affected area, it should be provided by local medical staff if possible, and it should be in keeping with pre-disaster care for that region.

*Access to Highly Specialised Care*

One of the features of conflict and catastrophes is the breakdown of the more specialised and expensive care regimens. This particularly applies to cancer therapy programmes, renal dialysis services and transplant programmes. Health care volunteers must be careful not to make rash promises, for example by referring patients to hospitals for the initiation or continuation of chemo- or radiotherapy for cancers when facilities no longer exist. In these settings, WHO advice is to concentrate on palliative care, particularly pain control.

# Venomous Bites and Stings

The prospect of being bitten by a venomous insect or reptile results in unnecessary fear and anxiety among expatriate health volunteers. The main risk is to indigenous populations, particularly if they are displaced or sited in a high-risk area.

## Classification

The classification offered here is pragmatic and based on common risks. The list of potentially dangerous creatures is impressive but the risk from vehicles exceeds all of these!

### On Land

Snakes
Spiders
Scorpions
Bees, wasps and hornets
Millipedes, centipedes and some caterpillars
Some beetles
Leeches

### Marine

Sea snakes
Fish (stingray, scorpion fish and stonefish)
Echinoderms (starfish and sea urchin)
Coelenterata (jelly fish)
Octopus
Sea snails

# Land-based Risks

## *Snakes*

Venomous snakes are likely to be present in areas where refugees and displaced people congregate. Health volunteers should, as part of their preparation, inform themselves of local risks and consider safety measures in advance of travel.
   There are five families of venomous snakes.

- Elapidae – cobras, kraits, mambas, coral snakes and Australian terrestrial venomous snakes.
- Viperidae – vipers, adders, pit vipers and rattlesnakes.
- Colubridae – African boomslang, vine snake.
- Atractaspidae – burrowing asps.
- Hydrophiidae – sea snakes.

Snake venoms are a complex cocktail of enzymes including cytolytic (causing cell breakdown), haemorrhagic, neurotoxic (toxic to nerves) and myotoxic (toxic to muscles) varieties. The clinical manifestations are both local and systemic. Local manifestations vary from trivial bruising to blistering and occasionally to frank necrosis over a wide area. Systemic manifestations depend on the quantity and nature of the venom injected. *Note that in up to 50% of cases, snakes fail to envenomate their target.* The major clinical sequelae are described below.

### *Haemostatic Disturbance*

Bleeding and clotting disturbances are associated with viper bites. Gastrointestinal or intracranial haemorrhage may be lethal.

### *Neurotoxic Signs*

Rapid onset of muscle paralysis commencing with the cranial nerves and then becoming widespread is typical of most Elapidae bites. Paralysis of the muscles of respiration may lead to respiratory arrest.

### *Rhabdomyolysis*

Widespread rhabdomyolysis is a feature of sea snake envenomation. This may lead to acute renal failure.

## *Case Management*

*Do:*

- reassure the victim;
- rest and immobilise the injured part in a splint or sling;

- consider pad and crepe pressure dressing for elapid bites;
- transport to a hospital or specialist centre if possible.

### Do not:

- suck the bite;
- incise the wound;
- apply ice or ice packs;
- apply an arterial tourniquet;
- give electric shocks.

Further management in hospital includes close observation for signs of systemic or severe local envenoming which would be an indication for the administration of an anti-venom.

Important aspects of management include:

- general wound care, including antibiotics, tetanus prophylaxis and dressings;
- surgical debridement of the bite if needed;
- observations for signs of systemic enuenomation.

If the snake has been positively identified, mono-specific anti-venom is appropriate. If the species of snake is unknown or uncertain, poly-specific anti-venom should be given. As anti-venom is hyperimmune equine or bovine immunoglobulin, the possibility of anaphylactic reactions must be considered. Note that anti-venom is unlikely to be available in the acute emergency phase of a conflict or catastrophe.

Patients presenting with or developing respiratory paralysis may require endotracheal intubation and mechanical ventilation. Other supportive measures include dialysis if renal failure supervenes. Later, surgery may be indicated.

## Spiders

While most spiders are venomous, few have significant clinical consequences. Bites by *Loxoscles* species (North and South America only) may cause local necrosis and gangrene which may extend to involve an entire limb. Bites from black widow, red-back, South American banana and Australian funnel-web spiders may all result in systemic signs including muscle spasms, headaches, vomiting and coma. Immediate action is similar to that for snake bite. Local anaesthetic infiltration is effective for pain. Anti-venoms are in use but are unlikely to be available for refugees or displaced communities.

## Scorpions

The risk of envenomation by dangerous scorpions is high in North and Southern Africa, USA, Mexico, the Caribbean, South America and India. In these high-risk areas, scorpion bites kill more people than snake bites. Envenomation results in severe local pain and swelling. A wide range of systemic signs and symptoms are possible and include vomiting and diarrhoea, neurotoxic signs and haemostatic disorders and signs of parasympathetic nervous system stimulation. General treatment measures are similar to those outlined for snake and spider bites. Local anaesthetic infiltration will control local pain. Anti-venoms are in use but are unlikely to be available.

### Bees, Wasps and Hornets

It is easy to underestimate the risks attached to envenomation by these insects. Single bites rarely cause problems unless the patient has previously been sensitised. In adults, envenomation by more than 100 bees or 30 wasps or hornets may be fatal. Considerably fewer may cause death in a child or baby. In a refugee or displaced community setting, treatment will depend on availability. General supportive measures including cardiopulmonary resuscitation should be applied based on clinical judgement. Sensitised volunteers should carry self-injectable adrenaline kits and should wear an alert bracelet.

### Marine Risks

Aid volunteers or vulnerable communities are very unlikely to be exposed to marine envenomation and the topic is not discussed further here. Readers wanting further detail are referred to the reading list at the end of this chapter.

## Miscellaneous

The conditions included here are not easily classified.

### Poliomyelitis

This condition is discussed here because it does not readily fit the classifications used in this chapter. For example, it may be spread by droplet infection or by contamination of food or water by infected faeces. It is an acute viral infection in which most of those infected remain asymptomatic. In a minority of people, disease is associated with acute flaccid paralysis. CFRs are low, and are quoted as between 2 and 10%.

Refugees and displaced communities are vulnerable to the spread of the disease and it should be considered as part of disease surveillance activity. The vaccine is cheap, safe and effective orally and should be part of the extended programme of immunisations.

### Rabies

The rabies virus is lethal in man, resulting in a progressive and untreatable meningitis and encephalitis. The disease is transmitted by the bites, licks or scratches of infected mammals. These include dogs, foxes, wolves, cats and bats. The most common cause of human rabies is the bite of a rabid domestic dog. The incubation period is usually between 20 and 60 days, but may extend for up to 4 years. The shorter the distance from the wound to the brain, the shorter the incubation period as the virus spreads along neurones to reach the central nervous system.

As the disease has no cure once symptoms have developed, the emphasis is on prevention, particularly for expatriate volunteers. Pre-exposure or pre-deployment regimens are widely available and effective. The most widely recommended regimen is the Merieux human diploid cell vaccine (HDCV). One ml IM or 0.1 ml intradermally (ID) is given three times: Day 0, Day 7 and Day 28.

Bites among refugees and IDPs require a post-exposure regimen which consists of wound cleaning, debridement, anti-tetanus measures and HDCV on Days 0, 3, 7, 14, 28 and 90. In addition, passive immunisation is achieved with human rabies immunoglobulin, 30 IU/kg body weight, with half infiltrated around the bite, and the remainder given by IM injection.

The best preventive measure in camps is health education and the destruction of stray dogs.

## Myiasis

Myiasis is the presence of the maggots (more correctly larvae) of tropical flies in human tissue. The maggots burrow into human tissue, and typical sites are below healthy skin, eyes, ears and the nasal passages. They may also infect open wounds. The condition is encountered in tropical Africa and South America, and in parts of Asia. Burrowing below healthy skin produces papules or boils which may ulcerate. Lesions may be multiple and resemble chicken pox, impetigo or scabies.

Treatment is by applying water or an oily substance such as vaseline over the surface of the lesion. This causes suffocation and the maggots can then be "shelled out".

Prevention is by the use of fly screens, careful attention to laundry (drying clothes indoors and ironing them), and by destroying any fly eggs which are encountered.

## Bugs, Ticks and Mites

Fleas and lice are associated with potentially lethal infections and have already been discussed. This section covers a wide variety of small creatures which, while largely of nuisance value, may cause alarm and considerable discomfort.

### Bed-bugs

As their name implies, these live in bedrooms and infest bedding material, including bed frames. They may also live under carpets and under wallpaper. They are nocturnal feeders and cause irritating bites which result in disrupted sleep patterns. They do not carry disease. Control is difficult – cleaning of bedding, insecticide sprays, moving bedding away from walls and leaving lights on at night are all recommended.

*Ticks and Mites*

These become attached to the skin of people walking through undergrowth in prevalent areas. They are easily seen and can become large when engorged. Removal is by grasping the head-end and disengaging the teeth by rocking the creature from side to side followed by removal, or by touching them with a lighted cigarette.

Ticks and mites are associated with a variety of diseases including scrub typhus and Rocky Mountain spotted fever. Volunteers should be aware of diseases endemic to their area of deployment. It is important to maintain a high index of suspicion and seek advice.

# On-going Health Care

On-going medical care must include attention to all the following points:

- health surveillance and reporting;
- continuing health needs assessment;
- establishment of a health clinic;
- acute medical care;
- preventive health measures;
- health education measures;
- maternal and child health measures;
- care of the elderly and other vulnerable groups;
- storing and dispensing medicines;
- a re-supply network;
- documentation and records.

A health information or surveillance system needs to be established early. Careful monitoring of trends in health and nutritional status is essential if problems are to be identified and preventive action taken. Mortality surveillance monitors changes in the crude mortality rate. Nutritional status, population movement and provision of health clinics should also be observed. The mortality caused by key illnesses can be studied using return forms. The forms used by most relief agencies vary little in content, but one type should be adopted by all organisations in the area to standardise the information collected.

## Mobile and Transitional Care

The focus of this chapter so far has been on the care of displaced people in established and static camps. However, you may have to care for victims prior to the establishment of a static camp.

This involves caring for individuals or a community on the move from their homes to a perceived place of safety, or at a transitional location prior to moving to a permanent location. Ideally, international organisations will be providing or guaranteeing safe passage. The safe passage may not be apparent to, or believed by, the community on the move, so reassurance coupled with transport assistance may be a primary task. In certain evacuations there may be control of the movement of certain categories of individuals, based on age, sex or nationality. This was particularly evident in the Balkans during the 1990s.

Depending on the transport available and the terrain and the distances involved, a form of sorting or triage may be needed to ensure that evacuees will survive the journey. For those prevented from travelling through illness or infirmity, medical care will have to be arranged.

Most displaced people who have been on the move for prolonged periods will arrive at their final destination in a highly vulnerable state. The measures outlined in the earlier part of this chapter are particularly appropriate here. Travel will usually have involved overcrowding, lack of sanitation, poor nutrition, thirst and exhaustion – the risk of early-onset communicable disease is very high.

You may be asked to advise on overcrowding or the suitability of transport. EU regulations on animal transportation are a good guide to the lowest acceptable level of provision. International law should generally be left to professionals. However, there is one rule which those assisting a mobile community need to be aware of. This is the principle of non-refoulment This states that:

> *No person (entitled to invoke Article 14 of the Universal Declaration of Human Rights) shall be subjected to measures such as rejection at the frontier or, if he has already entered the territory in which he seeks asylum, expulsion or compulsory return to any State where he may be subjected to persecution.*

## Transition from Acute Care to Long-term Development and Repatriation

This is a highly specialised field and beyond the scope of this manual. However, it is important to recognise the need to move towards long-term solutions when considering refugee care. As a rule, the post-acute phase begins when the excess mortality of the acute phase is controlled and basics needs are met. The commonly accepted marker which indicates the transition is a crude mortality rate of under one death/10,000/day.

### Other Aspects

#### Use of Local Staff

A displaced population will have a rich range of skills and attributes. Use them. Early utilisation of local skills will ease administration and is vital for surveillance. Pay scales must be standardised throughout if conflict is to be avoided. UNICEF may be a useful source of funding and advice on pay matters. A certain tolerance towards corruption may be necessary to ensure good labour relations and to prevent conflict.

*Relief Agency Rivalry*

It is sad to note that competition and rivalry do occur among relief organisations. In part, this is a matter of reputation, but there may also be funding and financial issues. Clear communication is vital to avoid misunderstandings and duplication of effort. The early establishment of regular meetings of representatives helps to defuse tension. Finally, each organisation should have clearly defined areas of responsibility and an atmosphere of cooperation should be fostered.

## Withdrawal and Return Home

This is discussed in various chapters in the manual. For most volunteers, withdrawal should be considered once the acute phase is over. Long-term care is best left to professionals. Withdrawal and hand-over should be planned and must avoid giving the impression of abandonment. If a successor is present, a formal hand-over is needed to ensure a smooth transition.

# Conclusions

This multi-part chapter may appear vast, yet it is merely an introduction to the myriad of medical and related conditions which may affect displaced populations. Readers are strongly recommended to read widely. Consult related chapters and use the Resources section in addition to the reading list below.

## Suggested Further Reading

Behrens RH, McAdam KPWJ, scientific editors. Travel medicine. British Medical Bulletin, Vol. 49. Edinburgh: Churchill Livingstone, 1993.
Cook GC, editor. Travel-associated disease. London: Royal College of Physicians, 1995.
Cowan GO, Heap BJ. Clinical tropical medicine. London: Chapman & Hall, 1993.
Dawood R, editor. Travellers health: how to stay healthy abroad, 3rd ed. Oxford: Oxford University Press, 1992.
Immunisation against disease. London: HMSO (updated annually).
Médecins Sans Frontières. Refugee health: an approach to emergency situations. London: Macmillan, 1997.
Perrin P. Handbook on war and public health, English ed. Geneva: ICRC, 1996.

EDITORS' NOTE – see also the Resources section at the end of this manual.

### Websites

The following websites are recommended. These can be used to search for current information on specific diseases and for links to related sites. Some contain journal articles and have question and answer sections.

Encarta:
http://encarta.msn.com/index/concise index

American Society of Tropical Medicine and Hygiene:
www.astmh.org

WHO Division of Control of Tropical Diseases:
www.who.int/health-tropics/idindex.htm

# 18. Women's Health

Charles Cox, John Duckett and N.K. Jyothi

**Objectives**

- To emphasise that in war and catastrophe, women are major victims.
- To highlight the problem of violence against women.
- To suggest a management approach to the ill or injured woman in a hostile environment.
- To discuss obstetric and gynaecological care in a hostile environment.

## Introduction

In conflict and catastrophe, women are major victims. Women experience these disasters differently to men, a phenomenon confirmed by those working in the field. This distinctive experience is related to the particular vulnerability of this group when disaster strikes, although its effects differ widely across cultures depending on the role of women in each society. Moreover, they are generally disadvantaged in terms of education and are considerably less mobile because of their traditional role in caring for others. Despite the prevailing situation, the "reproductive role" of the woman continues, and along with it the complications. Women are seen as a "sexual objects" and are often the victims of sexual assault.

In these areas, a variety of problems specific to women may be met and they depend on the length of the disaster. Many women will be pregnant or at risk of pregnancy. The infrastructure to care for pregnant women is likely to be severely compromised. Care for the woman, pregnant or not, will often fall on the inexperienced. The problems vary regionally and with the type of conflict or catastrophe. Pre-existing factors such as poverty, famine, chronic disease, anaemia and poor sanitation increase the risks associated with childbirth. The background mortality in terms of mothers and babies associated with pregnancy and childbirth is usually decreased. Infection is a major problem and is more frequent in areas where anaemia is prevalent, e.g. Somalia. These factors are to be borne in mind when dealing with trauma and obstetric emergencies in these areas. In western European countries, women affected by conflict are generally from a healthy population.

Culture and tradition influence medical management in certain parts of the world, especially those with a large Muslim population, e.g. Afghanistan and Bosnia. During the operation "Pacific Heaven", a humanitarian medical support mission in the

United States for Kurdish asylum seekers, even the provision of basic medical care was a challenge. The reasons for this were cultural norms and language barriers. The Kurdish women were unwilling to be examined or treated by male medical personnel. (Note the comments in Ch. 10 on keeping out of trouble.)

Women from all strata of society are vulnerable to human rights abuse in conditions of conflict and catastrophe. This may be because of their direct involvement in politics, or because of their association with people whom the authorities consider subversive. Women constitute the majority of the refugee and internally displaced adult population, and have been the victims of sexual abuse by police, soldiers or other government agents.

## Equipment and Resources

The equipment and drugs available depend on the agency involved, but are usually limited. There are various ready-made medical kits available provided, e.g., by the International Dispensing Association (IDA), the World Health Organisation (WHO) or the United Nations High Commission for Refugees (UNHCR). Most of them provide a special maternity or midwifery pack, which includes equipment necessary for conducting a normal birth and episiotomy suturing. Disposable gloves, plastic speculae, catheters and urine pregnancy detection kits are usually available. Intravenous fluids, antiseptics and routine antibiotics are also provided.

There may be a destruction of the local medical services and the previous infrastructure that provided the services. It is perhaps easier to cope when services have been more primitive than when there has been a complex medical service, as expectations are lower and local provision of basic midwifery is likely to be provided by traditional attendants. Technologically advanced systems are less portable when disasters occur and sophisticated equipment is more easily damaged. Simple obstetric forceps, for example, are more appropriate than the vacuum extractor as they are technology independent!

### Training

There are few formal training courses available to provide obstetric and gynaecological training for such disaster settings. The Royal College of Obstetricians and Gynaecologists runs a course with the Liverpool School of Tropical Medicine called the Diploma in Reproductive Health in the Developing Countries. The course is of 12 weeks duration and covers such areas as maternal care and safe motherhood, sexually transmitted diseases and family planning. The United Nations International Children's Emergency Fund (UNICEF) also publishes useful guidelines for pregnant women. The Advanced Life Support in Obstetrics (ALSO) course, which runs over 2 days, provides a good grounding in obstetric emergencies and is multidisciplinary.

### Rape and Sexual Assault

History confirms that the majority of refugees are women and children. The risks involved are great. Danger may come from armed factions, official or otherwise, who may attack refugees in flight.

On arrival at borders they may be turned back, or sexual favours may be demanded for allowing safe passage. Women who have been separated from male family members are especially vulnerable. In areas of civil turmoil or armed conflict, women are particularly vulnerable to human rights violations. They may be subjected to brutal treatment because of their country of origin or their particular ethnic group.

## Violence Against Women in Situations of Armed Conflict

Rape has been widely used as a weapon of war wherever an armed conflict arises. It has been used all over the world in Mexico, in Rwanda, in Kuwait, in Haiti and in Columbia. There may be victims of multiple rape committed by soldiers from all sides of a conflict. Such acts may be a demonstration of power to undermine the dignity of victims and reinforce a policy of ethnic cleansing, e.g. the former Yugoslavia. It has been estimated that between 20,000 and 50,000 rapes were committed during the fighting in the former Yugoslavia.

The so-called "comfort women", i.e. young girls of colonised or occupied countries, became sexual slaves to Japanese soldiers during the Second World War and others were forced into prostitution.

In Afghanistan, women are the main victims of the continuing human rights crisis. The Islamic fundamentalist faction, the Taliban, seized control over Kabul in 1996. This marked the beginning of a new era of repression, particularly for Afghan women. The Taliban policy of gender apartheid is disturbing. Assassination, abduction and rape are being committed with total impunity by government forces and armed political groups who are prepared to terrorise the civilian population in order to secure and reinforce their power bases. The rape of women by armed bodyguards belonging to the warring factions appears to be condoned by leaders as a method of intimidating vanquished populations and of rewarding soldiers. Armed men target women from ethnic or religious minorities they regard as their enemies. Party leaders and influential commanders have also reportedly forced families to sell them their younger daughters and sons, who have then been sold into prostitution, frequently in Pakistan and other countries.

In the case of Rwanda, it appeared that sexual violence constituted an integral part of the genocide, as evidenced by testimonies of genocide survivors. During the conflict, there was enormous propaganda in the Hutu militant literature against the Tutsi women, portraying them as "seductive spies". Thus, many Tutsi women were raped, humiliated, and told that they were too proud and arrogant. There are stories of rape of pregnant women by men known to have AIDS with the intention to pass on the disease. There are also instances of brutal sexual assault. There are reported incidences of gang rape where two men kept a woman's legs apart while others cut her genitalia with rusty scissors. Her clitoris was cut and labia were mutilated. This was then publicly displayed for everyone to see. There are other reports of sexual violence, including having a breast cut off, acid thrown on their genitals, or their reproductive systems permanently damaged as a result of large objects forced into their vaginas or through the sheer number of times they were raped. Other bodily damage incurred includes permanently tilted heads (where machetes had not succeeded in cutting the woman's head off) and missing limbs.

The health problems of the genocide survivors are a major concern. Rapes and sexual assault occurred on a large scale and many women bear permanent physical scars, deformities, major injuries to their reproductive organs and health problems including HIV/AIDS; 25–30% of the population in Kigali and 90% of the prostitutes were assessed to be HIV-positive, and this has risen since 1994. The vast majority, with their husbands now dead, have the full responsibility of bringing up their children. They harbour enormous feelings of hatred and revenge. Many have psychosomatic disorders such as palpitations, nausea, insomnia and frigidity.

Most women victims do not appear to report their ailments to medical professionals or attempt traditional treatments since the shame does not allow them to speak of the atrocities committed against them. According to many researchers and activists it is owing to deeply rooted Rwandan culture and tradition, the low status of women in society, and a deep sense of privacy that women victims of violence are reluctant to speak out about the traumatic experiences that they have suffered. In addition, there is the social stigma attached to being a rape victim or a victim of sexual violence.

The "culture" and traditional upbringing prevent women from speaking openly about such private matters. There seems to exist a cultural wall between the victims and witnesses on the one hand and the investigators on the other, as most of the investigators were male. The women are also frightened of repercussions and reprisals.

## Medical Management of the Sexually Assaulted Woman

The most important considerations, given the limited nature of the resources, are:

1. treatment of the physical injuries;
2. prevention of infection;
3. prevention of pregnancy.

### Treatment of the Physical Injuries

Sexual assault may result in a wide range of bodily injuries. Cuts on breasts or even a whole breast being chopped off, vaginal lacerations and bruises with concomitant damage to the internal pelvic organs may occur. Securing haemostasis and suturing the lacerations, along with assessment of the internal damage, is the priority in such cases. This is dealt with in the section on trauma in women. Appropriate pain relief should be given. Temporary catheterisation of the urinary bladder may be necessary if suturing involves areas close to the urethral meatus.

### Prevention of Infection

Two sources of infection should be considered. The local wounds can be infected, especially if they are extensive. Broad-spectrum antibiotics such as Augmentin, covering most common wound infections, can be used. Tetanus prophylaxis is important and readily available.

Screening for infection may not be practical. Depending on the resources available, various treatment strategies can be adopted. The important issue is the treatment of sexually transmitted diseases (STD) after rape and sexual assault – especially HIV/AIDS. It is unrealistic to expect to provide HIV prophylaxis to all rape victims.

### Post-exposure Prophylaxis PEP for HIV/AIDS

This is significant in places like Rwanda where the prevalence of HIV is high and rape is committed with the intention of inflicting disease. PEP is recommended if the assailant is known to be HIV-positive or of whom there is a strong clinical suspicion.

The risk of infection following exposure (male to female/female to male) is 1:300, and the risk following oral sex is 1:1000. PEP in HIV is most effective when started within 72 h of exposure.

The recommended regimen following a high-risk exposure is:

| | |
|---|---|
| Zidovudine | 200 mg tds |
| Lamivudine (3TC) | 150 mg bd |
| Indinavir | 800 mg tds |

The cost of a 28-day course of the combined treatment is £350. The risk of sero-conversion is reduced by 80% with the use of Zidovudine alone.

### Gonorrhoea, Chlamydia and Other Infections

The single most effective drug against gonorrhoea and chalmydia in terms of efficacy and compliance is a single dose of Azithromycin 1 g taken orally. This is also effective against chancroid, granuloma inguinale, lymphogranuloma venereum and non-specific urethritis. The cheaper option, but one needing compliance, is doxycyline 100 mg bd for 7–21 days for various infections. Erythromycin is also effective against chlamydia and most other STDs. Metronidazole 400 mg tds covers trichomonas and bacterial vaginosis.

### Hepatitis B Vaccination

Guidelines are available for vaccine-preventable STDs, including recommendations for the use of hepatitis A and hepatitis B vaccine. Hepatitis B immunoglobulin can also be given.

## Prevention of Pregnancy

The estimated risk of pregnancy following sexual assault is 2–4%.

### Yuzpe Method – PC4

High-dose combined oral contraceptive pills are provided in many of the package kits. These can be used as PC4 (two tablets of ethinyl estradiol 50 μg and two tablets of levonorgestrel 250 mg) administered two tablets at a time, 12 h apart, orally. This has the side-effects of nausea and vomiting.

*Progesterone-only Methods*

These have the advantage of a lower incidence of nausea and vomiting.

Mifeprestone, used as a single dose of 200 mg post-ovulation, has been shown to be very effective but is unlikely to be available.

Levonorgestrel, two doses each 0.75 mg 12 h apart, has a pregnancy rate of 1.1%.

PC50 consists of 25 microval tablets, the first dose given within 72 h of sex and another dose repeated 12 h later.

## Trauma in Women

The practical management of genital tract trauma, and the management of a normal delivery and common obstetric and gynaecological problems are described below.

### Genital Tract Trauma

Damage to the female genital tract is uncommon in trauma victims except when the trauma is inflicted deliberately. Occasionally damage can occur to the external genitalia with a straddle injury. This rarely damages internal organs, as penetrating injuries of this nature are uncommon and internal organs are protected by the bony pelvis. Treatment is control of haemorrhage with direct pressure or haemostatic sutures. Bruising and swelling may be gross, but will usually resolve with no specific treatment.

#### Deliberate Damage to the Genital Tract

This may occur as a result of intentional direct damage to the genital tract and may involve lacerations to the external genitalia with excision of the skin around the labia and clitoris. Lacerations around the perineum may bleed profusely and lead to exsanguination. Treatment is the application of firm pressure and haemostatic sutures if required. Penetrating injuries, e.g. the insertion of sharp implements such as knives or sticks, may cause damage to the perineal and intra-abdominal structures. The urethra, the bladder and the ano-rectal region may be damaged, and penetration may involve the peritoneal cavity leading to bowel damage with resulting peritonitis. It is therefore important to take as full a history as possible and to carry out an adequate examination, asking for experienced help if indicated. Examination of the abdomen may reveal tenderness and tenseness of the abdominal muscles (guarding). This suggests damage in the peritoneal cavity and surgical help is required.

Examination of the vulva, perineum and ano-rectal region should be carried out, and it will be helpful to place a urinary catheter in the bladder if possible. If there is a continued flow of *clear* urine then the bladder must be intact. Severe lacerations around the perineum will require a full examination under a general or regional anaesthetic. If this is not available, a urinary catheter should be inserted, haemorrhage controlled with direct pressure and transfer arranged. If this is not practicable, antibiotics should be started and the wound reviewed at regular intervals.

Damage to the bladder or bowel requires expert help. The mortality rate from damage to intra-abdominal structures leading to peritonitis is high, and damage to the anal sphincter, if unrepaired, will lead to loss of continence.

Antibiotics are mandatory, and Augmentin is particularly useful as it covers bowel organisms. If peritonitis is suspected, the patient should be kept nil by mouth.

In cases of rape, consideration should be given to contraception: "the morning-after pill" and an antibiotic to cover the common sexually transmitted diseases such as gonorrhoea and chlamydia. In areas where HIV is endemic, prophylaxis should be considered, as described above.

## Gynaecological Emergencies

Most of the acute gynaecological conditions encountered are likely to be complications of pregnancy. Spontaneous abortion occurs in up to 20% of pregnancies and is characterised by bleeding followed by pain. In most cases the pain and bleeding will settle, but on occasion there can be severe haemorrhage and shock may develop out of all proportion to the blood loss. This may be due to distension of the cervix by products of conception, which causes collapse due to stimulation of the autonomic nervous system (vaso-vagal shock). This can be simply treated by removing placental tissue from the cervix manually or with sponge forceps to relieve the stretching.

Septic abortion is not uncommon, especially after induced abortion carried out by an untrained person. If neglected, severe sepsis may result and the woman may develop a bleeding disorder and septic shock with a resulting high mortality. The treatment is to give high doses of a broad-spectrum antibiotic such as Augmentin and to remove infected retained products of conception from the uterus.

The technique for emptying the uterus of retained products of conception is comparatively straightforward and can be performed under sedation without the need for general anaesthesia. A speculum is placed in the vagina to expose the cervix. The cervix is grasped with a pair of forceps. Sponge forceps are quite satisfactory. Any products sitting in the cervix are removed and depending on the skill and experience of the operator, the cavity of the uterus can be explored gently with a finger or with sponge forceps or a uterine curette if available. An oxytocic agent (usually a combination of ergometrine and syntocinon, "Syntometrine" 1 ampoule) should be given if available; if not, then the uterus should be manually massaged to promote contraction. Antibiotic cover is appropriate. If the case is septic, great care must be taken not to damage the uterus, which will be soft and vulnerable to perforation.

## Pregnancy Occurring Outside the Uterus – "Ectopic" Pregnancy

It is a gynaecological maxim that all women between the ages of 10 and 55 should be assumed to be pregnant until proved otherwise! For a variety of reasons, women may choose to deny the possibility of pregnancy. This may be particularly so in the military environment where sexual relations are officially strongly discouraged! A urine pregnancy test will be helpful.

Massive internal haemorrhage may occur, and failure to consider the diagnosis may have fatal consequences. A high index of suspicion is required. Shock without an obvious source of major bleeding should be assumed to be due to ectopic pregnancy until proved otherwise. The treatment is to remove the fallopian tube from which the bleeding is occurring. There is no reason to remove the ovary except in the case of uncontrollable haemorrhage.

### Pelvic Inflammatory Disease (PID)

Acute pelvic inflammatory disease is generally due to a sexually transmitted disease except when occurring after childbirth. It is characterised by severe lower abdominal pain, fever and a purulent vaginal discharge. Broad-spectrum antibiotics should be administered and a high fluid intake maintained. Infection occurring after childbirth (puerperal sepsis or childbirth fever) should be treated aggressively, as untreated puerperal sepsis has a high mortality rate.

Rape victims should be offered antibiotics to reduce the risk of infection.

## Management of a Normal Delivery

The baby should be delivered by maternal effort unless there is a long delay between the delivery of the baby's head and the rest of the body. The birth canal can be widened by flexing the mother's hips onto her abdomen. Delivery may then be achieved by pushing the baby's head downwards, which will encourage delivery of the baby's anterior shoulder. This manoeuvre must be carried out during a uterine contraction. An episiotomy can be performed to widen the birth canal, but may produce considerable haemorrhage if not promptly repaired.

Once the baby has been delivered it should be dried. This will often stimulate respiration. The baby should be kept warm. Placing the baby to the mother's breast to suckle leads to the release of maternal oxytocin and encourages delivery of the placenta by causing the uterus to contract.

There is no hurry to ligate the cord. However, if the cord has snapped the baby's end of the cord should be ligated no nearer than 5 cm from the baby. When cord pulsations have ceased, the cord may be ligated.

The placenta should be inspected to check that it appears complete. The perineum should be checked for damage or bleeding. Uncomplicated tears of the perineum, which are not bleeding, do not require to be repaired.

## Obstetric Emergencies

Two patients are at stake. In developed countries, the unborn baby is afforded considerable priority and most women would not think twice about submitting to a Caesarean section if they thought it would improve the outlook for their child.

In developing countries, decisions regarding the management of obstetric problems are governed by the resources available at the time and the resources which are likely to be available to the woman in the future. In many countries, surgical facilities to carry out Caesarean section may be patchy, and a woman who is subjected to a Caesarean section which is not performed as a life-saving procedure for her will be left with a scar in her uterus and *a significant chance of scar rupture and death in a subsequent pregnancy.*

Therefore, in many circumstances, every effort should be made to avoid this potentially long-term life threatening maternal procedure (Caesarean section).

The feasibility of carrying out obstetric operations and procedures will be limited by the experience of the medical attendant and the facilities and equipment available. Remember the most important rule of medicine: "first, do no harm".

In the majority of cases the welfare of the baby will be at best of secondary consideration.

Life-threatening emergencies occurring in pregnancy are likely to be eclampsia, severe pre-eclampsia (toxaemia of pregnancy) and haemorrhage. Other conditions such as sickle cell anaemia are more likely to cause problems in the pregnant patient.

Toxaemia of pregnancy is characterised by fitting, swelling, especially around the face and eyes, the finding of protein in the urine and high blood pressure. The woman may pass very small quantities of urine which may be very concentrated (Coca-Cola urine). The management of the fitting mother is to protect her airway and to wait until the fit has stopped. Common drugs which may be useful in the control of fits include diazepam, magnesium sulphate and phenytoin. Opiates and promazine may be useful in the absence of the above. The definitive treatment for eclampsia or severe pre-eclampsia is to get the baby delivered, which will present problems if maternity facilities are not available! It is, however, very important to recognise the condition so that specialist advice may be sought.

Haemorrhage occurring in pregnancy may be from the site of the placenta and is almost always maternal blood. In one-third of cases, it may come from a normally sited placenta which has separated from the wall of the uterus (placental abruption). In another one-third of cases it comes from a placenta which is attached over the cervix (placenta praevia). The remaining third of cases of vaginal bleeding are due to other causes such as bleeding after intercourse, and the bleeding is not usually of a significant amount.

Bleeding from a significant placental abruption is almost always associated with pain and tenderness over the uterus. The baby is often dead. Delivery of the baby should be achieved as soon as possible, as problems with blood clotting and massive, often life-threatening, haemorrhage frequently occurs.

On the other hand, bleeding from placenta praevia is classically painless and the uterus is non-tender. The baby is usually still alive despite there often being quite considerable haemorrhage. A vaginal examination should not be carried out in cases of suspected placenta praevia as this may well precipitate massive vaginal bleeding. The diagnosis is confirmed by ultrasound, which is increasingly available, or by a *vaginal examination carried out in an operating theatre with the ability to carry out an immediate Caesarean section.* This condition carries a very high maternal mortality in the absence of obstetric facilities, as the treatment is Caesarean section to deliver the baby and an abnormally situated placenta.

Sepsis is more common in women who have pre-existing anaemia or chronic infection and in those women who have long difficult labours. If the baby has died or there has been retained products of conception after delivery, the risk is further increased.

Haemorrhage may be sudden and severe after childbirth, and many women will already be anaemic and be particularly vulnerable to further blood loss, especially those women who have had bleeding prior to delivery. (It is the ante-partum haemorrhage which weakens and the post-partum haemorrhage that kills.)

Bleeding can occur before, during or after delivery. If bleeding occurs before or during labour, a wait-and-see policy should be adopted. If labour has advanced to the second stage, low forceps delivery may be carried out if someone of sufficient experience is available.

Bleeding after delivery of the baby (post-partum haemorrhage) may be profuse. Has the afterbirth (placenta) delivered? Midwives and medical personnel will usually be familiar with "controlled cord traction", which involves gentle traction on the cord at the same time lifting the uterus in the other direction towards the patient's head. If this is unsuccessful and bleeding continues a hand should be introduced into the vagina to see if the placenta is sitting in the cervix. If so, the placenta may be grasped and removed. If not and bleeding is continuing, "rub up" a contraction. If the placenta does not deliver, an attempt should be made to deliver it by manual removal. This procedure requires adequate analgesia or anaesthesia, and involves the gloved hand being passed into the uterus to separate the placenta from the wall of the uterus. The uterus is steadied by the other hand controlling the uterus from above. The vaginal hand passes around the placenta in the plane between the placenta and the uterus, and when the placenta has separated, it is removed from the uterus. The uterus is then explored to check that there is no retained placenta. Blood clots should be removed, an oxytocic agent given and a contraction rubbed up.

## Obstructed Labour

Women may have been in obstructed labour for several days before they present for medical help. The baby will usually be dead, and the foetal tissues will then soften so that a macerated infant will usually deliver spontaneously or with the assistance of forceps. Obstructed labour in the Third World is a potent cause of maternal mortality and morbidity. It can lead to infection, haemorrhage and long-term damage to the bladder and the bowel, resulting in loss of bladder and bowel tissue, with fistula formation and resulting leakage of urine and faeces through the vagina. This leads to the woman being ostracised. Treatment consists of aiding delivery without causing further damage to the woman, dealing with infection and the reduction of long-term morbidity, for example by the use of in-dwelling urinary catheters to reduce the risk of fistula formation.

Obstructed labour in a woman who has delivered vaginally before is a particularly dangerous situation as there is a high risk of uterine rupture, with the subsequent death of the mother and baby. This situation requires experienced advice!

# Conclusions

Women will always be involved in catastrophe and conflict and are likely to make up a majority of the surviving population. It is not unusual to find that men have been killed in wars or deliberately killed in ethnic cleansing. The person on site must be able to contribute fully to the whole spectrum of disease affecting women. Life-threatening emergencies, gynaecological or trauma, are dealt with like any other surgical emergency. Obstetric emergencies need some specialist advice. The priority would be to save the mother's life. The foetus is secondary. In these areas,rape and sexual assault is wide-spread. In any society this is a difficult situation to manage, but it is often more difficult when operating in a different culture, particularly with language barriers. In some cultures, female medical personnel may be more appropriate.

## Acknowledgement

We acknowledge the contribution of Mr. Jonathan Duckett, whose personal experiences whilst serving with 23 Parachute Field Ambulance RAMC abroad have been invaluable in preparing this chapter.

## Further Reading

Chinkin C. Rape and sexual abuse of women in international law. Eur J Int Law 1994;326.
Coomaraswamy R. Report of the special Rapporteur on violence against women, its causes and consequences. UN Doc. E/CN.4/1998/54.
Gardam J. Women and the law of armed conflict. Int Comp Law Q 1997;46:74.
Gardam J. Women, human rights and international humanitarian law. Int Rev Red Cross 1998;324:421–32.
Guidelines for treatment of sexually transmitted disease1998. Centres for disease control and prevention. Morb Mortal Wkly Rep 1998;47(RR-1):1–111.
Human rights violation against women in Kosovo Province. Amnesty International Report, EUR 70/54/98, 1998.
Petter LM, et al. Management of female sexual assault. Am Fam Physician 1998;58:920–6,929–30.
Policy on refugee women. UNHCR, 1995; Sexual violence against refugees: guidelines on prevention and response. UNHCR, 1995.
United Nations Department of Public Information. DPI/1772/HR, February 1996.
Woman and War. International Committee of the Red Cross, 1995.

# 19. Children's Health

M. Gavalas, S. Nazeer, Claire Walford
and A. Christodoulides

**Objectives**

- To outline the physiological differences between children and adults.
- To discuss the impact of infectious diseases, malnutrition, starvation and environmental factors on the general health of displaced children.
- To emphasise the physical and psychological vulnerability of children facing adverse conditions.
- To highlight significant cultural and religious factors that may affect children at risk.
- To form strategies for the prevention of long-term sequelae.

## Introduction

In spite of the huge strides which have been made towards the improvement of health and education in developing countries, old problems are continuously confronting new generations. In addition to war, poverty, and other socio-political factors, the most vulnerable countries are also plagued by natural disasters. These disasters can strain resources and overwhelm even the most affluent of societies. However, the consequences in deprived societies can be profound, amounting to disaster in its true definition.

As always, children, the elderly and the infirm are particularly at risk.

This chapter is concerned with children; earlier chapters have covered other vulnerable groups such as lactating mothers, the elderly and the infirm (see Ch. 17). Plainly, many of the problems covered in earlier chapter are equally relevant to children. This chapter is concerned with important differences in assessment and care.

### Important Principles in Caring for Children in Adverse Conditions

Children are not small adults: they have unique anatomical characteristics. The skeleton is immature, and therefore bone and joint injuries merit especial care. Assigning low priority to fracture care in the midst of major disaster can lead to skeletal growth deformity, and this may have serious long-term consequences which will be further amplified in a vulnerable society. Growth can also be stunted due to metabolic and nutritional factors. Further, serious intra-thoracic and intra-abdominal injury may occur without evidence of bony injury – the best example is widespread contusion injury to the lungs with no evidence of rib fracture. This is quite unlike adult patterns of injury.

The ratio of body mass index to surface area (i.e. the size of the head is disproportionately large as compared with body size) predisposes children to the development of hypothermia and complications in fluid balance. This is complicated by low body weight, relative absence of adipose tissue for insulation and lack of glycogen storage, which can have profound effects on the physiological well being of children.

Drug dosages are dependent on body weight, and hence great attention to detail is essential when prescribing. Additionally, tubes, catheters, cannulae and other devices must be proportionally smaller when used in infants and children. This is particularly important when planning an aid mission where young children are numbered among the victims.

A child's psyche is as fragile as their physiological status. In the very young, emotional immaturity can be heightened by the added instability brought about by famine, natural disasters, war and strife. Separation from loved ones can lead to regressive psychological behaviour. Although children generally adapt well to adverse conditions and can easily bond with rescuers, they have a limited reserve when exposed to an unfamiliar, let alone hostile, environment.

Confounding issues that may disrupt the delivery of care need to be considered and may include:

- the nature of the disaster, i.e. natural or man-made;
- variations in climate;
- environment, i.e. urban or rural;
- infrastructure, which may be intact, compromised or destroyed;
- political situation;
- transport and communications.

The array of potential medical problems facing children is vast, and therefore a framework using the following headings is used.

- Water supply, food and sanitation.
- Mass gathering.
- Climate.
- Infectious disease.
- Pre-existing disease.
- Bites and stings.
- Trauma (physical injury).
- Miscellaneous.

Thse issues are not unique to children, and further details for all ages can be found in Ch. 17.

## Water Supply, Food and Sanitation

The provision of clean water and adequate food for growth and nutrition is a daily problem in the developing world. This is further complicated in conflict and disaster situations. Consequently sanitation poses an even more difficult problem, especially when vector control is a major health hazard. The well-being, growth and development of children depends almost entirely on access to a consistent and balanced intake of fluids and nutrients.

### Water

In considering water supply one must include not only drinking water, but also an adequate supply for preparing food, personal hygiene and, where possible, play. The physiological need for water is influenced by climatic conditions, and the presence of fevers and infectious diseases. The absolute minimum fluid requirements of children vary with age and weight. In children over the age of 1 year, weight may be estimated using the formula weight (kg) =2(age + 4). For the first 10 kg, the fluid requirement per day should be 100 ml/kg body weight. For the second 10 kg, the fluid requirement per day should be 50 ml/kg body weight, and for every subsequent kilogram the fluid requirement per day is 20 ml/kg body weight. So for a child of say 22 kg, the daily fluid requirement should be estimated as shown below.

> For the 1st 10 kg: 1,000 ml
> For the 2nd 10 kg: 500 ml
> For the last 2 kg: 40 ml

Therefore, the total fluid requirement for a child of 22 kg is 1,540 ml/day.

Fever increases the requirements by 12% per degree Celsius rise in temperature. Fluid loss due to vomiting, diarrhoea and burns needs to be replaced over and above the daily requirement given above. Total fluid needs are in excess of these figures in times of conflict or disaster. Aid organisations estimate that 20 litres/person/day is the minimum requirement if there is to be a positive impact on the health of compromised populations. It may be of value to remember native sources of fluids for oral consumption, e.g. coconuts contain a nutritious and sterile supply of "water", watermelons and melons have a very high fluid content, cacti and other succulents provide a source in desert conditions etc.

### Food

Infants and children are more vulnerable to under-nutrition than adults. Amongst the many reasons for this are low nutritional stores and high nutritional demands. The smaller the child the smaller the calorie reserve and the shorter the period the child is able to withstand starvation. At 4 months of age 30% of energy intake is used for growth, but by one year of age this falls to 5%, and by 3 years to 2%. There can be no doubt that breast milk is the best diet for babies, and it becomes even more important in situations of disasters and conflict when mothers should be encouraged to continue breast feeding well into the second year of life and beyond if nutritionally possible for the mother. Even amongst breast-fed children malnutrition can affect those aged between 6 months and 6 years. Dietary requirements of this age group are fairly stable throughout the world. On the basis of body weight, these children will require approximately 100 kcal/kg/day of energy and 1.5 g/kg/day of protein for normal growth.

### Sanitation

An undesirable, albeit inevitable, consequence of overcrowding and poor living conditions is faecal contamination of the water and food supply. For further detailed clarification see Ch. 17.

## Mass Gatherings

Large groups gather under normal circumstances for a variety of reasons including religious events and pilgrimage, political rallies, sport and music events. Large-scale planning and resourcing still do not prevent disease and illness even in an otherwise healthy population. The displacement of huge numbers of people is an inevitable consequence of major strife, conflict and disaster. Communicable diseases become an important problem in addition to trauma and separation.

Whereas previously much effort was put into the restoration of lost children to their family group, in recent times the emphasis has shifted towards the prevention of separation in the first place.

Preventing separation is important because:

1.  children have the right to be with their families;
2.  children are almost always better protected with and by their families;
3.  emotional disturbance is less if within a family unit during conflict and catastrophe.

Separation can be prevented by:

1.  involving non-governmental organisations (NGOs) such as Save the Children and Oxfam in forward planning;
2.  involving military agencies, particularly United Nations units who may be involved in the initial care of displaced populations;
3.  all agencies involved following agreed policies and strategies when children and their families are being evacuated from conflict and disaster zones.

*It is considerably more difficult and expensive to undertake replacement of lost children with their families. If lost children are to be adopted, then cultural and religious awareness is vital and should be done only after exhaustive investigations to locate surviving family members.*

# Climate

Unless relocation of the victim population is to a foreign environment, the effects of climate are largely a problem for the expatriate aid worker who lacks acclimatisation. More details on this topic can be found in earlier chapters.

## Infection and Immunity

Gatherings amassed following major disasters and catastrophes are prone to a wide range of illnesses. Various authors have used different classifications of communicable diseases. A simple and useful classification is presented in Ch. 17. This chapter highlights some specific conditions which present in childhood.

Infectious diseases, malnutrition and dehydration are by far the most serious threats to children in adverse conditions. Infections spread readily among children and may reach endemic proportions during war and natural and man-made disasters Diseases due to intestinal infections are very common in the developing world. Damage to water supply systems and leakage of sewage will significantly increase the incidence of infectious diarrhoeal diseases. Under normal circumstances, approximately 3 million children die of such diseases each year and roughly 10% of the world's population harbours *Entamoeba histolytica*, with many more carrying other gut parasites. Children suffer from the same spectrum of diarrhoeal diseases as adults, but are more susceptible to dehydration and therefore malnutrition. Further details of diarrhoeal diseases and their consequences can be found at the beginning of this chapter and in Ch. 17.

# Common Childhood Infections

## Measles

This common infection of children still kills over one million children in the world each year. It is a highly infectious disease caused by a paramyxovirus found throughout the world. Transmission is by droplets spread from nasopharyngeal secretions, with the port of entry being the respiratory tract. Because the disease is spread by active infection, massive vaccination programmes have the potential to eradicate the disease. In the Third World, measles is still endemic, but it can reach epidemic (almost pandemic) proportions and become the number one killer of children after trauma, given extra burden of strife, catastrophe and disaster. Following exposure a child will be symptom-free for 10–12 days, and having incubated the virus symptoms begin with a fever, cough and conjunctivitis. As early as 2 days later white spots appear inside the mouth (Koplik's spots) and by 4 days there is a high fever and the typical rash appears starting on the face, spreading to the trunk and arms and then reaching the feet. By this stage the fever begins to fall and the rash begins to fade, leaving a staining of the skin for several weeks. If the Koplik spots are not identified, the later rash can be difficult to see in children with darker skins. If the fever persists after the rash has cleared, bacterial infection, mainly of the respiratory tract, should be suspected and treated, as primary pneumonitis is uncommon but severe when it occurs. Other serious complications of measles include:

- diarrhoea, which can rapidly precipitate severe malnutrition;
- encephalitis, which can be severe and occurs in 1% of cases;
- xerophthalmia, a vitamin A deficiency combined with the effects of measles causing a rapidly progressive loss of vision and blindness;
- otitis media, which is common but can be overlooked in the presence of other more serious problems.

Management of a child with measles is in the main dependent on symptoms. Vitamin A therapy in high doses is imperative in compromised children. Secondary bacterial infections are treated with appropriate antibiotics when available. Breast feeding should not be interrupted, but if it is not available a lactose-free formula should be used to help the inflamed gut.

It is obvious that prevention is of the utmost importance, and therefore mass vaccination programmes for children aged 6 months to 15 years must be instituted as an absolute priority within the first week following a major disaster (see Ch. 21).

## Other Common Childhood Diseases

The incidence of many other childhood infections may not necessarily be affected by the extra consequences of disasters, but it is important to recognise the existence and significance of those listed below.

- Rubella (German measles), which is a less severe illness in childhood. Its main importance is in its ability to adversely affect the growing foetus inside a pregnant woman.
- Varicella (chickenpox), which is a viral condition often considered to be a benign childhood illness with significant complications in the older child and in the immuno-compromised individual.
- Poliomyelitis, which is uncommon in developed immunised countries, but can be a serious condition with high morbidity in unprotected mass gatherings.
- Mumps, in which orchitis (inflammation of the testicles) is the most feared complication but only has serious connotations after puberty.
- Impetigo, which is a bacterial skin infection that spreads rapidly in childhood.
- Tuberculosis (TB). Roughly 500,000 children die each year world wide from TB. Nearly half of infants and 90% of older children will show minimal signs and symptoms of infection. Initial droplet infection can occur as early as the first 2 months of life and causes a localised area of inflammation in the lungs (pneumonitis) called a Ghon focus. Organisms contained within this focus are not always killed and can be reactivated any time during the first year of life. Diseases such as measles, chickenpox, malnutrition and HIV infection all greatly increase the risk of reactivation. Also, other organs of the body such as kidney, brain and bone can be seeded by blood-borne organisms. Reactivation is also possible at these sites in early childhood (1–5 years of age). BCG vaccination should be part of the extended programme of immunisation for refugees and mass gatherings.

## Pre-existing Disability

Sadly most natural and man-made disasters occur in already vulnerable areas. The mortality and morbidity of children in developing countries are significantly higher than those in the developed world.

Pre-existing disability can be congenital or acquired. The higher incidence of consanguinity, the lack of formalised antenatal care and the inadequate provision of diagnostic and treatment facilities inevitably increases the incidence of significant congenital abnormalities. The social and cultural attitudes towards the more visible abnormalities may result in poor parenting owing to the already scare resources being targeted towards the more healthy members of the family. This may result in individuals who are less able to cope with the added consequences of disasters.

Previous to any disaster, a child can acquire almost any of the known diseases/traumas of childhood. Acquired illness may be acute or chronic. Acute illnesses, such as respiratory infections, urinary tract infections and food poisoning, are short-lived and can be managed at the time of presentation within the scope of limited resources. Acquired illnesses with the problem of chronicity, such as asthma, diabetes, osteomyelitis or eczema, require long-term management by specialists (paediatricians). Access to specialist resources may be seriously compromised due to breakdown of the infrastructure in areas affected by disasters. It is outside the remit of this chapter to present any details of congenital and acquired conditions of childhood. Good, readable books on childhood diseases are readily available, and more information can be gathered via internet sites referenced at the end of this chapter.

## Environmental Hazards

Children everywhere need a safe, healthy and loving environment in order to grow and develop normally. Children in the midst of disasters share the common hazards of children everywhere, namely accidents, poisons and abuse. The risk of environmental hazards is increased by:

- poverty;
- overcrowding and lack of adequate shelter;
- poor parenting skills, made worse by the disruption of family units.

Childhood accidents depend on the child's age and stage of development. Toddlers are explorative and inquisitive, and by their sheer nature are unaware of the consequences of their actions. They are prone to falls, burns and scalds, ingestion of harmful substances, drowning, stings and bites from various insects, snakes and animals. Older children experience a different range of accidents, such as falls from heights, deliberate self-poisoning and contact-sport injuries.

### Burns and Scalds

In situations of mass gatherings fires for cooking and warmth are mostly open and unguarded, increasing the incidence of burns and scalds in all children. Standard first aid measures, such as ice and cold running water to the affected part, may not be available. In fact help may be delayed due to the absence of parents and adults. It is common for babies and toddlers to be left in the care of older children whilst the adults forage for food and shelter. The complications of burns and scalds are:

- infection of the injured area;
- scarring, contractures and ensuing disability;
- fluid loss with severe extensive burns.

Management strategies are reliant on assessment and replacement of fluid loss, prevention of infection and attention to the positioning and placing of joints and limbs to avoid disabling contractures. Early input from specialists can reduce the level of disfigurement and scarring and enable the child to be rehabilitated sooner. Such specialists may be provided by organisations such as the Leonard Cheshire Centre of Conflict Recovery, Médecins Sans Frontières and many others. Further information may be found in the Resources section of this handbook.

Traumatic amputation of limbs due to land mines, bombs and incendiaries are common in children in war zones, but pose a different and difficult management problem from adults. For example, regular reassessment and refitting of limb prostheses will be required as the child grows. These children can become a huge economic drain not only due to extensive use of resources and specialist treatment, but also due to lack of earning power in adult life.

### Bites and Stings

The incidence of bites and stings may be higher in children, particularly toddlers. Most snake bites occur on the foot or hand, but painful bites at other sites may be from spiders or scorpions. The identification and treatment of bites and stings are outlined in Ch. 17. It is important to emphasise that envenomation is rare following a bite, and if envenomated, systemic spread of the venom can be delayed by immobilising the limbs with splints and a firm but not constricting bandage. Peripheral pulses should still be felt and the child should be kept as calm and quiet as possible.

## Trauma

Burns and scalds have been discussed, but it is now appropriate to discuss some particular problems surrounding paediatric trauma in general. While the injured child is approached in the manner described for adults in Ch. 17, there are some special features which need to be recognised.

### Airway

Maintaining and protecting the airway is the most critical element of overall management.

In managing the airway, the following key anatomical differences should be noted:

- small oral cavity and large tongue;
- large head which tends to flex when supine, resulting in "buckling" of the airway;
- large tonsils and adenoids;
- epiglottis at an acute angle, making visualisation difficult;
- short trachea with a risk of inadvertent bronchial intubation.

### Breathing

Children breath faster than adults – the smaller the child, the faster the rate. An infant breathes at a rate between 40 and 60 breaths per minute. With small tidal volumes (7–10 ml/kg) and delicate tissues, great care must be taken when assisting a child's ventilation.

Chest decompression must be performed with appropriately sized paediatric cannulae and chest tubes. Otherwise management is similar to that for adults.

### Circulation

The signs of blood loss may be cloaked for a time due to the child's excellent physiological reserves. When children finally decompensate, it is with precipitate speed. Consequently, diagnosis of hypovolaemic shock must be made as soon as possible and treatment commenced as a matter of urgency.

Resuscitation volumes vary with body weight. A useful formula for calculating resuscitation fluid boluses is 20 ml/kg body weight. This formula is for electrolyte solutions, which must be warmed. Two to three boluses may be required. For suspected significant bleeding, blood should be urgently cross-matched and a surgical opinion sought.

The good news is that, in the main, the time-honoured ABCD approaches works in infancy and childhood provided that medical attendants recognise some important anatomical and physiological variables.

## Miscellaneous

### Non-accidental Injury

Any physical action which results in, or may result in, a non-accidental injury to a child and which exceeds that which could be considered as reasonable discipline is classed as physical abuse. Child abuse may also be due to sexual abuse, emotional abuse or neglect, and may present as a combination of one or more of the above.

Child abuse is often the result of severe family stress, which is ever present in situations of strife and disaster. Accurate figures for child abuse are not available because the problem is only just being confronted in the developing world. Mass gatherings with young single parents coping in a setting of poverty and violence produce the ideal social setting for an epidemic of abuse.

# Conclusions

The most tragic consequence of conflicts and disasters is the loss of childhood. The Western world is beset by natural disasters that present their own sequelae, but the disproportionate incidence of natural and man-made disasters in the Third World makes the normal development and progression of childhood an almost unachievable target. Millions of children live in zones of conflict and become the main victims of those conflicts. UNICEF has estimated that in the last decade alone more than 2 million children have died as a result of war, and some 15 million children have been displaced. In these very same zones, children are exploited by both sides in the conflict as child soldiers, sex slaves and servants. Poor post-conflict communities need help in advance to prepare for returning soldiers, and programmes must include measures such as foster care to prevent recapture of the children by the armed forces. Girls require especially vigilant care following forced exploitations, and being shunned by their own community may drive them into further sexual exploitation and prostitution.

Education, vocational and employment opportunities are vital elements in the return to civil society. One example is the use of glove puppets in play therapy. Role playing exercises help children to resolve their feelings.

The authors would like to direct the reader to the many interesting and informative websites available on the internet. These are listed below, and include articles on easy access to weaponry, exploitation of children, children's rights and the effects on children of natural disasters such as famine, earthquakes and flooding.

## Further Reading

ABC of major trauma, 3rd ed. BMJ Publishing Group, 2000.
Monroe P, editor. What to do in a paediatric emergency. London: BMJ Publishing Group, 1996.
Lissauer T et al. Illustrated textbook of paediatrics. Tropical paediatrics. St. Louis: Mosby, 1997.
Valman HB. ABC of one–seven. London: BMJ Publishing Group, 1993.

## Web Sites

http://www.unicef.org/children
http://www.who.int/eha
http://www.savethechildren.org/crisis
http://www.ihe.org

NB. Readers are directed to the Resources section for further study.

# 20. Trauma: Surgical and Related Conditions

**Objectives**

- To indicate the range of common injuries and illnesses likely to be encountered across the spectrum of surgical disciplines.
- To describe a rational approach to the management of these conditions.
- To introduce the problems associated with ballistic and blast injury.
- To detail common surgical emergencies.
- To describe the principles of analgesia and anaesthesia in hostile environments.

## Part A – Introduction – Scene-Setting

Jim Ryan

The authors of this chapter include emergency physicians, surgical specialists and anaesthetists with experience of working in a wide variety of hostile environments. As with earlier chapters, the aim is not to "teach grandmothers to suck eggs". Senior surgeons with deployment experience will have their own tried and trusted methods for managing patients under austere circumstances, and some will belong to that dying breed the "general surgeon". This chapter is not aimed at the senior and experienced old hands. Rather, the purpose is to illustrate the range and complexity of conditions covered by our chapter headings for the more junior and often specialised health professional with a surgical interest in the widest sense

The chapter cannot be a complete discourse on surgery, trauma and anaesthesia. It is more of a vade-mecum, with the emphasis on conditions unique to, or modified by, conflict. A deliberate decision was taken to include advice on eye problems, ENT and maxillo-facial surgery, as these are areas where graduates from developed countries are often woefully deficient unless they practice within these fields. For example, how many general health professionals will be comfortable dealing with maxillo-facial, dental or ENT problems? Yet a surprising number of patients arriving at health centres in hostile environments will present with such conditions and will expect at least a rational consultation. To say "I do not do teeth!" is not good enough.

The topics covered in this chapter are:

- trauma and orthopaedics;
- ballistic and blast injury;
- acute surgical emergencies;
- dental, ENT and eye problems;
- anaesthesia and analgesia.

# Part B – Orthopaedics and Trauma

Jim Ryan, A. J. Thomas and Scott Adams

| Objectives | This section is concerned with raising awareness of trauma as a discrete disease which is often managed badly. The section also covers the general approach to the injured patient, and then moves on to give a brief outline of regional management of a variety of common injuries including soft-tissue wounds and fractures, and injuries to body regions. The section should be seen as an entry point into the topic, and it concludes with a guide to further reading. |
|---|---|

# Introduction

Trauma is the leading cause of morbidity and mortality during the first four decades of life and is the third most common cause of death overall. During catastrophe or conflict, trauma is often forced to the sidelines in the face of overwhelming public and environmental health risks. Yet it continues to afflict victims at each phase, and in war it may be one of the leading causes of death and long-term disability. It is worth noting that a leading cause of death and disability among humanitarian aid volunteers is a road traffic accident, often associated with over-indulgence in alcohol. Health professionals therefore have an obligation to provide assistance to the injured commensurate with their training and skill.

## Mechanisms

By convention, injuries resulting from physical trauma are classified as follows:

- penetrating;

- blunt;
- blast;
- thermal;
- chemical;
- miscellaneous (e.g. crush and barotrauma).

The physical effects to the tissues vary widely in nature and extent. Tissues may suffer any of the following effects, alone or in combination:

- compression;
- stretching;
- tearing;
- laceration;
- incision.

The severity will vary from trivial to irrecoverable. From a first health professional's viewpoint, the important factor to recognise is that injury severity and threat to life or limb may not be immediately obvious. Therefore, a systematic and didactic approach is called for.

## Management Philosophy

Management should be based on an "identify and manage life-threatening injury first, then reassess and manage other injures" philosophy. This is the basis of the American College of Surgeon's Advanced Trauma Life Support Programme©. While the programme was designed to be used by doctors working in the emergency room of a modern hospital, the approach holds good even in the austere setting of a refugee camp or in a conflict setting. The background to the approach is the recognition that death following injury occurs in a predictable manner. An obstructed airway will kill before a lethal chest injury, while a lethal chest injury will kill before a fatal circulatory problem. Death from all of the foregoing will kill before a life-threatening brain injury. Thus, the approach to an injured patient where major injury is suspected is as listed below.

- Primary survey: What is killing the patient?
- Resuscitation: treat what is killing the patient.
- Secondary survey: identify all other injuries.
- Definitive care: develop a definitive care plan.

*If you are likely to manage trauma victims during deployment, the authors strongly recommend that you complete some form of advanced trauma life support training appropriate to your speciality. A list of available courses can be found at the end of the chapter.*

In the pre-hospital or field setting the emphasis should be on the first two phases; the secondary survey and definitive-care phases are best conducted in a static health centre where the patient can be fully undressed and assessed in an appropriate environment. The primary survey and resuscitation phases are also described as the period of initial assessment. The elements of the primary survey, ABCDE, are described below.

A: Airway assessment while protecting the cervical spine.
B: Breathing and ventilation assessment.
C: Circulation assessment and control of bleeding.
D: Dysfunction of the central nervous system.
E: Environment considerations and exposure of the patient.

In the field setting, E also stands for evacuation (transfer) of the patient to an appropriate level of care – if such a place exists!

This ABCDE approach, or primary survey, constitutes a rapid and systematic approach in search of anything that may be killing the patient. It is a phase of urgency and crisis, which can be completed rapidly in a patient without serious underlying injury. In a patient with serious injuries, it may be lengthy.

## Initial Assessment in the Pre-hospital or Field Setting

Under normal circumstances, the aim of a pre-hospital health professional is to get the patient to the right hospital in the shortest possible time. This is known as "scoop and run". The approach recognises that the safest place for a severely injured patient is a well-equipped hospital. In the catastrophe or conflict setting this may not be possible for a whole raft of reasons – distance, lack of transport, destruction of physical infrastructure and so on. Under these circumstances it may be appropriate to carry out a more lengthy assessment and to initiate methods to stabilise the patient and then transfer to the nearest health facility, which may be very austere and many miles distant. This is the "stay and play" approach, and is best suited to either entrapment or lack of facilities.

The assessment is carried out with the patient supine (lying on their back).

### Airway Assessment and Management

The scope and extent of interventions will vary with skill, training and available equipment. Refer to the *ABC of Major Trauma* listed in the Resources section or an equivalent trauma life support manual for a full description of the options. Talk to the patient – someone who can reply in an effortless and coherent way has an intact airway and is breathing adequately.

Further action will be determined by skill and training. In totally untrained hands, a patient with an obstructed airway will die in 3–4 min and is best turned into the semi-prone or coma position. This risks further injuring an already damaged neck or spine, but in this setting there has to be a balance of risks. The old wartime adage still holds good for the injured in austere settings – "If I can see Heaven, I will soon be there".

A word on cervical spine control. Within peacetime life support systems, there is a near obsession with cervical spine protection by immobilisation during the early phases of management. This is right and reasonable, as most trauma victims in the developed world are involved in road traffic or industrial accidents where the incidence of unsuspected neck injury is high. During airway interventions in particular, the neck is protected from inadvertent movement by manual stabilisation or by the application of rigid neck restraints, reinforced with sandbags and forehead strapping. Under austere circumstances there may be insufficient personnel or lack of equipment. A valued judgement may have to be made. The best advice is to remember the risk and take as much care as is practical when managing injuries.

## Breathing and Ventilation Assessment

This requires exposure of the neck and chest and follows a "look, feel and listen" approach. Even in a field environment there is much that can be done and many lives may be saved. There is a finite list of lethal conditions that kill quickly, and a huge list of conditions that need not cause concern during the initial assessment phase. The lethal conditions which can, in most instances, be found with eyes, ears and hands are:

- tension pneumothorax,
- open pneumothorax,
- massive haemothorax,
- flail chest and pulmonary contusion,
- cardiac tamponade.

You are referred to the reading list in the Resources section if you wish to read a full account of these conditions. Only the principles of management can be covered in a manual of this nature.

### Look

- for wounds and bruises in the neck and over the chest,
- for evidence of distended neck veins,
- for evidence of excess respiratory effort,
- for chest symmetry or asymmetry,
- at the breathing rate – fast or slow, regular or irregular.

### Feel (Palpate)

- for the position of the trachea,
- for tenderness or evidence of rib fractures, and include the back,
- for wounds hidden around the back.

### Percuss

Percuss or tap the chest looking for resonance (air) or dullness (fluid). Percuss in the apices, axillae and bases.

*Listen*

Listen for the presence or absence of breath sounds. A stethoscope is valuable but not essential. You can listen by placing your ear over the patient's chest!

*Management*

Management of life-threatening conditions within the chest requires skills that cannot be obtained by reading a text or manual. If you are likely to manage chest injuries during deployment, you must attend a course appropriate to your role and abilities. See the course list at the end of the chapter.

## Circulation and Haemorrhage Control

This component of the initial assessment is concerned with shock. Shock is defined as a clinical state characterised by inadequate organ perfusion and tissue oxygenation. This definition covers shock irrespective of aetiology. In the trauma victim, the most common cause is blood loss. Other causes include:

cardiogenic or pump failure, associated with cardiac injury;

neurogenic, associated with high spinal injury;

septic, associated with neglected wounds;

anaphylactic, associated with an acute allergic response.

With the exception of septic shock associated with neglected wounds usually of more than 24 h duration, the other causes are rare in a hostile environment.

The key to successful management is early recognition. Haemorrhage or blood loss can be external and obvious or internal and concealed. Bleeding from an external site can usually be controlled by direct pressure and is often referred to as *compressible haemorrhage*; concealed haemorrhage is often very subtle in presentation and is referred to as *non-compressible*. For those working in hostile environments these are important distinctions, as by definition non-compressible haemorrhage requires a surgeon, and none may be available under these conditions.

Plainly, not every patient who bleeds will develop clinically significant shock. A careful clinical assessment is necessary. The following approach is recommended.

- Is there evidence of blood loss?
- Is there evidence of clinically significant shock?
- Attempt to classify the extent of shock (Table 20.1).
- Where is the source?
- Is field or pre-hospital management possible?
- Is evacuation to a surgical facility required?

The first question has been covered above. The next question concerns clinical evidence of shock. The general rule is: "an injured patient who is cool to the touch

**Table 20.1.**  Classification table for haemorrhage shock

|  | Class 1 | Class 2 | Class 3 | Class 4 |
|---|---|---|---|---|
| Blood loss | <15% 750 ml | 15–30% 750–1,500 ml | 30–40% 1,500–2,000 ml | >40% >2,000 ml |
| Systolic BP | Normal | Normal | Reduced | Reduced ++ |
| Pulse | Slight rise | >100 min | >120 min | >120 min, very weak |
| Respiratory rate | Normal | Increased | >20 min | >30 min |
| Capillary refill | Normal | >2 s | >2 s | Very delayed |
| Colour | Normal | Pale and cool | Pale and cold | Ashen |
| Mental state | Alert | Anxious | Anxious, panic | Drowsy and confused |
| Urinary output | Normal >30 ml/h | 20–30 ml/h | >20 ml/h | Little or absent |

and who has a tachycardia (pulse rate >100/min in an adult) is shocked until proven otherwise".

The next step is to make a best guess as to the extent of shock. Table 20.1 lists four classes of shock based on volume lost expressed as a percentage of actual amounts lost. Note that the classification is for adults.

Although a little artificial, the table should give a ballpark figure for the amount of blood loss. Note how unreliable the systolic blood pressure is as a guide to the extent of shock. Now ask, where is the source? A useful approach is the "blood on the floor and four more".

- Blood on the ground or on clothing – visible on examination.
- Blood in the chest – found during the assessment of breathing.
- Blood loss into the long bones – found when arms and legs are checked for wounds and deformity.
- Blood loss into the pelvis – look for tenderness and abnormal mobility (gently).
- Blood loss into the abdominal cavity – the silent reservoir – abdominal examination, the presence of wounds and the history may point to this site.

Having decided that shock is present, classified its extent and then diagnosed the source, it is possible to make decisions on management.

*Management*

Any health professional deployed should be able to render at least basic life support to a patient who is bleeding. The extent of intervention will depend on skill and training.

External blood loss is best managed by direct control and fluid replacement either orally or intravenously (or by the interosseous route in a child >6 years). The authors do not recommend the use of rectal fluids, although some people do. That route is unreliable and may be dangerous in the presence of intra-abdominal injury.

Remember, in a hostile environment oral fluid replacement should not be ignored provided that the patient is not vomiting for other reasons.

If haemorrhage into a body cavity or the pelvis is suspected, the key to survival is to get the patient to a medical facility where surgical control is possible. If no evacuation is possible, common sense should prevail. Remember that you cannot control concealed haemorrhage by giving large quantities of fluids intravenously. This is not to dismiss the use of these fluids. If available, vascular access should be obtained by someone trained to do so. Although hard evidence is lacking, medical opinion suggests that sufficient fluids should be given to maintain a radial pulse and a conscious patient. In most adults, a challenge of one or two litres of warmed (if possible) isotonic electrolyte will do no harm. Injudicious use of large volumes of intravenous fluids may inadvertently raise the blood pressure to levels sufficient to cause increased bleeding within a body cavity. A sense of realism must prevail; some of these patients will die.

### Dysfunction of the Central Nervous System

In the field setting, this component can be assessed quickly. There are two tasks. Use of the AVPU method to characterise the level of consciousness, and an assessment of the size and reactivity of the pupils.

The elements of AVPU are listed below.

A – Alert and orientated to the surroundings and the eyes are opened spontaneously.
V – Responds to the Voice of a medical attendant.
P – Responds to a Painful stimulus – squeeze an eyebrow.
U – Unresponsive to any stimulus.

The pupils are examined to assess equality and to check their response to light.

If any abnormality of the central nervous system is detected there is a limit on what can be done in a pre-hospital, hostile environment. What must be done, however, is to prevent secondary brain injury due to hypoxia. Pending transfer, if that is possible, medical attendants must ensure a clear airway. At its most austere, this may mean something as simple as lying the patient in the semi-prone position. In an unconscious patient, the gold standard would be endotracheal intubation and mechanical ventilation. In hostile field environments this will rarely be possible. Ingenuity and common sense must prevail.

## Critical Decision Making

At the end of the initial assessment phase decisions must be made concerning future care. The response of the patient and the local situation, including available resources, will all influence these decisions. A patient who has no life-threatening lesion, or one who successfully resuscitates, may be moved if that is possible. Others with more severe injury who fail to respond pose unique problems. If evacuation is possible, then this must be achieved safely and promptly. Where no evacuation is possible, reassurance and optimal nursing care, including pain control, is the minimum. Never move an unstable, dying patient when no destination is known. Have the moral courage to hold such people and care for them until they die.

## Secondary Survey

A brief word is appropriate here. A secondary survey is a full, head-to-toe assessment of a stable patient and takes place following a successful primary survey. It implies a stable, warm, safe environment, which means a hospital or medical centre. It cannot be done in the field in limited and austere circumstances.

# Multiple and Mass Casualties

Following natural disasters and during war and conflict, patient numbers may, for a time, exceed the capacity to deliver optimal medical care. Under these conditions, the normal medical approach to a single victim is inappropriate. The philosophy must be to do "the most for the most". A process of sorting is required to quickly identify the most severely injured for whom something can be done. Impacting factors will influence the size of the group and the nature of injuries that can reasonably be managed. This process is known as *triage*, from the French verb *Trier* which means to sift or to sort. The assessment requires skill and training and is usually carried out by a senior health professional who has the necessary skills and an overview of the overall situation. Failure to assign priorities correctly will result in an inappropriate use of resources to the detriment of those for whom survival is possible. It is a dynamic process and recognises that injured patients are inherently unstable and will deteriorate over time. This process underpins a successful outcome in all situations where patient numbers, at least for a time, exceed the capacity to deliver care.

There are a multitude of schemes in use. The following approach is increasingly recognised as the best and is recommended.

### Triage Sieve

A quick survey to separate the dead and the walking (lightly injured as a rule) from the severely injured.

### Triage Sort

Sorting the remaining (lying) injured into groups according to urgency. In an austere and hostile environment, four groups need to be identified.

- *Category 1:* critically injured and cannot tolerate delay. Examples of such patients include those with airway obstruction, lethal chest injury and catastrophic haemorrhage.
- *Category 2:* urgent with serious injury, but who can tolerate a delay of between 30 and 60 min.
- *Category 3:* less serious injuries where delay is unlikely to affect outcome.

- *Category 4:* severe multi-system injury where survival is unlikely – the expectant group.

Readers may have experience of other systems. If you are familiar with a particular system then use it, but make sure that it is appropriate to your environment.

## Wound Management

This section is concerned with the time-honoured principles governing open-wound management in a hostile environment. These are distilled from the lessons of war and disaster learnt over the last 200 years, often by hard example. They might appear at variance with what may be safely practised in a 21st century hospital in the developed world.

This section and the one that follows are in the main directed at health professionals who specialise in the management of traumatic wounds in hostile environments, but it should also help to inform all who may have to care for the injured.

The range of injury in hostile climates is considerable. The main features are:

- multiple open wounds, across multiple body cavities or systems;
- variable extent of soft-tissue injury;
- wounds associated with delay and heavy contamination;
- initial management rendered by relatively inexperienced personnel;
- poor working conditions and less than optimal equipment and environment.

### General Statement on Wounds

Prompt and appropriate initial management of all injury types reduces suffering and prevents unnecessary loss of life and limb. The majority of patients will present with conditions usually referred to as minor. Nonetheless, improperly treated soft-tissue injuries, wounds and other septic conditions can lead to prolonged or even permanent disability. Where possible one should document the history of the insult, including the circumstances, time and mechanism of injury (how, where and when), in addition to any treatment given.

A wound is any break in the continuity of the skin. The extent of tissue damage and therefore treatment required is related to the mechanism of injury. Most soft tissues react similarly to mechanical forces; five types of wound can usually be identified.

- Abrasion. A breach in the skin caused by friction.
- Contusion. Damage to the skin and deep structures caused by blunt force. Associated with bruising but no defect in the skin.
- Laceration. A breach in the integrity of the skin caused by the tearing effect of a blunt injury (includes degloving injury).
- Incision. Damage caused by a sharp object.
- Puncture. A penetrating injury involving deep structures.

Superficial abrasions, contusions and lacerations are often associated with similar internal injuries. In puncture or penetrating wounds, external evidence of serious internal damage may be minimal. The history of the injury is essential in estimating the extent of any damage, the likelihood of any contamination (chemical or infective) or the presence of foreign bodies. Minor wounds should be gently cleaned with antiseptic or sterile solutions and then covered with sterile dressings. Foreign bodies should only be removed if not adherent or penetrating. Large wounds, damage to special areas such as the eyes, hands or head, or wounds involving bones or internal organs need to be covered and reviewed by medically trained personnel.

## Principles

Open, penetrating wounds are usually obvious. What may be less obvious is the extent of concealed injury. Little can be determined from the wound's appearance and no assumptions can be made on the basis of appearance. Initial management when faced with patients with open wounds is as described in the preceding section. Apart from controlling compressible haemorrhage and covering the wound with a dressing, nothing further is appropriate until the primary survey has been completed and the patient is stable.

## Management Strategy

A suggested working management strategy is described below.

### Early Priorities

Take a history and examine the patient using the time-honoured ABCDE approach. Adopt life-saving measures prior to attending to a wound (other than controlling bleeding). Note any delays that point to the likelihood of impending sepsis. Cover the wound with a field dressing, wound pad or bandage. Record your findings and draw a diagram if possible.

### Pain Relief

If pain is a feature, small incremental doses of intravenous opiates are best. This will also allay anxiety.

### Control of Infection

While never a substitute for early and adequate surgery, systemic broad-spectrum antibiotics will control bacterial growth and colonisation for a time, perhaps up to 12 h if started in time (ideally within an hour of wounding). There is little evidence that the use of local antibiotic powders is helpful.

**The following sections are for surgeons who may be unfamiliar with wound management in hostile and austere environments.**

*Pre-operative Assessment*

Surgery should not be delayed for laboratory and radiological investigations if there is an immediate risk to life or limb. If time permits, some tests are appropriate. X-rays of the chest, pelvis and cervical spine are helpful in the multiply injured. In the case of ballistic injury, bi-planar X-rays are helpful in determining wound tracks and in locating metallic fragments. Some baseline laboratory tests are appropriate. These include a full blood count, blood for bacterial cultures, and serum for group and a cross-match of whole blood for transfusion.

*Surgical Technique*

Most surgeons will be familiar with techniques used in wound excision in the stable environment of a late twentieth-century hospital in the developed world. In a hostile and austere environment some modifications are appropriate.

Wounds in these environments are often old, neglected and contaminated. Further, many surgeons may not be familiar with injury caused by bullets, shell fragments or mines. Generous skin incision, wide fasciotomy and excision of devitalised tissue hold the key to success. In the field, neurovascular structures must be directly inspected for injury that may be subtle. At the end of the procedure it may be appropriate to leave the soft tissues open for a delayed primary closure at 4/5 days, a time-honoured lesson in these situations. Wounds should be carefully dressed as follows:

- lay on (do not pack) fine, fluffed gauze layers with overlying cotton wool;
- hold in place with a broad (6–inch), conforming crepe bandage;
- formal drainage is not required;
- for major limb wounds, splinting with plaster of Paris slabs or split casts is recommended;
- for associated fractures, external fixators are safer than internal fixation devices.

*Post-operative Care*

The wounded area should be rested and elevated if possible. Constant observation for impending vascular compromise and wound sepsis is mandatory. Soft-tissue swelling may require the readjustment of outer dressings. The inner wound dressings should be left undisturbed unless they are felt to be causing vascular compromise or are masking serious underlying bleeding.

Antibiotics should be continued for at least 72 h and changed if cultures indicate a resistant organism. Wounds under these circumstances often leak considerable quantities of blood and serum, even to the extent of requiring blood transfusion.

*Delayed Closure*

If wounds have been left open, the optimal time for inspection and delayed closure is between the 4th and 5th post-operative days. This usually requires a return to theatre and a general anaesthetic. If the wound is healthy and pink it may be closed, but this must be done by suture without tension and with minimal disturbance to the wound edges. In a case of tension, a combination of direct suture and split-skin grafting may be appropriate.

# Fractures and Dislocations

This section is aimed at health professionals with little or no exposure to treating fractures or dislocations, but who may encounter such patients during a deployment. It is not intended to be an exhaustive discourse on management, but rather an outline of the principles of early management. Experts in the field should manage such patients where possible.

## General Statement

A fracture is any crack or break in a bone. It can be associated with an open wound, and complicated by injury to adjoining muscle groups, blood vessels, nerves and organs. A dislocation is a displacement of a bone at a joint; there will always be associated sprains and tearing of ligaments around the affected joint. Deformed limbs should be gently returned to as normal a position as the patient will allow. Any further movement should then be restricted by splinting, since it may cause additional injury or pain. Splint devices need not be tailor-made; blankets or belts, for example, can be used to restrict unnecessary movement. The definitive treatment of any fracture or dislocation requires specialist medical input.

## Biomechanics and Pathophysiology

Fractures and dislocations occur when the bony skeleton fails when a load or force is applied. The skeleton rarely fails in isolation – surrounding structures such as soft tissue and neurovascular structures may also suffer injury. The principle that should apply is not to manage bones and joints in isolation. The affected limb or limbs should be assessed as a whole. In managing these injuries, the approach outlined earlier should be applied. Start with the primary survey and work through it in the usual way. Injuries to bones and joints will normally be encountered either as part of the 'C' of the ABCDE paradigm (life threatening), or during a detailed secondary survey (limb-threatening).

# Management Strategy

The recommended approach is outlined below.

### Primary Survey and Resuscitation

Check for and manage any life-threatening injury. In the context of limb injury, this will be recognition and control of external haemorrhage and placing the injured limb in rough alignment and length. Doing this is a very effective measure in controlling bleeding and reducing the risk of further injury. It also reduces pain. Do not do this against resistance!

## History

The history (road traffic accident or gunshot wound, for example) gives important information on the extent of injury. Road traffic accidents are typically associated with multiple and multi-system injuries. Ambulance paramedics refer to this as "reading the wreckage". Falls from a height suggest foot, ankle, leg, pelvic and spinal injury. Gunshot wounds inevitably mean injury to multiple structures and wound contamination. The history may also give an indication of the delay between injury and management.

## Limb Examination

A systematic approach is necessary. The time-honoured way is known as look, feel, move, stability.

Look at the skin, soft tissues and bone.
Feel the skin, surrounding tissues and over the bone (gently!).
Movement: first ask the patient to move the limb, and then move it yourself (gently!).
Stability: gently check the stability of the affected joint.

In a field setting there is much that can be learnt by this simple approach. The general vascular state of the limb can be ascertained, and the extent of swelling will be noted. The range of movement will also be noted actively and passively. The complete examination will not only give an indication of the extent of injury, but also a guide to the necessity of urgent intervention and the need to get the patient to a hospital or higher level of care.

## Treatment

Treatment should be divided into immediate and early.

### Immediate

This means save life, then limb. For example, if the patient is unconscious, clear the airway and then attend to the limb. If there is vascular compromise, pulling the limb out to length and roughly realigning it may restore circulation. If not, urgent hospitalisation is required. External haemorrhage should be dealt with by external compression over a wound pad. Only as a last resort should a tourniquet be applied, and someone familiar with the technique should perform this. The time of application should be noted and the patient moved to hospital.

*Early*

In the field, there should be no attempt to perform definitive reduction. Returning the limb to length and alignment should now be attempted if this was not done earlier. It is usually possible to do this with fractures but not with dislocations. Do not use force! An expert may perform reductions of dislocations to shoulder and ankle in the field. As a rule, some form of intravenous analgesic and anxiolytic agent are required. *Do not attempt reduction if you are not trained in these procedures.*

Having achieved length and alignment and attended to wound dressing, some form of splint is required. In the field setting ingenuity may be required. Use any materials in the immediate surroundings such as pieces of wood or tree branches. *No matter what your discipline or area of expertise, you should acquire some basic knowledge in the management of wounds, fractures and joint injuries.* Many humanitarian agencies will insist on such training. If not, approach organisations such as St. John Ambulance or the Red Cross societies.

Many of these injuries are very painful and frightening. If available, opiate analgesia is best, given in small intravenous boluses rather than a single dose by intramuscular injection. Repeated small intravenous increments maintain a plateau of pain relief and overall less analgesia may be required.

# Other Injuries

## Sprains and Strains

Sprains are stretching injuries of joint-related structures, whereas strains involve damage to muscular tissue. The acronym PRICE summarises the initial treatment priorities for both problems.

- Protection and pain relief. The injury and the individual should be protected from further harm; simple analgesia should be given if available.
- Rest. The initial injury may be exacerbated by any undue exertion. Pain and swelling will also restrict the amount of activity possible.
- Ice. A cold compress made from crushed ice, bags of frozen peas etc. should be wrapped in a towel to protect the skin from cold injury and placed next to the injured area for 20 min per hour for the first 24 h.
- Compression. Where possible, the injured area should be compressed by a layer of bandaging. Care needs to be taken not to constrict the circulation; an increase in pain may indicate a dressing that has been applied too tightly.
- Elevation. Raising the injured area above the level of the heart can reduce swelling and pain.

After 2 days, or when tolerated, gentle mobilisation of the injured area can begin. Continued pain or swelling may be an indication of a more serious underlying condition requiring more specialised medical help.

# Burns

Burns are injuries caused by heat, but by convention, and since the treatment is similar, damage caused by irradiation and chemicals are also included. The source of the injury is usually outside the individual, and as a result the surface layers of the body are commonly affected first. Exceptions to this are electrical burns where extensive damage can affect deep structures with little damage to the skin. The initial management of any burn is to remove the source of the injury; this may involve stripping the patient. The damaged area should then be flushed with cold water; this cools the burn, removes any residual chemical contaminant and provides pain relief. Minor burns, as assessed by depth and area, can be treated by sterile dressing and observation. Larger, deeper burns or burns to a special area (face, hands, genitalia) need more intensive resuscitation or treatment and are best looked after in appropriate medical facilities. Since burns are initially sterile, antiseptic preparations should only be used if the wounds have become infected, if sterile dressings are not available or if evacuation is likely to be lengthy.

# Bites and Stings

Trauma is caused by the mouth or hind parts of animals. Problems with these wounds arise either from infection associated with the germs harboured in the mouths of all animals (e.g. human, dog), or by envenomation (e.g. spiders, snakes). Bites from sharp, pointed teeth cause penetrating or puncture wounds while others, human teeth for example, can lacerate or contuse tissues. The vast majority of stings or poisonous bites, although painful and alarming, are not life- or limb-threatening. In allergic individuals or in cases of multiple stings, anaphylactic reactions can occur rapidly and require immediate medical help. Stings to the mouth and throat can result in swelling that can impede the airway and should be taken very seriously. The initial management of simple bites or stings is similar to that for sprains and stains, although the injured area should be kept dependent rather than elevated. If possible, patients stung in the mouth should be given ice to suck. Where there is thought to be a risk of envenomation, an attempt should be made to identify the species responsible. This should be abandoned if it puts any further people at risk of similar injury.

# Injuries to Special Sites

Certain injuries are beyond the scope of this manual. They require highly specialised training and expertise. Included here are serious head injuries and spinal injuries. Readers who are likely to encounter such injuries during their deployment should ensure a level of training appropriate to their seniority and field of work.

# Part C – Ballistics and Blast
Peter Hill

This section is concerned with unique injury mechanisms – ballistics and blast. Although not unique to the hostile environment, most aid workers will not have encountered injuries of this nature. This section serves to introduce and de-mystify the topic.

## Ballistic Injuries

Ballistic wounds are produced by penetrating missiles. These cause injury by giving up their energy to the body, which results in laceration, contusion and disruption of tissue.

### Mechanism of Injury

#### Energy Transfer

When the body is struck by a missile, the damage inflicted depends upon the characteristics of the missile and the tissue through which it passes. The amount of damage caused is related to the amount of energy that the missile transfers to the tissues. Injuries can broadly be classified into low-energy-transfer and high-energy-transfer injuries. The greatest amount of tissue damage is caused by high-energy transfer, which is related to the retardation of the missile.

The retardation of the missile is an important factor in the creation of the wound, for the more rapidly a missile is retarded, the greater will be the energy release and consequent tissue damage. Retardation depends upon missile factors such as shape, stability and composition, and tissue factors such as density and elasticity.

#### Fragments and Bullets

Penetrating missiles can be classified into two major groups, fragments and bullets. Fragments are the most common wounding agents in war, accounting for between 44% and 92% of all surgical cases. Anti-personnel fragments from military munitions tend to be small and numerous and are fairly regular in shape to ensure adequate range and consistent performance. Most military anti-personnel fragments have poor penetrating power and limited effective range. The energy available for wounding is low and so a low-energy-transfer wound is created.

In civilian practice, bullets are the predominant penetrating missiles, although fragmentation injuries can occur following terrorist bombings, as the blast produces fragments of irregular shape and size by disrupting the surrounding environment. Bullets have a greater range and penetrating power than fragments. Hand-gun bullets tend to have a lower velocity than rifle bullets, but both can produce a spectrum of high-energy-transfer and low-energy-transfer wounds, depending on the amount of energy transferred to the tissues.

*Wound Track*

When a projectile hits the body, it produces a wound track. As already stated, the nature of the wound track will depend upon the amount of energy transfer. Low-energy-transfer wounds are characterised by the injury being confined to the wound track. Injury results from a simple cutting mechanism, and the severity will be determined by the nature of the tissue penetrated.

*Cavitation*

High-energy-transfer wounds are characterised by the formation of a temporary wound cavity, as well as by cutting and laceration in the path of the missile. This phenomenon is called "cavitation" and occurs because the tissues surrounding the missile track are accelerated away. The velocity and momentum imparted causes the tissues to continue to move after the passage of the missile and create a cavity that is 30–40 times the diameter of the missile. Due to the elasticity of the tissue, this cavity expands and contracts several times. It is this cavitation effect which leads to the devastating injuries seen in high-energy-transfer wounds.

*Indirect Injuries*

As the effects of a missile are not confined to the missile track, indirect injuries can occur. For example, the spinal cord may be involved when the wound track passes close to the vertebral column, or a long bone may fracture in a limb even if it is not hit by the missile itself.

*Entry and Exit Wound Size*

The sizes of the missile entry and exit holes are governed by the size and shape of the penetrating missile and the degree of energy transfer at the site. Although a large tissue defect is the result of large energy transfers, the corollary that small entry and exit wounds imply low-energy transfer is not true, as high-energy transfer may have occurred internally. This is particularly true of long wound tracks, such as those occurring in abdominal wounds. Significant injury may have occurred within the abdominal cavity due to a large amount of energy dissipation, although the projectile only retains a small amount of energy at the end of its track and so produces a small exit hole, or may even remain lodged within the tissues.

## Wound Contamination

*Pattern of Spread*

Contaminants can enter the wound track from both entry and exit wounds. Low-energy-transfer wounds have contamination which is limited to the wound track itself, whereas high-energy-transfer wounds have contamination spread throughout the boundaries of the temporary cavity. Contaminants include skin bacteria from the normal skin flora, pieces of clothing, fragments of the projectile and material from the external environment (e.g. mud and dirt).

*Bacteria*

Clostridium welchii causes gas gangrene and has a rapid onset which is quickly fatal. *Staphylococcus aureus* and *Streptococcus pyogenes* infections develop in the first 3 days, followed by gram-negative bacilli infections (e.g. *Pseudomonas aeruginosa*, *Escherichia coli*).

## Principles of Treatment of Ballistic Injuries

### Basic Principles

#### Staged Surgery

The surgical treatment of a ballistic wound is a two-stage operation. The first part is concerned with saving the life and the limb, and the prevention of serious sepsis by primary wound excision. The second is the closure of the wound, which is carried out 4 or 5 days later.

#### Timing of Surgery

All wounds are contaminated by a mixture of organisms. Infection remains latent and superficial for about 6 h, after which time it becomes established and invasive. Therefore, surgery should be carried out as soon as possible after wounding.

#### Resuscitation

Patients should receive adequate fluid resuscitation before surgery, although surgery may be part of the resuscitation process.

#### Débridement

The wound should be thoroughly débrided. There should be generous surgical access, extensive wound débridement with decompressive fasciotomy for limb wounds, control of haemorrhage, excision of devitalised tissue and debris, and dressing of the wound opening in preparation for delayed primary closure at 3–5 days or more definitive surgery.

It may be necessary to excise some viable soft tissue when there is extensive soft tissue contamination.

#### Antibiotics

Antibiotics are only an adjunct to, and not a replacement for, surgery. They should be used early in the treatment for maximum effect and should be discontinued as quickly as possible (5–7 days) to prevent the emergence of resistant strains of bacteria.

*Dressings*

Once dressed, wounds should only be inspected in the operating theatre or a special dressing area.

## Blast Injuries

An explosive is a substance that undergoes chemical decomposition into gaseous products at high pressure and temperature.

### Physics

#### Blast Shock Wave

The explosive substance, when detonated, is rapidly converted into large volumes of gas, which results in the formation a blast shock wave. The blast shock wave rapidly expands as a sphere of hot gases with an instantaneous rise to peak pressure (the overpressure) that travels at supersonic speed. The overpressure falls as the speed of the shock wave declines, ending as a phase of negative pressure. This change in pressure results in blast winds, which blow alternately away from, and then back to, the epicentre of the explosion. Blast waves may be reflected by buildings or other fixed structures, causing complex interactions of pressure changes. Injuries following blast are traditionally divided into primary, secondary and tertiary types, although a victim may exhibit components of all three.

## Injuries Due to Blast

### Primary

The overpressure associated with the shock or blast wave is responsible for the primary blast injuries. The most vulnerable sites are the air-containing organs such as the ear, lungs and bowel.

#### Ear

The ear is the most sensitive organ, with rupture occurring at modest pressures. Blast damage may result in tympanic membrane rupture, disruption of the ossicles and inner-ear damage. The usual symptoms are tinnitus and deafness. The orientation of the ear relative to the shock wave is important in determining whether ear damage will occur.

#### Blast Lung

Lung contusion (blast lung) is rare, and occurs in less than 10% of survivors. Damage occurs at the alveolar membrane, resulting in haemorrhagic contamination of the alveoli and pulmonary oedema. Although usually mild, it may take the form of rapidly progressive respiratory distress syndrome.

*Bowel Injury*

Bowel injury is rarely a cause of clinically apparent injury when the blast occurs in air, but is an important mechanism of injury in underwater blast. The most usual injury is haemorrhage into the bowel wall, but there may also be visceral disruption.

*Sudden Death*

Sudden death may occur with no apparent evidence of external injury. This is believed to be due to cerebral or coronary embolism, although fatal dysrhythmias have also been suggested.

## Secondary

*Fragment Injuries*

Secondary blast injury is caused by the impact of missiles from the explosive device or from other debris generated and propelled by the explosion. There are primary fragments from the explosive device itself and secondary fragments from surrounding objects. Casualties will have multiple penetrating wounds, most of which will be relatively superficial, widespread bruises, abrasions and lacerations, and severe bacterial contamination of wounds. In fatalities, the principle cause of death is from head injury arising from penetrating missiles and blunt impacts. Thoracic and abdominal wounds account for the majority of the remainder, and the pattern can extend from multiple very high-energy-transfer wounds, to injury in a vital organ from a small, low-energy-transfer projectile with good penetrating power.

## Tertiary

*Blast Wind*

Tertiary blast injuries are caused by the blast wind. Victims may be thrown through the air, sustaining impact injuries particularly to solid organs. Such injuries have been estimated to occur in 25% of the victims in a confined space. Traumatic amputation can occur as parts of the body are torn off and long-bone fractures and head injuries can occur. The bodies of victims very close to the explosion may be completely disrupted. Traumatic amputation of limbs by blast occurs only very close to explosions.

*Anti-personnel Mines*

The most common explosive wounds of limbs in modern conflicts are those inflicted by anti-personnel mines, which cause a typical pattern of injury. There is traumatic amputation or disruption of the foot with mud, grass and fragments of the mine, shoe and foot being driven upwards into the patient's genitals, buttocks and arms. The other leg is normally severely injured. Massive contamination occurs throughout the limb, even though only the foot has been amputated. Similarly, if a hand is traumatically amputated, tissue damage extends beyond the forearm, especially along the tendon sheaths.

### Crush Injuries

Tertiary injuries may also result from building collapse. Crush injuries can result from falling masonry. In prolonged entrapment, amputation at the scene may very occasionally be required.

### Burns

Thermal injury may result from exposure to the fireball. These are usually flash burns affecting the exposed parts of the body. They are usually superficial, but airway damage and oedema may occur. If the interior of a building ignites, flame burns may also occur. An additional hazard in confined spaces is inhalation of smoke and toxic gases.

### Psychological Problems

Approximately 40% of those involved in a bomb incident will develop psychological sequelae. As well as the victims of the bombing, health care workers will also be psychologically traumatised, but this appears to be less troublesome amongst trained rescue personnel, especially if their actions had a beneficial result.

## Treatment of Blast Injuries

### Non-limb Injuries

All those suspected of having been exposed to a significant blast effect should be observed for 48 h. Patients with no injury other than a ruptured eardrum should be considered to have been exposed to a significant blast effect and should be observed accordingly.

### Blast Lung

Blast lung will usually occur within 6–12 h, but may take up to 48 h to develop and so the patient needs careful observation. Chest X-rays, if available, will reveal bilateral diffuse shadowing. There will be hypoxia and hypercapnia on blood gas analysis.

There is a risk of bilateral pneumothorax and so consideration should be given to the insertion of prophylactic bilateral chest drains. Vigorous chest physiotherapy is required during the severe phase of blast lung. The role of corticosteroids remains controversial.

Resuscitation should be with colloids or blood. Crystalloids may exacerbate pulmonary oedema, as will over-infusion of fluids.

*Tympanic Perforations*

The majority of uncomplicated tympanic perforations will recover with conservative management.

*Abdominal Injuries*

Abdominal injuries may present as mild abdominal pain due to multiple small haemorrhages. Conservative treatment is appropriate, although should the patient develop signs of peritonitis, significant gastrointestinal haemorrhage or radiographic evidence of free gas under the diaphragm (where X-ray facilities are available), a laparotomy should be performed.

### Limb Injuries

Survivors with limb wounds from blast alone are amongst the most severely injured patients. The amputated limbs have been torn away from the torso and nerves, blood vessels and tendons are often avulsed at a proximal level. After resuscitation, surgery is confined to wound toilet with extensive débridement of dead and possibly infected tissue. There will be multiple fragment wounds, which will also need débriding.

## Further Reading

Coupland RM. War wounds of limbs: surgical management. Oxford: Butterworth–Heinemann, 1993.
Greaves I, Porter K, editors. Blast and gunshot injuries. In: Pre-hospital medicine: the principles and practise of immediate care. London: Arnold, 1997.
Greaves I, Dyer P, Porter K, editors. A handbook of immediate care. London: W B Saunders, 1995.
Kirby NG, Blackburn G, edtors. Field surgery pocket book. London: HMSO, 1981.
Ryan J, Cooper G, editors. Ballistic trauma. London: Arnold, 1997.
Skinner DV, Whimster F, editors. Trauma. A companion to Bailey and Love's short practice of surgery. London: Arnold, 1999.

# Part D – Abdominal Pain and Acute Surgical Emergencies
Adam Brooks

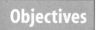 **Objectives**  This section deals with non-traumatic surgical emergencies. It describes the range of conditions which may present and suggests a management approach suitable for the hostile environment.

# Introduction

Acute surgical patients fall into two broad categories – those who require urgent surgery and those who can be managed, at least initially, without surgery. Once a provisional diagnosis has been made there are two questions that need to be answered taking into account local medical skills and available facilities:

- surgical or non-surgical management ?
- treat or transfer?

Once these questions have been answered, a treatment plan can be started. Frequent re-evaluation allows the detection of improvement or deterioration, and if either is found the treatment should be altered accordingly.

It is vital to know the capabilities of local hospitals, NGOs and military facilities so that informed decisions on treatment and evacuation can be made.

# Abdominal Pain

The diagnosis of abdominal pain relies on three factors – history, examination and to a lesser extent investigation.

## History

The patient's history should be ascertained in the following areas.

### Age

Some conditions are more common in certain age groups, e.g. appendicitis in children and young adults and diverticulitis in the elderly.

### Sex

In women, it is important to remember the common causes of gynaecological pain and emergencies, e.g. ectopic pregnancy, ruptured ovarian cyst.

### Pain

- Site. Where did the pain start, and has it moved?
- Radiation. Is the pain also felt in other areas of the body?
- Time and mode of onset. Was onset sudden or more gradual?
- Progression and duration of pain. Is the pain steady, gradually worsening or fluctuating?
- Character of the pain. Is it a burning or stabbing pain, or the intermittent cramping pain of intestinal colic?
- Severity of the pain. Is it a mild ache or the most severe pain imaginable?
- Aggravating and relieving factors: position, pain relief.

## Bowels

- Appetite.
- Time of last meal.
- Flatus (wind).
- Constipation. A history of absolute constipation (no flatus or bowel movements) and colicky abdominal pain is strongly suggestive of intestinal obstruction.
- Diarrhoea: frequency, blood, mucus.

## Vomiting

- How often?
- What is being vomited: bile, blood, faeces, altered blood (coffee grounds)?

## Genito-urinary Tract

- Frequency of bowel movements.
- Is there burning and pain?
- Is there vaginal discharge? When was the last menstrual period?

## Past Medical and Surgical History

- Has the patient had previous surgery, e.g. obstruction from adhesions, previous appendectomy?
- Has there been any medical illnesses masquerading as surgical pain?

# Examination

- Take into account the whole patient and do not just concentrate on the abdomen, e.g. yellow colour in the eyes (jaundice) may have an abdominal cause; a pale colour (anaemia) may be because of loss of blood from the gut.
- Pneumonia may cause abdominal pain if at the base of the lung.

## General Signs

- Is the patient comfortable or rolling around in agony, e.g. ureteric colic, or lying still but in pain, e.g. peritonitis?

## Pulse and Temperature

- A raised temperature (pyrexia), increased heart rate (tachycardia) and abdominal pain are strongly indicative of underlying pathology.

## Abdominal Examination

Most surgeons divide the abdomen into nine areas to allow an easy description of the site of pain, but it is simpler and has become acceptable to use abdominal quadrants – right and left upper and lower quadrants (Table 20.2). In this way, the site of the pain and elicited tenderness may lead straight to a differential diagnosis.

- *Look*
  - Scars, distension, hernial orifices (lumps in the groin), abdomen moving freely on respiration.
- *Feel*
  - Guarding and rigidity of peritonitis.
  - Localised pain and guarding, e.g. pain in the right upper quadrant on examination in cholecystitis.
  - Rebound tenderness.
  - Abdominal masses and hernias.
- *Percuss*
  - Percussion tenderness in peritonitis.
  - Drum-like (tympanic) note of intestinal obstruction.
  - Dullness over the distended bladder in acute urine retention.
- *Listen*
  - High-pitched tinkling of intestinal obstruction.

**Table 20.2.** Site of abdominal pain: generalised pain; peritonitis; bowel obstruction

| Right upper quadrant | | Left upper quadrant |
|---|---|---|
| Peptic ulceration and perforation | | Peptic ulceration |
| Acute cholecystitis | | Splenic infarct |
| Cholangitis | | |
| Upper gastrointestinal bleed | | |
| Lower lobar pneumonia | | |
| Hepatitis | | |
| | **Central** | |
| | Acute pancreatitis | |
| | Small-bowel obstruction | |
| **Right lower quadrant** | | **Left lower quadrant** |
| Appendicitis | | Diverticulitis |
| Mesenteric adenitis | | Ovarian cyst |
| Renal colic | | Ectopic pregnancy |
| Ovarian cyst | | Pelvic inflammatory disease |
| Ectopic pregnancy | | |
| Pelvic inflammatory disease | | |
| **Lower abdomen and groin** | **Loins** | |
| Obstructed and strangulated hernia | Renal colic | |
| Testicular torsion | | |
| Acute urinary retention | | |

- Silence of peritonitis.

Internal examinations should be performed only by qualified health professionals.

### Rectal Examination

- Pain and tenderness in the space between the rectum and the bladder or uterus in peritonitis, e.g. appendicitis.

### Vaginal Examination

- Discharge.
- Tenderness of the cervix in pelvic inflammatory disease.

## Investigations

- Investigations should be directed towards confirming or rejecting a clinical diagnosis and not performed simply as "routine".
- Where access to tests is very limited there is a greater emphasis on the history and examination.

The investigations can be divided by type and performed in a step-wise manner.

### Urine

- Dipstick test. This is a valuable investigation which can reveal blood, protein, ketones, white cells, glucose and bilirubin in the urine and help in the diagnosis of renal colic, urinary tract infection, diabetic ketoacidosis causing abdominal pain and differentiating obstructive jaundice from other causes etc.
- Urine microscopy gives an accurate diagnosis of urinary tract infection.

### Blood

- Haemoglobin. Low haemoglobin (anaemia) may be acute or chronic.
- White cell count (WCC). A raised white cell count may be indicative of infection or impending bowel strangulation.
- Urea and electrolytes. Dehydration may be detected by raised urea, and vomiting may lead to dehydration accompanied by low potassium.
- Liver function tests. Raised bilirubin will be found in obstructive jaundice.
- Amylase. Very high amylase is diagnostic of pancreatitis, although many intra-abdominal problems may cause a limited rise.

More specialised investigations are often not available in the field, and if necessary the patient will need to be evacuated to a facility that can offer them. If specialised investigations are required, then transfer/evacuate to a higher level of care because on-going management is likely to be necessary.

## X-rays

- Plain X-rays can provide confirmatory evidence of a diagnosis.
  - On a chest X-ray look for free gas, or basal consolidation.
  - On an abdominal X-ray look for renal calculi, distended obstructed bowel and fluid levels in erect films, or the calcification of aneuryms.
- Contrast
  - On as intravenous urogram look for a delayed renogram and ureteric obstruction with a distended collecting system with renal calculi.
  - With a barium enema look for obstruction, diverticular disease or inflammatory bowel.

## Special radiological investigations

- Ultrasound is used for an assessment of gallstones and cholecystitis, renal pathology, aortic aneurysms, and gynaecological pathology.
- Computerised tomography is used for acute abdominal pain and surgical emergencies, but the detail that it provides is infrequently required.

## Special investigations

Endoscopy. Endoscopic instruments allow visualisation of the lumen of the bowel and require special expertise and occasionally sedation. They can be either rigid, e.g. the sigmoidoscope used for detecting rectal tumours and the source of rectal bleeding, or flexible, e.g. the colonoscope or gastroscope which will help detect the source of gastrointestinal bleeding.

# Management

## General

- Initially most causes of abdominal pain can be treated with:
  - adequate pain relief,
  - intravenous fluids,
  - nil orally.
- Recording the fluid balance, especially urine output, is vital, and nasogastric aspiration should be commenced where vomiting continues.
- Broad-spectrum antibiotics should be started where indicated, e.g. peritonitis, or where a diagnosis has been made and the patient is waiting for theatre, e.g. appendicitis. However, antibiotics are not a substitute for the surgical release of pus.

It is of vital importance to remember that the patient who presents with several days' history of vomiting, fever or intestinal obstruction will have lost several litres of fluid. They will require significant extra resuscitation fluid in addition to their daily maintenance intravenous intake.

*Indications for Surgery*

Each case must be assessed individually, but general conditions where surgical intervention is likely include:

- generalised peritonitis;
- progressive distension;
- localised guarding and rigidity;
- spreading tenderness;
- free gas on X-ray;
- shock with bleeding or infection and pus in the abdomen.

# Acute Surgical Emergencies

## Associated with Generalised Pain

### Peritonitis

Peritonitis is not a diagnosis but the result of an intra-abdominal infective or inflammatory process. It may be localised, as in appendicitis, or generalised, such as a perforated ulcer. It presents with a rigid abdominal wall and severe pain.

#### History and Examination

The history is that of the underlying condition, and the signs depend on the severity. However, systemic signs of tachycardia and fever will be present and the patient will be unwell. The abdomen will be rigid, and movement and coughing will exacerbate pain.

#### Investigations

The diagnosis of peritonitis is clinical, but investigations are directed towards the under lying cause.

#### Treatment

Urgent surgery is required, which may require the patient's evacuation. Initial fluid resuscitation, antibiotics, analgesia and general management principles must be started (Table 20.3).

## Associated with Bowel Obstruction

Mechanical obstruction of the bowel arises from a number of causes. If the blood supply to the bowel is compromised it is a strangulating obstruction and leads to the death of the bowel. The causes include:

- outside the wall, hernias, adhesions from previous operations, volvulus (a twist of the bowel);

**Table 20.3.** General treatment of acute surgical emergencies

Adequate pain relief
Intravenous fluid – resuscitation to make up for losses and maintenance
Nil orally
Nasogastric aspiration
Urinary catheter
Accurate recording of fluid balance
Broad-spectrum antibiotics if peritonitis or sepsis
Frequent re-evaluation
Surgery as indicated

- in the wall, tumours;
- in the lumen, gallstone ileus.

*History and Examination*

Small-bowel obstruction tends to present with colicky central abdominal pain with waves of pain every 2–3 min, vomiting and absolute constipation. Large-bowel colic is less frequent and may be lower abdominal. Absolute constipation is frequently found, and prolonged cases may present with faeculent vomiting. Distension occurs with high-pitched obstructive bowel sounds. Localised tenderness with fever and a tachycardia suggest actual or impending strangulation and require operation.

*Investigations*

Raised WCC may be indicative of strangulation. An X-ray may show distended loops of bowel and erect films fluid levels. An unprepared contrast enema may provide some information in large-bowel obstruction.

*Treatment*

Initial "drip and suck" conservative regime of intravenous fluids, a nasogastric tube and close observation unless there are signs of peritonitis. Signs of impending strangulation or failure to settle within 12–24 h demand surgery.

## Associated with Central Abdominal Pain

### Acute Pancreatitis

The commonest causes of this acute inflammation of the pancreas are gallstones and alcohol, although there are numerous rarer causes including drugs, mumps, hypothermia and scorpion stings.

*History and Examination*

The patient presents with severe epigastric pain radiating through to the back, nausea and vomiting and in severe cases shock. There is upper abdominal tenderness.

*Investigations*

The diagnosis is made on blood tests by a significantly raised amylase. Further investigation is required to determine the severity of the attack, including blood glucose, liver function tests (LFTs), WCC, arterial blood gases, urea and electrolytes (U&E) tests and calcium.

*Differential Diagnoses*

These include perforated peptic ulcer and cholecystitis.

*Treatment*

The clinical course depends on the severity of the attack. A mild case can be managed with a combination of intravenous (IV) fluids, nasogastric aspiration, nil orally, analgesia and antibiotics. Monitoring of fluid balance and blood tests on a daily basis is required. The mortality from a severe attack is significant, and these patients are best cared for in a high-dependency or intensive-care environment where the severity is staged by Ranson criteria, close attention is paid to monitoring and fluid balance, and support for the cardiovascular and respiratory systems is available.

# Associated with Right Upper Quadrant Pain

## Perforated Peptic Ulcer

This can be a burst stomach or duodenal ulcer. Exacerbating factors include non-steroidal anti-inflammatory drugs and steroids.

*History and Examination*

A sudden onset of epigastric/right upper quadrant pain, occasionally with a background of indigestion symptoms. Patients may occasionally say they felt something burst. Examination will reveal tachycardia, and often fever and peritonitis.

*Investigations*

Erect chest X-ray shows free gas under the diaphragm.

*Differential Diagnosis*

Diagnosis of free gas includes a perforated diverticulum or caecal perforation from obstruction.

*Treatment*

Surgical intervention, with fluid resuscitation, antibiotics, all other general principles and intravenous ranitidine prior to theatre.

## Acute Cholecystitis

This is acute inflammation of the gall bladder. This common complication of gall-stone disease is more common in middle-aged, overweight women, but is certainly not exclusive to this group. The length of symptoms and raised WCC differentiate it from biliary colic.

### History and Examination

Right upper quadrant pain associated with nausea, fever and vomiting. Examination will elicit tenderness and guarding in the right upper quadrant.

### Investigations

Raised WCC. Ultrasound will usually show the gall stones and inflammation of the gall bladder wall.

### Differential Diagnosis

Pancreatitis and peptic ulcer perforation.

### Treatment

A conservative regime including antibiotics will usually result in the symptoms settling in 24–48 h. If symptoms do not settle, emergency surgery and cholecystectomy may be required.

## Cholangitis

This condition of an obstruction of the flow of bile, leading to jaundice and ascending infection, requires prompt action.

### History and Examination

Right upper quadrant pain with fever, rigors and jaundice (Charcot's biliary triad).

### Investigations

Raised WCC. Ultrasound will show biliary obstruction.

### Treatment

IV antibiotics and surgical or endoscopic decompression of the biliary tract.

## Upper Gastrointestinal Bleeding

The source of upper gastrointestinal bleeding may be peptic ulceration, oesophageal varices, Mallory Weiss tear, cancer or rarer causes. It is important to make a diagnosis of the source so a management plan can be made.

*History and Examination*

The bleed may vary from old blood (coffee grounds), to a small bleed (Mallory Weiss tear), to a catastrophic bleed of a peptic ulcer or oesophageal varices. The history may allow differentiation between the likely aetiology.

*Investigations*

Urgent haemoglobin test to determine anaemia and clotting, and to cross-match the blood, and upper gastrointestinal endoscopy to determine the source of bleeding.

*Treatment*

The initial treatment is resuscitation with fluid and blood as appropriate, and correction of any underlying clotting abnormality. Further management depends on the cause, as varices may be managed by endoscopic injection or in an emergency situation the use of a Sengstaken tube to produce tamponade. Surgical intervention is required where there is massive uncontrolled bleeding, a re-bleed, especially if a bleeding vessel or clot was found at endoscopy, or a bleed of more than four units over 24 h.

## Associated with Right Lower Quadrant Pain

### *Acute Appendicitis*

Acute inflammation of the appendix.

*History and Examination*

Despite all the advances in modern surgery, appendicitis remains a clinical diagnosis and one that is often difficult to make. It is the commonest cause of an acute abdomen in the UK, and is more common in children and young adults and rare (but does occur) at the extremes of age. The classical presentation is with an initial period of cramping central abdominal pain associated with nausea, loss of appetite and occasionally a vomit. This is followed by a sharp pain in the right lower quadrant (classically right iliac fossa), a low-grade fever, white furred tongue and a characteristic sweet smell to the breath. There will be tenderness and guarding in the right lower quadrant with anterior tenderness on rectal examination.

*Investigations*

White cell count will usually, although not always, be raised.

*Differential Diagnosis*

As appendicitis rarely presents in its classic form, the differential of right lower quadrant pain is varied and includes a number of gynaecological conditions.

*Treatment*

Appendicitis requires urgent surgery. Once this decision has been made, antibiotics specifically to cover anaerobic bacteria should be started, along with general surgical management.

## Mesenteric Adenitis

Inflammation of the glands in the abdomen as the result of non-specific infections, often colds etc. Common in children.

*History and Examination*

Abdominal pain associated with a high temperature and a recent upper respiratory tract infection.

*Investigations*

None

*Differential Diagnosis*

Needs to be differentiated from appendicitis.

*Treatment*

General supportive treatment with pain-killers and fluids.

# Associated with Left Lower Quadrant Pain

## Diverticulitis

Diverticulae are out-pouchings of mucosa through the large bowel wall and are common in elderly Western patients. They can become inflamed (diverticulitis), bleed or perforate.

*History and Examination*

Generally colicky left lower quadrant abdominal pain, occasionally with diahorrea, constipation or distension.

*Investigations*

Raised WCC; gentle sigmoidoscopy to exclude cancer; plain film to exclude perforation.

*Differential Diagnosis*

Colonic carcinoma, Crohn's disease.

*Treatment*

Conservative measures with analgesia and antibiotics and oral fluid only. Increasing tenderness or the development of generalised peritonitis indicates perforation and requires surgery.

## Associated with Lower Abdomen Pain and Groin Signs

### Obstructed and Strangulated Hernia

Whilst uncomplicated hernias require only elective repair, obstructed (the hernia contents become obstructed but the blood supply remains intact) and strangulated (blood supply is compromised) hernias require emergency surgery for their relief. All common hernias – inguinal, femoral, umbilical – are susceptible to becoming complicated, as are a number of the less common hernias.

*History and Examination*

Symptoms of obstruction, i.e. absolute constipation and vomiting, or infarction of bowel, fever, tachycardia, associated with a tender, irreducible swelling at a hernial site.

*Investigations*

Look for obstruction with X-rays, dehydration in U&Es and a raised WCC.

*Treatment*

Complicated hernias require surgical reduction, repair of the underlying defect and attention to the viability of the bowel involved. Forced attempts at closed reduction should not be made.

### Testicular Torsion

This is a true surgical emergency, as delay to surgery threatens the future viability of the testicle. The incidence is highest in males aged between 10 and 20 years, and the twist is of the spermatic cord.

*History and Examination*

Sudden onset of severe pain in the scrotum, often radiating to the lower abdomen. Examination reveals a swollen painful testis and any manipulation leads to further severe pain.

*Investigations*

This is a clinical diagnosis.

*Differential Diagnosis*

The main differential is epididymo-orchitis, but doubt must err on the side of exploration.

*Treatment*

Surgical exploration, untwisting the testicle and if it is viable fixation of both testicles.

## Acute Urinary Retention

Although far more common in men with prostatic hypertrophy, acute retention can occur from local causes, e.g. stones or a blood clot, or general causes such as drugs.

*History and Examination*

There is often a history of chronic retention or progressive difficulty in voiding, poor stream, frequency or urinary tract infection (UTI). Examination will reveal a tense, tender, distended bladder.

*Investigation and Treatment*

Gentle insertion of a catheter will provide not only evidence to support the diagnosis but instant relief. The U&Es should be checked as obstructive renal impairment can occur.

## Urinary Tract Infection and Acute Pyelonephritis

A urinary tract infection is common, especially in young females. It can present in many guises and is common where there is an abnormality to the flow of urine, e.g. pregnancy or bladder outflow obstruction. Progression to acute pyelonephritis requires more urgent treatment.

*History and Examination*

Symptoms of burning on passing urine, frequency and urgency are found in UTI. When associated with abdominal or loin pain, haematuria, fever and rigors with tenderness in the loin or flank it is suggestive of acute pyelonephritis.

*Investigations*

Ward testing of urine and microscopy. Raised WCC. Ultrasound after commencing treatment to look for renal damage.

*Treatment*

Fluid orally and intravenously if required. Antibiotics to cover possible organisms.

## Ruptured Ectopic Pregnancy

All women of child-bearing age who present with abdominal pain should have a pregnancy test to exclude ectopic pregnancy, and a high index of suspicion needs to be maintained in the shocked woman with abdominal pain who is proved to be pregnant.

### Investigations

Pregnancy test.

### Treatment

Fluid and blood resuscitation and emergency surgical intervention.

## Associated with Loin Pain

### Renal Colic

The pain of renal colic is said to be worse than that of childbirth. The cause of kidney stones is often unknown. Unfortunately, people who have suffered from renal colic are likely to have subsequent episodes.

### History and Examination

Severe colicky loin pain, often radiating round into the groin and associated with sweating, nausea and vomiting. Patients may have loin tenderness, fever and blood in the urine on ward testing.

### Investigations

The stone may be visible on a plain abdominal X-ray taken to include kidneys, ureters and bladder (KUB). An intravenous urogram will show any obstruction.

### Differential Diagnosis

The pain of left-sided renal colic must be differentiated from that of a stretching or leaking abdominal aortic aneurysm.

### Treatment

Initially conservative with analgesia (often non-steroidal) and oral fluids. In the majority of cases the symptoms will settle, but stones that are causing obstruction or that fail to pass may require specialist treatment. Evidence of infection and an obstructed renal system warrant intervention and drainage of the kidney by a specialist.

# Abscesses

## Breast Abscess

These are commonly associated with breast feeding and following acute mastitis.

### History and Examination
Often a red, inflamed, tender swelling which may become fluctuant.

### Investigations
Clinical diagnosis.

### Treatment
Surgery – incision and drainage.

## Anorectal Abscess

Abscesses in the peri-anal region are common, and in up to 30% of patients they may give rise to a fistula in-ano.

### History and Examination
Initial diagnosis can often be made from the end of the bed as sitting aggravates the condition. A constant throbbing pain with a tender mass in the peri-anal area clinches the diagnosis.

### Investigations
None.

### Treatment
Surgery – there is no alternative to the surgical release of the pus.

# Other Surgical Emergencies

## Acutely Ischaemic Limb

Acute arterial occlusion may be the result of embolus from a distant source or thrombosis on under lying atherosclerotic disease. The cause must be sought and treatment instituted urgently if the limb is to be saved.

*History and Examination*

The five 'P's:

- pain,
- pallor,
- pulse-less,
- paraesthesiae,
- paralysis.

A history should be sought for atrial fibrillation, or recent myocardial infarct that may be the source of emboli, or intermittent claudication where thrombosis is likely.

*Investigations*

Look for a source of emboli, an electrocardiogram and urgent arteriography. Baseline clotting studies.

*Treatment*

Transfer to an appropriate facility. Systemically anticoagulate. Surgical embolectomy should be performed where arterial embolus is suspected. Where available, intra-arterial thrombolysis is the preferred management for thrombosis, followed by treatment of the underlying disease by balloon angioplasty.

## Tropical Diseases Presenting with Abdominal Pain

More remote places in the world not only have fewer medical facilities, but also provide a collection of diseases that are seldom seen in European practice (Table 20.4). In such environments these conditions must always be thought of

**Table 20.4.** Some tropical causes of severe abdominal pain and symptoms

| Site | Cause |
|---|---|
| General peritonitis | Amoebic colitis perforation<br>Ruptured hydatid cyst<br>Typhoid perforation<br>Abdominal TB |
| Right lower quadrant | Ileocaecal TB |
| Right upper quadrant | Helminth infection of the biliary system |
| Left upper quadrant | Splenomegaly – malaria<br>Splenic abscess |
| General pain | Intestinal obstruction, e.g. *Ascaris lumbricoides*<br>Infective diarrhoea – *Vibrio* cholera, *Salmonella, Giardia* etc. |

and perhaps a specialised text be consulted for the management, although the basic principles of treatment still stand.

## Summary

The management of abdominal pain and acute surgical emergencies remains simple.

- History and examination.
- Working diagnosis.
- Surgical or non-surgical management.
- Treat or transfer.

### Further Reading

Cook GC, editor. Manson's tropical diseases. 20th ed. London: WB Saunders, 1996.
Ellis BW, Paterson-Brown S, editors. Bailey & Love emergency surgery. Hamilton Bailey's emergency surgery. 13th ed. Oxford: Butterfield–Heinemann.
Raftery AT, editor. Churchill's pocket book of surgery. London: Churchill Livingstone.

# Part E – Dental and ENT
Peter V. Dyer

# Dental

## Introduction

Those conditions involving the mouth and oral structures may be divided into two groups:

- hard tissues (including the teeth and bony anatomy of the face);
- soft tissues.

### Nomenclature

The mouth is divided into four quadrants to identify the teeth and the site of intra-oral lesions. Both the upper and lower arches are divided into the patient's left and right as viewed from looking directly into the mouth. The teeth are named as follows, starting at the midline:

- incisors,
- canines ,
- premolars (only found in adults),
- molars.

There are *20 primary* teeth (deciduous teeth) in children. When looking into the mouth, the teeth are sequentially lettered a – e starting from the midline in each quadrant, e.g. "⌊d" is the upper left first deciduous molar.

In adults there are 32 permanent teeth which are sequentially numbered from 1 to 8 starting from the midline in each quadrant, e.g. "3̅⌋" is the lower right canine.

# Examination of the Mouth

The mouth should be examined in a good light and with the aid of a dental mirror. The patient will normally be able to point to the affected side of the mouth and may be able to identify the exact location of the problem.

Tapping a tooth with the handle of the mirror may elicit a painful response if there is a significant problem with that tooth. If in doubt, apply a cold stimulus such as ethyl chloride on a pledget of cotton wool to the tooth suspected of being the cause of the pain.

## Hard Tissues

### Toothache

1. *Pulpitis* (inflammation of the pulp) is the commonest cause of dental pain. The main causes are:

- dental caries;
- fracture of the tooth;
- dental treatment (exposure of the nerve).

The symptoms of pulpitis are:

- pain (sharp and stabbing in nature);
- hypersensitivity to hot and cold stimuli;
- patient kept awake at night because of pain.

Examination of the mouth may reveal a carious (decayed) tooth. The main treatment is either to remove the pulp (nerve) from the tooth or to extract the tooth. Dental cement containing oil of cloves can be applied to the tooth as a temporary analgesic measure.

2. *Periapical periodontitis* is inflammation of the periodontal membrane around the apex of a tooth. It is due to spreading infection following the death of the pulp. The symptoms are as follows:

- pain on biting on the tooth (which can be extruded out of the socket);
- worsening pain (throbbing in nature);
- hot and cold stimuli have no effect.

Treatment is again aimed at either saving the tooth or extracting it.

3. A *dental abscess* occurs when infection persists around the apex of the tooth following periapical periodontitis. Pus may spread directly into the surrounding tissues and emerge into the mouth or onto the face. The patient may complain of pain and swelling in the mouth or on the face. Examination may reveal an unwell patient with pyrexia. They may not have eaten or drunk recently due to trismus (difficulty in opening the mouth). The position of the swelling will indicate the tooth that is the source of infection. This is illustrated below.

*Name of tooth and position of swelling*

*Upper teeth*

| | |
|---|---|
| Central incisor | Upper labial sulcus |
| Lateral incisor | Anterior palate |
| Canine | Inner canthus of eye |
| Premolars | Upper buccal sulcus |
| Molars | Upper buccal sulcus |

*Lower teeth*

| | |
|---|---|
| Central incisor | Lower labial sulcus |
| Lateral incisor | Lower labial sulcus |
| Canine | Lower buccal sulcus |
| Premolars | Lower buccal sulcus |
| Molars | Lower buccal sulcus |
| 2nd and 3rd molars | Submandibular space |

These patients may need intravenous fluid replacement and antibiotics. The antibiotic currently suggested is a broad-spectrum penicillin, although metronidazole is also effective. The source of the infection should be extracted and the abscess drained.

### Post-Extraction Haemorrhage

The causes of bleeding following the extraction of a tooth are listed below.

- Trauma to the bone socket.
- Soft-tissue trauma.
- Bleeding disorder.
- Anti-coagulant therapy.
- Infection.
- Failure to follow post-operative instructions.

The patient should be examined in a good light and preferably with an assistant to suck away any blood. The tooth socket should be examined for signs of excessive trauma. The treatment is described below.

- Reassure the patient and instruct them to sit down quietly.
- Ask them to bite on a rolled-up piece of gauze placed over the socket for half-an-hour.
- If the bleeding persists, the socket should be sutured using a local anaesthetic (2–4 ml 1 in 80,000 adrenaline and 2% lignocaine) infiltrated around the area.
- The patient should avoid hot drinks for 12 h.

*Injury to the Teeth*

Teeth may be *avulsed* (completely lost from the socket), *extruded* (partially lost from the socket), *intruded* into the socket or *subluxed* (displaced in a forward, backward or sideways direction).

Injuries to the tooth may be confined to the enamel, the dentine and the enamel, or extend below the level of the gum. A fracture of the tooth may involve the pulp and be painful.

A tooth which has been completely avulsed (usually a front tooth) should be managed in the following way.

- Instruct the patient to reinsert the tooth into the socket immediately and hold it in place until seen.
- Alternatively, advise the patient to place the tooth into a container of milk and to bring it to the carer as soon as possible.
- Under local anaesthetic, wash the socket using saline and re-implant the tooth.
- Temporarily hold the tooth in place using wire from a paper clip and a dental adhesive.
- Antibiotics should be prescribed.

If a tooth or a fragment of a tooth is missing, a chest radiograph is necessary to exclude the possibility of inhalation.

Fractured teeth involving the pulp may be dressed using a calcium hydroxide paste on the exposed surface.

*Injuries to the Bones of the Face*

Injuries to the face are usually assessed during the secondary survey. However, some injuries may be life-threatening and should be managed during the primary survey and resuscitation phases.

## Mandibular Fractures

- Mobile fragments of jaw.
- Teeth not meeting properly (malocclusion).

- Sublingual haematoma.
- Step deformity along the line of the jaw.

### Maxillary Fractures

- Mobile maxilla.
- Teeth not meeting properly.
- Bilateral facial swelling.
- Bilateral periorbital haematoma.

Life-threatening injuries in the face which may compromise the airway, particularly in a patient with an associated head injury, are listed below.

- Displacement of the fractured maxilla.
- Loss of tongue control (occurs with a bilateral fracture of the mandible).
- Foreign bodies, e.g. teeth, dentures, bone fragments, vomitus or haematoma.
- Haemorrhage.
- Soft-tissue swelling and oedema.
- Direct trauma to the larynx and trachea.

*Cervical spine* injury occurs in 2% of facial trauma cases and must always be considered. The spine should be protected with a cervical collar and appropriate radiographs obtained.

### Dislocation of the Jaw

This may follow trauma to the jaw or be caused by simply yawning widely. The symptoms are:

- the mouth is fixed open,
- the patient is unable to speak,
- drooling saliva,
- considerable pain.

The jaw can be relocated by seating the patient in a low chair with the clinician standing in front. Both thumbs are placed over the posterior lower teeth and pressure is applied in a downward and backward direction. The clinician can feel the jaw move back into the correct position and the patient has immediate relief. Occasionally sedation may be required, particularly if the patient is anxious or if the dislocation happened some time before.

## Soft Tissues

There are a number of conditions which commonly affect the soft tissues of the mouth. The gingivae (gums) may be affected by:

- chronic periodontal disease;
- acute necrotising ulcerative gingivitis (ANUG);
- acute pericoronitis;
- Ludwig's angina;
- Trauma.

1. *Chronic periodontal disease* is very common and is caused by plaque or calculus (tartar) building up around the teeth. The main reason for this is inadequate brushing of the teeth. The patient usually complains of bleeding from the gums on brushing. Treatment is to improve the cleaning of the teeth.
2. *Acute necrotising ulcerative gingivitis* (ANUG) (trench mouth) may occur in epidemic form, especially in institutions. It is often preceded by:

- viral respiratory infection,
- fatigue,
- immune defects.

The symptoms are:

- widespread soreness of the gums,
- spontaneous bleeding of the gums,
- characteristic halitosis,
- pyrexia and malaise,
- cervical lymphadenopathy.

The appearance of the gums is diagnostic. The papillae (between the teeth) are ulcerated, tender and bleed to the touch. ANUG is managed by gentle cleansing with a toothbrush and diluted hydrogen peroxide. Metronidazole is the appropriate antibiotic.

3. *Acute pericoronitis* is an infection of the gum around a partially erupted lower wisdom tooth (3rd molar). The symptoms are:

- pain ranging from mild to severe,
- bad taste in the mouth,
- halitosis,
- difficulty in opening the mouth,
- cervical lymphadenopathy,
- occasionally pyrexia and malaise.

The immediate treatment is antibiotic therapy with penicillin or metronidazole. Hot salt mouthwashes are helpful. If the patient is unwell, intravenous fluids should be commenced. There is a potential airway risk if the infection is not treated. Extraction of the tooth will prevent further episodes of infection.

4. *Ludwig's angina* is a rare but life-threatening spreading infection, usually from a lower molar tooth. Both sides of the floor of the mouth become swollen and the tongue is raised up against the roof of the mouth. Swelling spreads below the lower jaw on both sides to compromise the airway. This must be treated

immediately with high-dose antibiotics and drainage of all the infected tissue spaces. Occasionally tracheostomy is needed.

5. *Trauma.* Bleeding from the soft tissues of the mouth, face and scalp may be profuse due to the good blood supply in that the area. Fractures of the facial bones can also produce considerable haemorrhage. Life-threatening bleeding due to airway obstruction or hypovolaemic shock must be managed in the primary survey.

- Open wounds should be assessed for blood loss.
- Open wounds should be cleaned using chlorhexidine solution (0.05% chlorhexidine gluconate) and covered with a sterile dressing.
- Simple nose bleeding (epistaxis) may be controlled by direct digital pressure to the lower nose.
- Closed wounds may produce bleeding from the nose and mouth. The nose may be packed using ribbon gauze anteriorly and a 12/14 G Foley catheter and balloon posteriorly.

# Eye Injuries

- Periorbital haematoma (black eye) may be due to soft-tissue injury or an underlying fracture of the cheek bone (zygoma) or maxilla.
- The eye must be examined and the visual acuity (ability to see) tested.
- Foreign bodies should be left in situ and the eye covered with a non-compressive pad.
- Penetrating foreign bodies must not be removed.
- If the globe is disrupted, the eye should be covered with a non-compressive pad.
- If chemicals enter the eye, copious amounts (500–1,000 ml) of normal saline, sterile water or Hartman's solution should be used to wash the eye.

N.B. Patients with foreign-body injuries should be referred to an appropriate surgical team if one is available.

# Ear, Nose and Throat

Examination of the patient should be in a good light, preferably using a mirror. Common problems include:

- infections,
- foreign bodies,
- trauma (see above).

## Infections

1. *Acute otitis externa* is inflammation of the ear canal and may be due to trauma or eczematous ear canal skin. The symptoms are:

- mild irritation to severe pain,
- discharge from the ear canal,
- hearing loss.

Treatment consists of gentle removal of ear canal debris and application of antibiotic/steroid drops, ointment or spray.

2. *Acute otitis media* is inflammation of the middle ear and is common in children. Symptoms include:

- recent upper respiratory tract infection,
- severe earache, which may be bilateral,
- pyrexia and malaise,
- rupture of eardrum produces relief of pain.

Treatment consists of bed-rest, antibiotics and painkillers.

3. *Acute mastoiditis* may occur if acute otitis media is inadequately treated. It is often seen in young children and the symptoms are:

- severe pain,
- pyrexia and tachycardia,
- swelling and redness behind the ear.

Intravenous antibiotics are necessary for treatment.

4. *Acute pharyngitis* commonly occurs following a viral infection. The patient will complain of:

- difficulty in swallowing,
- feeling unwell.

Treatment is aimed at relieving the symptoms and includes fluids and painkillers.

5. *Acute tonsillitis* is seen in children and the symptoms include:

- sore throat,
- difficulty in swallowing,
- pyrexia and malaise,
- cervical lymphadenopathy.

Treatment includes bed-rest, painkillers, antibiotics and fluid replacement.

6. *Quinsy (peritonsillar abscess)* occurs as a complication of acute tonsillitis and is more common in adults. An abscess forms around the tonsil causing the patient to complain of:

- sore throat on the affected side,
- difficulty in swallowing and dribbling saliva,
- change in the voice (hot-potato quality),
- malaise,
- difficulty in opening the mouth (trismus)
- earache,
- cervical lymphadenopathy.

Intravenous antibiotics and drainage of the abscess are essential for treatment.
7. *Supraglossitis* affects children between 3 and 7 years of age and requires urgent management. It is characterised as follows:

- stridor (noisy breathing resulting from an upper airway obstruction),
- sore throat,
- mouth breathing and dribbling.

Immediate treatment with intravenous antibiotics (chloramphenicol) is essential.

## Foreign Bodies

1. Ears.

- Commonly occurs in children.
- Earache may be the presenting complaint.
- Can be removed either by grasping the foreign body with forceps or by gentle syringing (providing that the item is not vegetable matter which may swell).
- General anaesthetic may be required for children.

2. Nose.

- Commonly found in children.
- Foul discharge from a nostril may be the presenting symptom.
- Can be removed by visualising the object and grasping it with forceps.
- General anaesthetic may be required for children.

3. Throat.

- An object may lodge anywhere in the pharynx or laryngo-tracheo bronchial tree.
- May cause scratching, tearing or perforation of the mucosa.
- Differentiation must be made between inhaling and swallowing the foreign body.
- Inhalation may be suggested by a sudden onset of coughing. Chest infection may be the presenting symptom.
- If the airway is compromised, a sharp blow to the back may dislodge the item.
- A general anaesthetic may be needed to remove a foreign body.

## Suggested Further Reading

Andreasen JO, Andreasen FM. Essentials of traumatic injuries to the teeth. Copenhagen: Munksgaard, 1994.

Dhillon RS, East CA. Ear, nose and throat, and head and neck surgery. Edinburgh: Churchill Livingstone, 1994.

Greaves I, Porter K, editors. Pre-hospital medicine. The principles and practice of immediate care. Maxillofacial injuries. London: Arnold, 1999; Ch. 24.

# Part F – Anaesthesia and Analgesia

Paul Wood and Peter F. Mahoney

- To discuss pain relief in a hostile environment.
- To discuss the principles of treatment.
- To describe the range of agents and techniques available.
- To discuss local and general anaesthesia in a hostile environment.
- To discuss the options and to describe techniques.

# Introduction

Treating an injured person's pain is an important humanitarian task. Throughout this chapter, the term *analgesia* is used to mean relieving pain, whereas *anaesthesia* is used to mean the absence of sensation. Anaesthesia may involve general anaesthesia (the patient is put to sleep, usually to allow a surgical procedure to be performed) or local anaesthesia (where a body part is deprived of sensation). Some anaesthetic drugs provide analgesia (e.g. ketamine) and some analgesic drugs (e.g. certain opioids), if given in large doses, will cause unconsciousness and general anaesthesia. All of these drugs have effects other than analgesia and anaesthesia. Depending on the drug and the dose given, this can include decrease in blood pressure, stopping a casualty breathing and other toxic effects.

## Principles of Treatment

- Talk to patients, reassure them, explain what is happening, and assess their injuries and pain.
- Resuscitation comes before attempts at pain relief. Sorting out problems with a casualty's airway, breathing and circulation (ABC) helps to correct hypoxia and hypovolaemic shock. This in turn helps to relieve the pathophysiology of uncontrolled pain.
- Simple physical measures to relieve pain should be tried first. This includes splinting limb fractures and cooling burns.

- The use of pain-relieving drugs and techniques will depend on a number of factors:
  - what medicines and equipment are available (either locally in personal kits, or in packs supplied by an aid agency or the military);
  - the training, skill and experience of the person(s) managing the casualty or casualties;
  - the number of casualties involved, their clinical condition and the circumstances of injury (including threats to the safety of both casualties and carers).

## Clinical Assessment

Clinical assessment will be modified in the light of the situation and the number of casualties. Where practical, it is valuable to find out about the past and present history. Before giving a drug, contraindications (such as pregnancy or allergy) should be ruled out.

Clinical assessment relies on clinical observation and regular measurement of consciousness level, blood pressure, pulse rate and respiratory rate (these findings should be charted in a manner which will be understandable to personnel both in the field and following reception in hospital). After giving a drug, any or all of these parameters may change and appropriate resuscitative action may be required.

Clinical assessment may be supplemented with electronic monitoring apparatus such as pulse oximetry, which measures the arterial oxygen levels, but this does not remove the need for continued clinical assessment.

## Routes of Administration

Drugs can be given by a number of routes. The choice of route will depend on how the drug is formulated and the condition of the casualty.

### Orally

Oral analgesics are effective after minor surgery and in the less seriously injured. After serious injury or major surgery, gastric emptying and gut motility are likely to be delayed and patients may vomit so alternative routes for giving drugs are needed.

### Intramuscular Injection

Intramuscular injection of drugs may be necessary when carers lack cannulation skills, resources are limited, and casualties are inaccessible or presenting in large numbers with minor injuries. Intramuscular (IM) injection has a number of limitations. Onset of drug action is unpredictable and will be delayed in the shocked and cold patient. Subsequent fluid resuscitation and re-warming following an IM injection can result in the drug being rapidly "washed" out of the muscle into the circulation. This may in turn produce cardiovascular and respiratory depression.

## Intravenous Injection

Intravenous injection (IV) provides a faster onset of analgesia and is best done by giving small amounts of the drug slowly into an intravenous cannula and monitoring the patient's response.

## Infiltration and Nerve Blockade

This will be discussed under "local anaesthetics" later in this part of the chapter.

## Inhalation

The drug is absorbed across the large surface area of the lung. This will be considered further under "Entonox" later. An advantage is the rapid onset of drug action. A disadvantage of Entonox is the weight and bulk of the equipment needed to administer it.

## Choice of Drugs for Medical Kits

In many situations it will be a case of what is available. If a medical kit is being put together (see Resources section), make sure that the analgesics:

- are familiar to the people who will be giving them;
- are non-addictive;
- can legally be taken into the country or area of work;
- can be supplied or purchased locally;
- will withstand the temperature and conditions likely to be encountered;
- have a predictable action and minimal side effects;
- have effects which can be reversed in the event of an accidental overdose.

## Individual Pharmacology and Techniques

### Oral Analgesics

For treating musculoskeletal and soft-tissue injuries, the authors recommend individual or combined use of paracetamol, diclofenac (see non-steroidal drugs below) and codeine phosphate (see opioids below).

## Paracetamol

This drug has a good analgesic action and unlike aspirin causes minimal gastric irritation. For adults, 500 mg to 1 g is taken up to four times a day. In the correct dosage, other side effects are rare. Paracetamol is dangerous in overdose and can cause fatal liver damage.

## Non-Steroidal Anti-Inflammatory Drugs (NSAIDs)

This group of drugs is used in hospital to treat musculoskeletal and post-operative pain. They have been shown to have opioid-sparing effects. A range of drugs is available, but they differ in terms of recommended dosage, dosage interval, licensed route of administration and severity of side effects. They have been used effectively in a variety of circumstances. Intramuscular ketaprofen has been used successfully in battle casualties with minor fragment wounds, while in emergency department practice, oral ibuprofen and intramuscular ketolorac have supplied comparable analgesia for musculoskeletal injuries. In the authors' experience, diclofenac is one of the most effective analgesics of this group when used in trauma patients.

At present, out-of-hospital injectable use of NSAIDs may be restricted by the conditions of a particular drug's license.

There are also a number of disadvantages and limitations to the use of NSAIDs.

- They can inhibit platelet aggregation and prolong bleeding time, resulting in an increase in bleeding during surgery.
- Post-operative haemorrhage has been reported.
- They have been implicated in acute renal failure, particularly in patients with diminished renal function.
- They may exacerbate asthma.
- They may cause gastric irritation and should not be used in aspirin-sensitive people.

This means that their use is limited, particularly in cases of major injury associated with haemorrhage and shock.

## Opioid Analgesics

These drugs remain the gold standard by which other analgesic agents are judged, particularly for treating severe visceral pain. Many synthetic and semi-synthetic drugs are available, but certain comments are relevant to all opioids.

- In severe pain, small incremental doses should be administered by the intravenous route where possible, and patient response should be observed closely both to assess pain relief and to check for adverse effects (particularly for signs of respiratory depression).
- The opiate antagonist naloxone must always be available, as should facilities for advanced airway management.

- Anti-emetics will frequently be necessary when opioids have been used.
- Certain of these drugs are controlled and subject to the Misuse of Drugs Regulations.

The above disadvantages have been partially offset by certain synthetic opioids such as nalbuphine, which are characterised by a low potential for respiratory depression and addiction.

*Morphine*

This is the standard narcotic analgesic against which all other opioids should be assessed. Its classic actions of analgesia with euphoria (and ultimately physical dependence) and respiratory depression depend upon an agonist (positive) action at central nervous system opioid receptors. These effects are reversible with the opiate antagonist naloxone.

In the field, a 1 mg/ml solution can be used to provide an adult bolus injection of between 2 and 5 mg followed by 1-mg increments according to patient response. Intravenous analgesia may be expected in some 5–10 min. Cardiovascular effects include a lowering of blood pressure from systemic vasodilatation following histamine release. Morphine is generally avoided in head injuries as hypercapnia may occur and papillary assessment during neurological examination may become more difficult.

*Nalbuphine*

This is an injectable (subcutaneous, intramuscular or intravenous) synthetic opioid characterised by its minimal abuse potential. A dose of 10–20 mg is given every 3–6 h as necessary. Its analgesic effect and degree of respiratory depression are stated to be similar to those of morphine, while nausea and vomiting may be less. Reports of its clinical effect in hospital are varied, but pre-hospital use is reported to be safe and effective.

*Codeine Phosphate*

This is an opioid with good analgesic activity; 30–60 mg is given orally or intramuscularly every 4–6 h up to a maximum of 240 mg per day. Constipation and drowsiness may occasionally be problems.

## Inhalational Analgesia

Pre-mixed 50:50 nitrous oxide and oxygen (Entonox) has been a traditional analgesic in UK pre-hospital care for some 30 years. Its popularity is owing to its ease of administration and safety. The mixture is provided from on-demand valved cylinders and administered via a mask or mouthpiece. Overdose is unlikely as once a patient becomes drowsy they release the mouthpiece and their level of conscious-ness recovers.

Analgesia will peak some 2–5 min after inhalation, and this fact needs to be respected when Entenox is used to assist procedures such as patient extraction. Size D cylinders allow 20–30 min continuous use, the efficiency of which is improved by locating the demand valve at the patient's mouthpiece.

During storage, care must be taken to ensure that the temperature of the gas is not allowed to fall below –7°C because at this point separation of the gases can permit delivery of a hypoxic mixture.

When necessary, a cylinder can be re-warmed at 10°C for 2 h and then completely inverted three times (to mix the gases), or rapidly re-warmed by immersion in water at 37°C for 5 min and then inverted three times.

Entonox is contraindicated in decompression illness. It should also not be used in the presence of a pneumothorax unless there is a functioning chest drain in situ. Nitrous oxide diffuses out of the blood stream into gas-filled cavities (and bubbles) faster than nitrogen can be removed, causing an increase in pressure and volume within these spaces. Theoretically similar considerations apply to air collections within the cranial cavity of head-injured patients. In practice, Entenox should be safe for a casualty with mild concussion and pain from other injuries, particularly since it is likely to be given for a short time period.

### Combination Therapy

Drugs and techniques may be used in combination as they are in UK hospitals to manage post-operative pain. For example:

- for a casualty with a sprained ankle, use appropriate bandaging and support and supplement with regular oral analgesics;
- for a casualty with a fractured femur, use splinting to reduce pain and blood loss and a femoral nerve block with supplemental intramuscular or intravenous morphine.

## Anaesthesia

This chapter is not attempting to train people in providing anaesthesia. In the UK, anaesthesia is given by doctors who have undergone a period of specialised training. In parts of Europe and the USA, nursing staff are also trained as anaesthetists. In remote-area work in conflict and disaster settings, it is likely that non-specialists will be called on to provide anaesthesia. Recommended reading and sources of training are given in the reading section at the end of this chapter and in the Resources section.

Untrained people should not attempt anaesthetic techniques for the following reasons.

- Giving a general or regional anaesthetic to an unresuscitated patient may produce a catastrophic fall in blood pressure. Equipment for, and expertise in, resuscitation must be available.
- Drugs and techniques that alter a patient's consciousness level may result in the patient being unable to maintain their own airway, and becoming vulnerable to aspirating on regurgitated gastric contents or debris in their mouth or nose. Practitioners must have expertise in airway management and airway protection, and have equipment to hand to perform oro- and naso-pharyngeal suction.

## Local Anaesthesia

Local anaesthetic techniques can provide safe and effective analgesia in acute trauma. Regional anaesthesia is a local anaesthetic technique that removes sensation from a particular body region, e.g. using a nerve block for a limb or using spinal or epidural injections to numb the abdomen and legs.

There are a number of limitations to anaesthesia in pre-hospital and field conditions:

- personnel with the appropriate anatomical knowledge and training may not be available;
- preparation of the patient (resuscitation, positioning and access) is difficult;
- there may be insufficient time to perform the technique and wait for it to work;
- inadvertent toxic problems may be difficult to manage.

In practice, local anaesthesia will be used for certain specific purposes.

- Infiltration. Direct injection of local anaesthetic into the skin and subcutaneous tissues for wound exploration and suturing, or to assist practical procedures such as chest drain insertion.
- Nerve blocks. Certain blocks such as femoral nerve block (which can be performed quickly and safely, in some instances even during transport to hospital) or intercostal block to assist with chest drain placement or moving a casualty with fractured ribs.
- Haematoma blocks. Direct injection of a fracture haematoma is useful for certain limb fractures, particularly at the wrist.
- Specialised blocks. Less common and more specialised techniques such as caudal, epidural and spinal anaesthesia.

Local anaesthetic safety is a complex subject. The potential danger will vary according to the technique proposed, the patient's condition and the local anaesthetic selected.

Safety is maximised by ensuring that:

- an intravenous cannula has been sited in the casualty (to allow fluid resuscitation and treatment of allergic and toxic reactions to the local anaesthetic);
- accidental intra-vascular injection of local anaesthetic does not occur;
- the recommended maximum safety doses (MSD) relevant to nerve block and infiltration techniques are not exceeded.

Where practical, the use of solutions containing adrenaline (used to prolong the duration of action of a local anaesthetic) are best avoided, so that complications from systemic absorption of the adrenaline or incorrect injection into areas of vascular compromise cannot occur.

## Individual Local Anaesthetics

The figures given for MSD are approximations, and in practice they may need to be reduced depending on the condition of the patient and the techniques being used.

### Lignocaine

Lignocaine is a rapid acting synthetic amide available in 0.5, 1 or 2% concentrations with or without adrenaline (1:200,000 = a final concentration of 5 µg of adrenaline per ml). The MSD is 4 mg/kg body weight without adrenaline and 6 mg/kg body weight with adrenaline; 1% solutions are suitable for most infiltration and nerve block techniques.

### Bupivacaine

Bupivacaine is a long-acting amide with a slow onset of action. It is available in 0.125, 0.25, 0.5 and 0.75% concentrations with or without adrenaline. The MSD is 2 mg/kg body weight. Bupivacaine is widely used in hospital practice, but the advantage it affords by being long-acting must be balanced against its toxicity. *Cardio-respiratory collapse following accidental intravenous injection of bupivacaine may prove fatally resistant to resuscitation.*

## Selected Local Anaesthetic Procedures

Exact details of anatomy and technique should be studied from any of the standard texts on nerve blocks and regional anaesthesia.

### Femoral Nerve Block

This technique may be used to assist splinting or movement of an injured during leg extrication. A 3-cm, 23-gauge needle will be sufficient for non-obese patients. The nerve is frequently more superficial (1–1.5 cm deep) than is taught in some trauma skills courses. As a quick-onset analgesia is required, lignocaine is a suitable anaesthetic and bi-lateral blocks are permissible within the MSD. The local anaesthetic should be deposited in a fan-shaped distribution in order to accommodate the variable distances of the nerve lateral to the femoral artery. Careful aspiration prior to and during aspiration will ensure that inadvertent vascular injection does not occur.

### Peripheral Hand Blocks for the Hand

Ring blocks of digits or single nerve blocks at the wrist or ankle may occasionally be of value for individuals whose limbs are trapped in machinery. Do not use adrenaline.

### Haematoma Block for Reduction of Closed Fractures

This is useful when dealing with large numbers of casualties. Attention to sterile techniques is important to avoid introducing infection in the haematoma, and adrenaline-containing solutions should be avoided.

### Intercostal Nerve Block

This technique can be used to treat pain from fractured ribs. The practical danger is the risk of pneumothorax, and short, small-gauge needles must be employed. The authors have found intercostal nerve blocks helpful when placing chest drains in alert casualties.

### Caudal, Epidural and Spinal Anaesthesia

Caudal and epidural techniques have been used in field settings to provide post-operative analgesia. Spinal anaesthesia has been used to provide anaesthesia for lower-limb surgery. This should only be carried out when the patient has received adequate fluid resuscitation and can be given regular monitoring of pulse, blood pressure and consciousness level by a trained individual during the procedure.

## General Anaesthesia

The ability to conduct general anaesthesia in adverse conditions is limited both by the availability of trained personnel and by the lack of essential drugs and equipment, particularly in respect of inhalational anaesthesia with controlled ventilation. Preparation for these situations depends on specialist training courses, studying the experiences of others and personal experience.

Equipment for general anaesthesia broadly divides into:

- what can be carried by the anaesthetist (e.g. the man-portable Military Triservice Anaesthetic Apparatus);

- what can be found in-country (which will depend on the state of the hospital infrastructure, the state of maintenance of the equipment, and whether the anaesthetist is able to use this equipment);
- what can be imported for use, e.g. modular operating theatres brought in for a particular incident.

## Intravenous Anaesthesia

### Ketamine

Ketamine given intravenously produces dissociative anaesthesia. This is a pharmacological state characterised by dissociation from the normal conscious condition, associated in this case with intense surgical anaesthesia. When using ketamine, the upper airway reflexes remain more competent than with other sedative agents, but airway competence and protection cannot be assumed. Salivation increases after ketamine and suction may be required.

Respiratory depression is not usually a problem, although caution is necessary when narcotics or other potential central nervous depressants have been given.

Muscular relaxation is not pronounced and muscle tone may increase. This may limit the scope of surgical procedures that can be performed using ketamine alone, but otherwise the drug produces good conditions for moving patients, or performing surgery on musculo-skeletal injuries, or when repeated painful procedures such as dressing changes are necessary.

Ketamine's action on the sympathetic nervous system produces a tachycardia and hypertension. Blood pressure is usually maintained on induction of anaesthesia, although hypotension may occur in shocked patients.

Ketamine can cause an abrupt increase in intracranial pressure (ICP) in patients with intracranial pathology unless blood carbon dioxide levels can be controlled by artificial ventilation.

Ketamine given intravenously (1–2 mg/kg body weight over 60 s) normally produces some 10 min anaesthesia. An intramuscular dose of 10 mg/kg body weight should, after 5–10 min, produce 12–25 min surgical anaesthesia.

Using a solution of 10 mg/ml, the authors have used intravenous boluses of 10–20 mg (1–2 ml) in pre-hospital situations to allow gradual release and splinting of trapped limbs.

Recovery from ketamine anaesthesia can be associated with distressing emergence phenomena. These can be prevented or obtunded with small doses of short-acting intravenous benzodiazepines.

## Preparation and Further Reading

### Preparation

1. Anaesthesia in the UK for doctors.
   The Royal College of Anaesthetists, 48–49 Russell Square, London WC1B 4JY.

2.  Training for anaesthetists in anaesthesia for difficult locations.
    Courses run by the Departments of Anaesthesia at Frenchay Hospital, Bristol, and the Radcliffe Infirmary in Oxford.
3.  The recommendation is for qualified medical and nursing staff who are unfamiliar with pain management to arrange to spend time in a hospital post-operative recovery unit.

## Further Reading

Atkinson RS, Rushman GB, Alfred LJ. A synopsis of anaesthesia. 10th ed. Bristol: Wright, 1987.
British Medical Association and The Royal Pharmaceutical Society of Great Britain. British National Formulary (BNF). Updated every 6 months.
Dobson MB. Anaesthesia in the district hospital. Geneva: World Health Organisation, 1988.
Eriksson E. Illustrated handbook in local anaesthesia. 2nd ed. London: Lloyd-Luke, 1979.
Fenton PM. Africa anaesthesia. Malawi: Montford Press, 1993.
King M, editor. Primary anaesthesia. Oxford: Oxford University Press, 1986.

The Society of Apothecaries of London who run the Diploma in the Medical Care of Catastrophes examination have a library of candidate dissertations. Several of these are on the subject of anaesthesia under adverse circumstances.

## Related Topics in This Handbook

Part E of Ch. 20.
Part B of Ch. 8.

# Conclusion to Chapter 20

In this multi-part chapter we have tried to cover the more important issues likely to be encountered during a deployment. The potential of volunteers in terms of age, experience and specialist field has influenced the layout and content. To reiterate, the chapter is an attempt to heighten awareness and to act as a spur to further reading and study. A final word: field deployments in hostile environments are not places for the inexpert or inexperienced to "give it a go". If in doubt, always seek help – "first do no harm".

**EDITORS' NOTE** – see also the Resources section at the end of this manual.

# Trauma Life Support Training Courses

Advanced Trauma Life Support (ATLS©) courses. These courses are for physicians working in an emergency room (ER) environment.
Pre-Hospital Trauma Life Support (PHTLS) courses. These courses are for paramedics working in the pre-hospital or field environment.

Battlefield Advanced Trauma Life Support (BATLS©) courses. These courses are run by many NATO countries and are for military medical officers deploying on humanitarian and conflict missions.

Battlefield Advanced Resuscitation and Trauma Skills (BARTS©) courses. As above, but for non-medically qualified students.

Pre-Hospital Emergency Care (PHEC) course. A starting course for training in medical and trauma emergencies in the pre-hospital setting. For medical and non-medically qualified personnel.

Advanced Trauma Nursing Course (ATNC). Specifically for qualified nursing staff engaged in trauma care.

There are a myriad other advanced life-support courses concerned with care of children, burn victims and care of injured pregnant women.

# Aftermath

# 21. Conflict Recovery

Jim Ryan, Matthew Fleggson and Caroline Kennedy

| Objectives | • To introduce the concept of conflict recovery. |
|---|---|
| | • To describe transitions from acute response to long-term recovery. |
| | • To illustrate the situation with case examples. |
| | • To summarise the work of a university-based centre for conflict recovery. |

## Introduction

The bulk of this manual is concerned with activities during the acute phase in a hostile environment, whether it is as a result of war, conflict or a natural disaster. In a sense, this is the most attractive or glamorous period. There is typically widespread media coverage, and a myriad of aid organisations deploy and begin their work in the full glare of TV news cameras. The immediate aim of these agencies is to drive down mortality rates in ways that have been described in earlier chapters. These activities are exciting and telegenic, and occur at a time of maximum international interest and attention. This phase passes, and along with it goes media interest. Further, many of the aid agencies which specialise in acute-phase activities depart very quickly when the situation stabilises.

There now follows the post-emergency phase, which includes the transition to recovery. Money, equipment and skilled personnel, so abundant during the emergency response, become scarce. Budgets are cut, volunteer numbers are scaled down and vital equipment items are no longer supplied. The reasons for this are complex. The post-emergency phase is difficult and long-term, has little media attraction, may be dangerous and is usually hugely expensive. Yet this unattractive and open-ended phase is at least as important as the emergency response. It is this neglected aspect of medical care in hostile environments that this chapter attempts to examine.

This is a manual for health professionals, and this chapter reflects that. However, medical readers should be aware of the great importance of the many non-medical aspects of recovery. Key examples include major engineering projects and the restoration of civic structures.

The transition from acute response to recovery will vary and no one model exists. It may be lengthy, difficult, dangerous and multifaceted depending on the nature of the disaster or conflict. To simplify matters here, the recovery period will be divided into four phases and each of these will be illustrated with a single country case example. The periods are:

- transition phase;
- early phase;
- medium-term;
- long-term.

# Transition Phase

It is often a moot point when the emergency ends and recovery begins. The transition may be short and clear cut, or may be protracted with the distinctions blurred. An example of the problems encountered in the phase of transition is the Falkland Islands, a region with just over 2,000 inhabitants, in June 1982.

## Background

Prior to the Argentine invasion, medical care in the Falkland Islands was unique. A senior medical officer provided care with four general practitioners and 16 nurses and midwives, all based in the territory's only hospital, which was in the capital, Stanley. An outreach service was provided, and there was radio contact between the hospital and outlying community settlements. All doctors and nurses had specialist interests such as obstetrics and gynaecology or paediatrics, but there were no hospital specialists. Prior to the war, specialist consultation and treatment was provided from South American mainland hospitals in Buenos Aries and Montevideo.

## Falkland Islands – 1982

Readers should also refer to Dr. R. Diggles' work on the Falkland Islands in Ch. 5.

The situation in the Falkland Islands in early June 1982 is summarised below.

- Argentine troops invaded the Falkland Islands in April 1982, taking complete control of the territory.
- All public utilities, including medical, continued to function but under Argentine military control.
- The Governor and all officials were arrested and deported and a military ruling body was installed.
- The health service was taken over by military medical personnel.
- The only hospital was taken over and run as a joint civil/military hospital and a trauma surgical service was provided by military surgical teams.
- Some of the civilian medical staff were interned or deported; others were allowed to work.
- Control of estates, utilities and re-supply was vested in the Argentine military.

Following an invasion and a number of battles on land, sea and air, the Argentine military force surrendered, was briefly interned on the islands and later returned to Argentina.

With the cease-fire, the territory quickly entered a transition to recovery phase. The problems encountered are summarised below.

1.  Security and safety: in the absence of a local police or military force, security became the responsibility of the British military.
2.  Public and community health: the provision of clean water, food and shelter for the locals became the responsibility of environmental health specialists from the British Defence Medical Services (DMS).
3.  Primary health care was provided by joint DMS and civil primary care medical personnel working from the island's hospital. Medical advice to outlying settlements was provided over short-wave radios.
4.  Hospital utilities and health care: the DMS provided surgeons, anaesthetists, physicians and specialist nursing staff. The DMS also provided professionals allied to medicine (PAMs) in pharmacy, physiotherapy and environmental health. DMS nurses made good civilian nursing shortages.
5.  Other services and utilities: as an interim arrangement, British military personnel became responsible for other utilities such as engineering, communication, policing and education.

Transition back to civilian administration and government began within days and was largely uneventful. However, fundamental differences from the pre-war position were evident.

Three of the more striking differences were:

- the islands were now garrisoned with a force exceeding the indigenous population;
- the islands' hospital became de facto a joint civil and military facility with all secondary care provided by military medical teams;
- it was no longer possible to refer patients to Buenos Aires for a specialist opinion.

We will return to the Falklands in the final section of this chapter, and look at later conflict recovery problems.

# Early Phase

## Kosovo – 1999

Kosovo in the summer of 1999 is a good case example of the problems encountered during the early phase. There was a fairly clear-cut transition from the emergency phase (NATO entry and consolidation) to a well-defined early phase.

The situation in Kosovo in 1999 is summarised below.

NATO peacekeeping forces entered Kosovo in summer 1999.

The region had suffered from civil warfare, large-scale population displacement and a limited NATO bombing campaign.

Although de jure a part of the Federal Republic of Yugoslavia, it became de facto an independent state under international supervision.

The returning population faced damaged and destroyed housing and an infrastructure which was unable to cope.

There were many pressing tasks related to security, engineering, justice and medical care, to name but a few.

In the absence of a structure for governing the region, the UN Interim Administration became the government, with the World Health Organisation (WHO) taking over the health portfolio.

In this section we look at one particular problem by way of illustration – medical care provision at the region's only teaching hospital, the University Hospital Pristina. The measures taken are summarised below.

1. Securing and demilitarising the hospital and related facilities, which included the removal of blockades and occasional booby traps.
2. Restoration of power, water and sanitation. This included cleaning up a massive collection of dumped clinical waste, and a mortuary with bodies which had been dumped in corridors and in the entrance.
3. Dealing with medical and ancillary staff. Some unique problems existed:
   - most pre-existing staff (Serbs in the main) had fled;
   - most in-coming staff (Albanian) had no proof of identity or training, having been sacked by the Serbs in 1991;
   - most public records had been destroyed;
   - most clinical case records had been taken or destroyed;
   - a non-existent management structure;
   - medical school in a similar state.
4. Establishment of a hospital management and administrative system. Most key posts were initially held by ex-patriots to avoid conflict. Key appointments included:
   - Medical Director;
   - Hospital Administrative Officer;
   - Estates and Facilities Manager;
   - Management board.
5. Establishment of a medical provision and re-supply system.
6. Establishment of a post-graduate training programme.

The immediate task was to create a new health care system out of the surviving remnants of the pre-1999 Eastern European centralised model.

In parallel, the UN established other interim government departments to oversee the establishment of other vital services such as the provision of water, food and power. Later, an education department reintroduced schooling at primary, secondary and tertiary level.

These early-phase activities attracted considerable overseas and media interest, but not for long. There was a demand for early transition from external government to local control. In Kosovo this is not yet possible as the region remains without local structures and is also highly unstable.

In summary, the early recovery phase often involves a complete take-over of the levers and instruments of state, resulting in an almost totally dependent population. The length of this phase varies from very rapid in the case of the Falkland Islands in 1982 to protracted and unpredictable in the case of Kosovo and East Timor in 1999.

## Medium Term

It is not possible to give an accurate time scale for any of the phases under discussion. However, by medium term we mean that a phase has been reached where the afflicted region or territory has a government, however unstable, with a working (however poorly) infrastructure. Further, hostilities will have been at least suspended, although a long-term solution may not be in sight.

An example from the Caucasus is the Republic of Azerbaijan.

### Azerbaijan 1997–2001

This former Soviet republic, which is now independent, is situated on the western edge of the Caspian Sea. Surrounded by Russia to the north, Armenia to the west, Iran to the south and Turkey to the south-west, Azerbaijan faces the Caspian Sea but is otherwise a landlocked and partly blockaded country with a population of 7.7 million. Its problems are summarised below:

- 70 years of Soviet control;
- a territorial war with Armenia, which lasted about 5 years and is yet to be resolved;
- 20% loss of national territory;
- destruction of its industrial, agricultural and medico-social infrastructure;
- nearly 1 million refugees and internally displaced persons (IDPs) within its borders.

In 1997, the government of Azerbaijan requested the Leonard Cheshire Centre of Conflict Recovery (LCC), at University College London, to undertake a conflict recovery study focussing on medical conditions in three IDP camps in the south of Azerbaijan. The LCC's investigation revealed the difficulties experienced by refugees and IDPs in accessing secondary and tertiary hospital care, and a concomitant need for surgical aid.

The collapse of Azerbaijan's health system meant that patients could not gain access to free treatment. In addition, most regional hospitals were in dire need of the equipment and resources necessary to carry out routine operations. Primary health-care was available in the camps, but there was no provision for surgical treatment. In response to this situation, the LCC developed the Fast Track Referral System (FTRS) – an enabling programme for IDPs requiring general and traumatic surgery. This system had two principal, interrelated aims: to provide operations to patients who would otherwise be unable to afford them; to collate data regarding the medical conditions and requirements of a post-conflict setting in order to develop appropriate models of care.

Originally, the LCC sought to focus on life- and limb-saving operations. The programme later expanded to include a wider variety of conditions, such as hernias and burns, as it became apparent that such cases would otherwise remain untreated, and that surgery would dramatically improve the patients' quality of life. The LCC had to retain a flexible approach to case selection, and update its criteria regularly.

Inevitably, the LCC also had to realize the limits of its scope. Complex cardiac or cancer cases, for example, could not be taken on by the LCC – the costs of the treatment would have been prohibitive, and it was also doubtful whether the facilities for treating such cases effectively existed in Azerbaijan. Similarly, the LCC could not become involved in referring patients out of the country.

The FTRS depended on close links with government departments, teaching hospitals in Baku and NGOs. Foremost among this last group were the International Federation of Red Cross and Red Crescent Societies (IFRC) and the United Methodist Committee on Relief (UMCOR), which managed the IDP camps involved with the FTRS. These organisations cooperated closely with the LCC, referring patients for treatment and providing logistical support.

Patients were examined by visiting LCC medics in cooperation with local camp doctors. The LCC logistician, the only LCC expat in Azerbaijan, arranged operations for pre-selected patients at one of the FTRS's partner hospitals in Baku. The LCC paid for all the necessary medicines and consumables, as well as transport to and from the hospitals. Surgeons provided their services free of charge. The goodwill and cooperation of directors, surgeons, anaesthetists and nurses at the partner hospitals was essential to the running of the programme.

Local surgeons performed most FTRS operations. Where the expertise was unavailable within the country, the LCC arranged for specialist surgeons to visit Azerbaijan. Even in these cases though, visiting surgeons worked alongside their Azeri counterparts, as well as with local teams of anaesthetists and nurses. Visits by physiotherapists were also arranged.

One of the essential features of the FTRS was that it enabled local medical staff to treat their own population. Many patients in Azerbaijan cannot afford hospital treatment; consequently hospitals tend to be underused, and morale among medical staff is low. The FTRS also provided contacts between local and visiting nurses, physiotherapists, anaesthetists and surgeons – a stimulus both for Azeri health professionals, largely isolated from medical centres in other countries, and their visitors, who gained experience of practising their profession in a post-conflict setting.

Medical decisions regarding the FTRS were not imposed from outside, but worked out within the context and constraints of the local health system. This had several benefits – the decisions were more likely to be viable, easier to implement over a longer period, and cheaper, ensuring the optimal use of donor money. Also, having evolved within a post-conflict setting (rather than having been developed within the UK), the FTRS could be adapted to similar situations in other post-conflict countries.

Once the programme had been well established, the daily management of the FTRS was handed over to a new organisation composed of former local employees. In preparation for the handover, the new Programme Manager and Coordinator travelled to London to receive appropriate management training. A transition period followed, during which the LCC provided managerial and financial support to the new organisation, giving it time to adapt gradually to its responsibilities.

The surgical aid programme has been amended to make the most of local medical contacts in the hospitals and IDP camps. Surgeons from partner hospitals now conduct surgeries in the camps themselves, giving them a greater degree of responsibility and involvement. This arrangement has also made the system of referring patients more effective.

The hand over of the programme to a local organisation was vital for its sustainability. The LCC lacked the necessary resources to run the programme indefinitely, and the FTRS had developed to such an extent that it could only be managed effectively within the country. The programme needed to be allied more closely to the local health system, through contacts with government departments and local hospitals, in order to improve its chances of long-term survival. In effect, it was important that all those involved with the FTRS shared a sense of ownership of the programme.

As well as being of immediate humanitarian benefit, the FTRS also has the potential to be a useful model for those involved with conflict recovery. In accordance with its original aim, the LCC has begun work on an academic paper on the FTRS. This paper will constitute a useful source of reference and information on the medical requirements of an IDP population, and contribute towards the study of conflict medicine in general.

The project described gives some insight into the often intractable problems which remain after the acute phase has passed.

In summary, the LCC's mission in Azerbaijan emphasised the importance of the following tasks.

- Conducting an initial needs assessment, including a survey of services already provided by NGOs.
- Developing and maintaining good contacts with local government departments and NGOs.
- Promoting contacts between UK and Azeri medics.
- Keeping the programme's aims flexible, and recognising its limitations.
- Planning in advance a phased withdrawal, including a period of long-distance monitoring and support.
- Training local staff to take over the programme.
- Considering the programme's sustainability from the outset – for example, by involving local medical and non-medical staff as much as possible.

# Long Term

Long-term recovery should have as its end point a return to *pre-conflcit* or *pre-catastrophe* conditions, or perhaps a move towards an improved position. That process may take years, and in some cases the target is never reached. The long-term effects of conflict or catastrophe can be manifested in unusual and unexpected ways. To illustrate a long-term problem which was not anticipated, we return to the Falkland Islands in spring 2000 to close the loop, not only on the Islands, but also on this chapter.

In the years following the war, the Falkland Islands were restored to normality. A major re-building programme removed most of the scars of war, and a new 32-bed hospital was built to provide a national health service. The hospital continued to be a mixed civil/military facility, with the surgical, anaesthetic and intensive care support provided by military teams on roulemont tours of 4–6 months. This appeared to remove the pre-war problem of the provision of surgical support from abroad, and few people now required transfer to South America. The system worked well and was backed up by specialist visits from the United Kingdom and by an aero-medical evacuation facility for those requiring tertiary care.

This civil/military model of secondary health care seemed set to continue long-term. However, problems surfaced in the mid-1990s following a defence costs study which closed most of the military hospitals in the UK, and resulted in a drastic reduction in the numbers of secondary-care medical personnel. By 2000, the Falkland Islands government was forced to accept the complete withdrawal of military personnel from the hospital. At first sight, replacing military medical personnel with civilians was expected to be easy, but on more careful study, serious problems surfaced.

A return to the pre-war medical system could not be contemplated. A population which by now was highly sophisticated and well informed expected a standard of health care which was equivalent to that of the National Health Service in the UK. The recruitment of civilian equivalents was not straightforward.

- Subspecialisiation in the developed world had removed a previously existing group of multiskilled doctors, nurses and professionals allied to medicine (PAMs).
- Other than military medics, few doctors would wish to take on single-handed posts with a 24-hour on-call commitment.

A novel solution was reached, and the main points are summarised below.

- The appointment of medical advisors with a background in medicine in conflict and catastrophe situations to advise the government.
- An acceptance that single-handed secondary-care specialists cannot provide the level of care found in the developed world.
- An agreement on the minimum standards to be provided. For example, any surgeon appointed should be able to deal with most common life- and limb-threatening emergencies.

- A world-wide advertising campaign, in recognition of the fact that few people in the developed world would have the necessary skills and training for such posts.
- The establishment of a telemedicine consultation link to tertiary centres in the UK.
- Tours of duty should be limited to 4–6 months in recognition of the fact that the provision of 24-hour cover for longer periods is unacceptable in the twenty-first century.
- An audit process should be built in to assess performance.

The Falklands example highlights some important principles which are common to the late recovery phase.

- What may be acceptable to a population during and immediately after a conflict may not be acceptable in the longer term. Populations are increasingly well informed and have high expectations.
- In planning a model of health care, distinctions need to be made between the "wants" of a population and their actual "needs".
- The reliance on military assistance with recovery programmes is fraught with risk. Aid agencies have little control over military assets and they may be withdrawn with little or any notice.
- Medical training in developed societies is increasingly less suited to the needs of medical personnel in conflict and conflict-recovery settings.

## Development

Before concluding, a word about development. This is a huge topic which deserves a book in its own right. There is pretty well universal agreement within the humanitarian aid community that the transition from emergency aid programmes to long-term development programmes is fraught with difficulty.

Part of the problem is reaching an agreement on meaning and definition. So far in this chapter we have talked about the early, medium and late phases of conflict recovery. Where does development fit into this construct? Are recovery and development the same thing?

The United Nations Declaration on the Right to Development, resolution 41/128, 4 December 1986, provides a definition of development.

> *Development is a comprehensive, social, cultural and political process, which aims at the constant improvement of the well-being of the entire population and of all individuals on the basis of their active, free and meaningful participation in development and in the fair distribution of benefits resulting therefrom.*

It would therefore seem that for the development phase to commence, a high degree of stability must exist, and the restoration of institutions and instruments of government must have occurred. There is the risk that development will be attempted before recovery is sufficiently complete. This was well illustrated in Kosovo during

1999. The beginning of the medical development programme had to be delayed because insufficient recovery had taken place. This situation will cause friction. Donor and Western governments are keen to move to development programmes as soon as possible, and long term, they may be cheaper than acute recovery programmes. However, if begun too soon, they will fail.

# Conclusions

This chapter has highlighted a neglected topic, i.e. care beyond the acute and exciting emergency phase. Yet recovery and development are mandatory if the affected society is to have any hope of a return to normal.

## Acknowledgements

The following individuals and organisations have been involved in the LCC's conflict recovery missions. The authors of this chapter wish to acknowledge their immense contribution and support.

UK

Mr. John Beavis
Richard Black
Mr. Peter Budney
Dr. Richard Bunsell
Gwen Burchell
Ms Jamila Christie
Ms Annie Cornforth
Dr. Judith Darmady
Sister Alison Finch
Ms. Sally Forrest
Cameron Gazijev
Edward Harris
Velda Harris
Namik Kamranov
Caroline Kennedy
Sister Shirley Ludlow
Staff Nurse Elizabeth Ludlow
Cara Macnab
Dr. Peter Mahoney
His Excellency Ambassador Mahmud Mamed-Kuliev
The nursing staff of Stoke Mandeville Hospital
Dr. Annie McGuinness
Mr. Anthony Roberts

Emma Ryan and all involved with the Drama Education Programme
Sister Catherine Ryan
Sister Zeb Seers
Richard Slater
The Lord and Lady Swinfen
Katrina Vaughan
Sir Patrick Walker
A Trust wishing to remain anonymous
Azerbaijan Airlines
Leonard Cheshire and Leonard Cheshire International
The Anglo-Azeri Society
The Swinfen Charitable Trust
University College London and University College London Hospital

AZERBAIJAN

Dr. Fuad Abasov
Dr. Seving Abduayeva
Fazil Alekperov
Mehriban Alekperova
Dr. Humar Annagiyeva
Professor Akshin Bagirov
Shahnaz Bakhshaliyeva
Ramsan Gasimov
Dr. Bayram Gorchiyev
Ali Hasanov
Dr. Qafar Jafarov
Dr. Vagif Jafarov
Dr. Fariz Jamalov
Professor Fikret Kafarov
Professor Alekber Kerimov
Dr. Sannam Kerimova
Dr. Azer Khudiyev
Dr. Cafar Mammedov
Ilham Mazanli
Sevinj Rzayeva
The nursing and anaesthetic staff of partner hospitals in Baku
The doctors and nurses in the camps
IFRC – Azerbaijan
UMCOR – Azerbaijan
United Aid for Azerbaijan

# 22. Hard Knocks and Hard Lessons

Jim Ryan, John Beavis and Tony Redmond

- To heighten awareness of traps and pitfalls.
- To describe common and recurring problems.
- To emphasise the need for an avoidance strategy.

## Introduction

This section of the handbook concludes with a chapter describing the more important pitfalls that face the health professional deployed in a hostile environment. No attempt is made to list or describe every single adverse event that might occur – that would merit a complete text in its own right. What we describe are "the big ones"! These are the problems that beset aid operations again and again. Most of these events are predictable and preventable. The other ambition in this section is to emphasise that lessons can be learnt from taking hard knocks, and these lessons need wide dissemination to the vast number of youthful and inexperienced volunteers waiting in the wings for their first overseas deployment.

## Hard Knocks and Hard Lessons

To give a sense of structure the lessons are listed and described in roughly chronological fashion, starting with hard knocks relating to poor planning and preparation, moving to adverse events during the emergency phase, and concluding with risks relating to the transition to recovery, the post-emergency phase and the return home.

### Pre-Deployment Phase

#### Square Pegs in Round Holes

Two surgeons were recruited by an aid agency for an emergency deployment to Central Africa. On arrival, there were other surgeons in the field but only one anaesthetist. Worse, there were no suitable facilities with which to operate. The aid agency redeployed the surgeons as primary care doctors, where they were required to see and manage ill children, provide antenatal care in advanced pregnancy, and manage

> **Lesson:** The lesson here is to ensure that if you are deployed as a specialist, the appropriate specialist infrastructure and logistic support is in place. Surgeons deprived of their operating theatres are like fish out of water!

ill and vulnerable elderly patients. In an age of specialisation, neither surgeon felt competent, which led to ill will and a wasted trip.

### Squeezing Blood out of a Stone

This case example relates to a consultant physician who wished to do something for his fellow human beings during the Bosnia crisis. An aid agency despatched him to a hospital in Bosnia with the aim of providing short holidays for local physicians who had worked for months without a break. A 4-week tour of duty was agreed. No political or situation brief was given, and no equipment of any kind was provided. On arrival, he was taken to the designated hospital. This was a front-line hospital subject to daily shelling and sniper fire. He was warmly welcomed and was presented with a holiday roster indicating that the local doctors would each in turn take 2 weeks' leave. The roster covered a 3-month period, which was the period they expected the visiting doctor to stay. He indicated that a 4-week tour of duty had been agreed in London. This led to anger and hostility. Trouble was avoided when he compromised and agreed to stay for 6 weeks and to find a colleague to come for a further 6 weeks. During his 6 weeks' deployment he worked a 12-h day, 7 days a week. On return home he developed a stress-related illness and was on sick leave for a period.

> **Lesson:** The lesson here is not to deploy without a full briefing on the nature of the deployment, the working conditions and the end-of-tour date. Ideally, get a return ticket before you go. Finally, avoid deployment as a singleton – go with a mate or mates if you can.

## Travelling and Arriving

### "Papers Please"

A volunteer arrived in part of the former Soviet Union to join an aid mission. He had among his possessions a comprehensive medical pack for self-use. Included in this was a range of prescription medicines, syringes and needles. While his passport and visa were in order, he had neither a packing list for the medical equipment nor a letter of authorisation. He was accused of smuggling medicines into the country and was threatened with arrest and imprisonment. The equipment was confiscated, and he was only allowed to leave after a considerable delay and following intercession by his deploying agency.

> **Lesson:** Documentation requirements vary from country to country. With medicines and medical equipment, have full packing lists, a letter of authorisation, and, if necessary, import licenses.

### Lost and Abandoned!

A medical advisor arrived to join his agency in the Balkans. On arrival at the airport his instructions were to wait for an agency vehicle and driver. Impatient after an hour-long wait, he hailed a taxi despite being unfamiliar with the territory. He was driven around for a considerable period, and then driven down a side street where he was robbed of his money, credit cards and passport.

> **Lesson:** Before travelling to potentially hostile destinations, make sure you have local addresses and contact telephone numbers. If a driver fails to turn up, phone the agency. If it is out of hours, contact the airport authority or the police. If all else fails, look for vehicles from other agencies. (In conflict settings, aid agency vehicles are usually easy to identify.) Do not travel alone in taxis in unfamiliar environments, and do not take lifts from strangers.

## Deployment

### Promise Nothing

Aid agency personnel are frequently shown hospitality by government agencies and other officials. In the Balkans and the Caucasus, such hospitality takes the form of lengthy dinners and liberal amounts of alcohol. Officials may take the opportunity to cajole agency personnel to widen their projects or promise additional input to their activities. The authors of this chapter have all experienced this. Remember, an offer to think about it will be misconstrued, and statements like "I will try" become "I promise". This can, and has, led to embarrassment and confrontation in the following days.

> **Lesson:** When under pressure from local officials, stay on guard and watch your language. If possible, decline hospitality associated with lengthy meals and copious quantities of alcohol. Try to avoid accepting gifts from officials. If pressed, accept on behalf of your agency and report the gift to your headquarters. Drink moderately or not all – if necessary, blame a stomach upset.

### Sweets for the Children

One of the authors was on a joint mission with an aid agency from the Far East. On a visit to a large group of internally displaced persons (IDPs) situated in an inner-city slum, agency personnel loaded the boot of their vehicle with sweets. At the end of the visit they attempted to get the children into orderly lines to hand out sweets. Hundreds of children appeared and formed an unruly mob. There were not enough sweets for all of them. Older boys grabbed the lion's share and took sweets from girls and smaller children. A riot ensued, joined by hostile parents. Buckets of water and rotting garbage were thrown over the well-meaning agency personnel who had to beat a hasty retreat. The noise of crying children was unforgettable. A distressed agency member said: "children in our country would have queued and shared equally".

> **Lesson:** Beware of giving or promising gifts. In displaced communities, the strong will often take from the weak, leading to distress and fighting. If you must, give small gifts or sweets to camp leaders who will know how best to allocate them.

### Failure to Communicate – Mission Creep

Many agencies will deploy outreach teams, and problems with communication and "command and control" may arise. An agency with a long-term medical development programme had personnel deployed in an IDP/refugee camp a considerable distance from their headquarters and logistic base. Communication with the base was impossible. Resident agency volunteers, on their own initiative, organised an income-generating activity involving local women knitting and weaving products for sale. It was a worthy activity, but no market research was possible and in the end no outlets could be found for the products. Disappointment and embarrassment ensued.

> **Lesson:** Have clear aims and objectives from the outset. Consult with agency coordinating personnel before embarking on any new activity. While fully appreciating local pressure "to do something", departure from the original mission nearly always ends in tears.

### Do not Become a Casualty Yourself

A middle-aged doctor deployed into a remote setting. He had long-standing peptic ulcer disease, but had been free of symptoms for years and was not on any medication. During a particularly stressful period he developed severe abdominal pain and after some days had an episode of haematemesis (vomiting fresh blood). He had to be evacuated under very arduous conditions. Fortunately, he arrived home safely for treatment of his reactivated peptic ulcer disease.

> **Lesson:** Chronic diseases are prone to relapse under stressful conditions. Ideally, such personnel should not deploy, particularly to remote settings where access to medical help is difficult. If deployment is essential, take appropriate medication. Careful medical screening should be routine before any deployment.

## Medevac

This is a perennial and often heart-rending problem. After wars and conflict where normal medical resources are destroyed, large numbers of individuals will require reconstructive surgery or treatment for lethal conditions such as cancer, and will seek to be sent abroad for treatment. The emotional pressure can be overwhelming. We are aware of one child, a double amputee, who was evacuated through unofficial channels. On arrival in the receiving country, few of the promised arrangements were in place and a cascade of problems ensued, encompassing interpreters, accommodation, treatment costs and long-term care.

> **Lesson:** Casevac is not just a question of taking someone out of a country. There is a whole series of events that need to be considered. Leave casevac to the experts. An international organisation, notably the World Health Organisation, will normally take this task on. Avoid involvement and make no promises.

## War Tourism

On longer deployments it is usual to grant volunteers some mid-mission rest and recreation. A young volunteer took the opportunity to join a locally employed colleague to tour the mountains by car. Without his knowledge, they approached the border area adjacent to a neighbouring country where special travel permits were required for foreigners. Frontier Police arrested him, which was fortunate as the area was notorious for assaults and kidnapping by local warlords. After a brief incarceration he was released unharmed.

**Lesson:** Aid agencies routinely work in hostile environments. Aid agency personnel are increasingly vulnerable to attack, which is often politically motivated. If you wish to visit other parts of the country in which you are deployed, take expert advice and be aware of restrictions and prohibited places. Plan a route and inform your agency – provide them with route maps and expected timings. You should always travel with a radio and keep in contact at regular intervals.

## Map Reading

This connects with the lesson above. A group of medical aid workers with some time off decided to explore the local countryside. One of them had been in the military and fancied his map-reading skills, and he offered to guide the group to a local beauty spot. Within a very short time the group were hopelessly lost, and without realising it they drove into an area which had been the scene of recent fighting. They were directed out by a friendly military patrol.

**Lesson:** Overconfidence can lead to trouble. Know your limitations and do not attempt to explore in potentially dangerous areas.

## No Place for Rambo

A group of aid workers were stopped at a roadblock. Some of them were wearing military-style clothing, which led to a confrontation with the police. The aid personnel became aggressive towards the police, leading to a brief period of arrest.

**Lesson:** Aid workers should avoid military-style clothing, particularly in countries with militias and irregular groups which are similarly attired. In addition, when stopped at roadblocks or checkpoints, behave in a quiet and civil manner and obey all reasonable instructions. Carry a radio and inform your base.

## Unwelcome Souvenirs

Conflict and catastrophe environments are often associated with pandemic venereal disease, including HIV. There are countless reports of aid workers visiting prostitutes, often after consuming alcohol. The price is often a multi-drug-resistant venereal disease, and at worst, AIDS.

> **Lesson:** Pre-deployment briefings must include a risk analysis for venereal disease. Sexual contact with strangers during deployment must be avoided. Any form of sexual contact should be accompanied by avoidance measures such as the use of condoms.

## Alcohol and Driving

The greatest risk to a deployed volunteer is a road traffic accident, and these are usually associated with alcohol. All major agencies have experience of personnel being injured and sometimes killed in road traffic accidents. Equally, the boorish and noisy behaviour often associated with alcohol consumption will cause offence and resentment. Such behaviour may also lead to arrest and imprisonment.

> **Lesson:** Let locally employed personnel do the driving. They will know the roads and local driving conditions. If you must drive, abstinence from alcohol is mandatory. The local police usually take an extreme view of foreigners who are involved in driving incidents.

## Baring the Flesh

Many societies afflicted by war and disaster will have social norms and taboos concerning dress and public behaviour. Not only may people wearing inappropriate clothing cause scandal and offence, they may also undermine the status and projects of other aid workers.

> **Lesson:** Be aware of local customs and taboos before deployment. Behave with dignity and humility. Exhibitions of group drunkenness should be particularly avoided.

## Professional Preparation

A surgical team, consisting of two consultants, a specialist registrar and theatre staff, arrived in a Bosnian city during the recent war. They had expected to deal with acute major trauma, but were confronted with complex delayed complications of severe war injuries. The problems included nerve reconstruction, tendon transplants and severe bone non-union with infection. Much of this work was outside their experience and they could offer only theoretical advice in many cases. The local surgeons were not impressed and it took several visits, with increasing activity by one of the consultants, before their confidence was restored. A decision was made to deploy the returning consultants to assess patients each time before other specialists visited the city.

> **Lesson:** Reconnaissance is essential before sophisticated medical teams deploy to a war or disaster area. The individuals within teams are representatives of their country, their profession and their agency. It is imperative that the teams are made up of people with precise and relevant skills.

## Going Home

### Mission Endpoint

Withdrawal from a mission is often fraught with difficulty, particularly after longer-term development deployments. All too often, missions appear to end abruptly, with agency personnel appearing to retreat to the departure airport with indecent haste. Quite apart from local disappointment and disillusionment, agencies and individuals may suffer considerable loss of reputation and prestige. The authors have experience of some agencies virtually fleeing in the night.

> **Lesson:** All missions should have a clear endpoint and a departure strategy planned in advance. Careful thought must be given to handing over an on-going mission to another agency or to a local group. This requires considerable planning, has financial implications and may involve "long reach" support for a period of time following the return home.

### Overwhelmed

Deployments are often hazardous and fatiguing. Youthful and enthusiastic volunteers frequently overstretch themselves without realising they are doing so. An immediate return to work and normal activity is often associated with illness, including both physical and stress-related disorders.

> **Lesson:** Pace yourself. Be aware of post-deployment fatigue and stress. Take a significant break, even a formal holiday, after a mission. Seek expert help – see below.

## Debrief and Health Check

Most major agencies have a policy on post-deployment debriefing and health checks. Individuals deploying alone who are not picked up on their return home face the greatest danger. Many conditions, including stress reactions, may take time before manifesting. One of the authors of this chapter developed malaria 3 weeks after returning home from a mission in East Africa.

> **Lesson:** The mission does not end on your return home. Debriefing and post-mission health checks are vital. Check that these will happen before deployment. Many illnesses have long incubation periods, requiring continuing prophylaxis and review.

## Post-deployment Visits, or "Return Matches"

This links to the "promise nothing" tale above. Many local health professionals will ask for an opportunity to visit your home country or institution. A senior medical colleague on a visit to a major hospital in a conflict area mentioned that it would be nice for local colleagues to attend a forthcoming medical conference in his home country – a perfectly reasonable consideration. He provided a letter of invitation to facilitate visa applications. A number of surgeons arrived with no money and very little luggage. The doctor who issued the invitation found himself picking up bills for hotel accommodation, travel and conference fees running into thousands of dollars.

> **Lesson:** Visits to overseas conferences are important for impoverished and isolated colleagues. They often have much to teach us. Plan invitations properly and arrange funding. Do not make idle promises – much disappointment and resentment will result when the promise cannot be met.

## No Partner, No Job

We are familiar with individuals who have arrived home to be faced with irate partners and/or employers. Cases of separation, divorce and sacking are not uncommon.

# Conclusions

Aid missions in hostile environments are fraught with traps and pitfalls. Most are well known and you should be aware of them. They may involve individuals,

**Lesson:** The lesson begins before deployment and continues during deployment. In our experience, it is of the utmost importance that your partner consents to your mission. Agree not just on the deployment, but also on the duration and means of access in an emergency. Put all your administrative affairs in order before you go. If necessary, arrange for power of attorney in legal and business areas. Work out means of regular communication – modern technology allows contact even in the most remote settings. Also seek the consent and support of your employer and consider the impact of deploying on professional training programmes. Finally, if mission overshoot is beyond your control, communicate that fact early.

an agency or even groups of agencies. Careful preparation and pre-deployment briefing will prevent most of the pitfalls. An avoidance strategy and a high degree of awareness are recommended.

Further reading on this subject can be found in the Resources section. A browse through the relevant web sites is particularly recommended.

## Acknowledgements

The editors would like to thank the following people for their input and advice with this chapter: Jack Beavis, Richard Black, David Childs, Matthew Fleggson, Ed Harris, Alan Hawley, Caroline Kennedy, Pete Mahoney, Tony Redmond, Jim Ryan, Zeb Seers and Richard Slater.

# Resources

**Objectives**

- To direct the reader to specialist literature.
- To advise on essential check-lists for medicines and equipment items.
- To direct the reader to a growing number of useful web sites.

## Introduction to Section Five

This handbook has already been described as a point of entry to the topic of medical care in hostile environments, which is a vast subject. It is hoped that the handbook will raise awareness of the topic, and direct readers to acquire in-depth knowledge of areas particular to their current or future deployments. Knowledge in depth has traditionally been found by consulting standard textbooks. However, there are now a myriad sources. This section is intended to act as a guide for readers in their quest for further information.

# 23. Publications

Jim Ryan, Peter Mahoney and A. J. Thomas

## Introduction

The publications listed here are over and above the references and further reading lists found at the end of many of the chapters in this handbook.

A browse through a specialist bookshop will indicate the sheer volume of publications dealing with the subject matter of this manual. The questions are what to read, what to buy, and perhaps what to take on deployment. Publications covering topics in the field of medical care in hostile environments subdivide into clearly recognisable categories.

## Categories

The following classification is fairly universal.

### Reference Texts

These are usually large, specialised, often hardback and frequently expensive. Larger, multi-author texts may be 3–4 years in preparation, and some information may already be out of date on publication. Nevertheless, they are usually the best source of core knowledge and in-depth information. For the impecunious aid worker they are best not purchased, but consulted in a local medical or general library.

### Handbooks, Manuals and Vade Mecums

These may be specialist or general. They are usually affordable, but are often hard to access. Many are weather-proofed and suitable to take on deployment. Shorter production times mean they are usually up to date.

### Journal Articles

These include reviews, and scientific and evidence-based papers. Also included are editorials and reviews on single topics. As a rule they are the best source of most recent information. Many are listed at the end of individual chapters.

## Monographs and Position Papers

Many of these are produced by individual aid agencies, often in-house, and may be difficult to access. They tend to be mission- or specialist-topic-related.

## Mission Reports

These are usually produced by aid agencies and cover the period of a specific mission. They are not always widely available, but are increasingly found on agency websites.

## Guidelines and Schedules

A huge and increasing spectrum is covered. They come from a variety of sources, including academic, government and agency sources, and are increasingly available.

## Pamphlets and Booklets

These are produced by a variety of agencies, including government and non-government organisations. They typically contain general advice on specific topics such as vaccination requirements and protection against communicable disease.

# Recommended Publications

These are in addition to the reading material suggested at the end of some of the chapters. We do not recommend that every health worker about to deploy should spend their time perusing every publication recommended. People's skills and needs vary, as will their need for further reading. The list includes material that the authors and their colleagues have found useful, but it is far from complete. It is very satisfying to see the literature in this field grow, almost by the week.

We recommend that the reader merely browse and pause where they wish.

## Reference Texts

### Politics

World politics – trends and transformation, 7th edition. C.W. Kegley, E.R. Wittkopf. Macmillan, London, 1999. ISBN 0 312 16657 5.

### Preventive Medicine

Disease control – priorities in developing countries. A World Bank Book. D.T. Jamison et al., editors. Oxford Medical Publishers, Oxford, 1993. ISBN 0 19 520990 7.

## Psychological Medicine

Critical incident stress debriefing. F. Parkinson. Souvenir Press, London, 1998. ISBN 0 285 63372 4.

## Terrorism

Protecting against terrorism: analysis and counter strategies. A. Scotti. Butterworth–Heinemann, Oxford, 1994. ISBN 0 75069212 X.

## Torture

Guidelines for the examination of survivors of torture, 2nd edition. Produced by the Medical Foundation for the Care of Victims of Torture, 96–98 Grafton Road, London NW5 3EJ, UK. No ISBN number. Web address: www.torturecare.org.uk

## Trauma

Ballistic trauma – clinical relevance in peace and war. J.M. Ryan, N.M. Rich et al., editors. Arnold, London, 1997.

Emergency care – a textbook for paramedics. I. Greaves, T. Hodgetts, K. Porter. Saunders, Philadelphia, 1997. ISBN 0 7020 1975 5.

Short practice of surgery, 23rd edition. R.C.G. Russell, N.S. Williams, C.J.K. Bullstrode, editors. Arnold, London, 2000. ISBN 0 340 75924 0 (hb).

Trauma care manual. I. Greaves, K. Porter, J.M. Ryan, editors. Arnold, London, 2001. ISNB 0 340 75979 8.

War wounds of limbs – surgical management. R.M. Coupland. Butterworth–Heinemann, Oxford, 1993.

## Tropical Diseases

Atlas of medical helminthology and protozoology, 4th edition. P.L. Chiodini, A.H. Moody, D.W. Mansen. Churchill Livingstone, Edinburgh, 2001. ISBN 0 443 06267 6.

Lecture notes on tropical medicine. Bell. Blackwell, Oxford, 1991. ISBN 0 63202455 0.

Manson's tropical diseases. G.C. Cook et al., editors. Saunders, Philadelphia, 1996. ISBN 070201764 7.

Medical zoology for travellers, 3rd edition. J. Hull Grundy. Noble Books, Lyd, UK, 1979. ISBN 0 906949 00 9.

## Handbooks and Related Publications

ABC of AIDS. M.W. Adler. BMJ Publishing, London, 1997. ISBN 0 72791137 6.

ABC of healthy travel, 5th edition. E. Walker et al., editors. BMJ Publishing, London, 1997. ISBN 0-7279-1138-4.

ABC of major trauma. P. Driscoll et al., editors. BMJ Publishing, London, 2000. ISBN 0 7279 1378 6.

ABC of sexually transmitted diseases. M.W. Adler. BMJ Publishing, London, 1998. ISBN 0 72791368 9.

Acute medicine – a practical guide to the management of medical emergencies, 2nd edition. D. Sprigings et al. Blackwell Science, Oxford, 1997. ISBN 0-632-03652-4.

Control of communicable disease manual. J.E. Chin. American Public Health Association (APHA), USA, 2000. ISBN 0 87553 242 X.

Engineering in emergencies – a practical guide for relief workers. J. Davis, R. Lambert. IT Publications, London, 1997. ISBN 1 85339 222 7.

Major incident medical management and support. Advanced life support group. BMJ Publishing, London, 1995. ISBN 0-7279-0928-2.

Questioning the solution – the politics of primary health care and child survival. D. Werner, D. Sanders. Healthwrights, California, 1997. ISBN 0-9655585-2-5.

Refugee health – an approach to emergency situations. Médicins Sans Frontières. Macmillan, London, 1997. ISBN 0333 72210 8.

Surgery for victims of war. D. Dufour et al. ICRC Publications, Geneva, 1988. ISBN 2-88145-010-5.

The medics guide to working electives around the world. M. Wilson. Arnold, London, 2000. ISBN 0 340 76098 2 (pb).

The Oxfam handbook of development and relief. 3 volumes. Oxfam, Oxford, 1995. ISBN 0 85598 274 8.

The Sphere Project: humanitarian charter and minimum standards in disaster response. 1st edition. Sphere Project, Geneva. ISBN 92 9139 049 6

The travel and tropical medicine manual, 6th edition. J. McCullen. Saunders, Philadelphia, 1995. ISBN 0 7216 4214 4.

The travellers good health guide. T. Lankester. Sheldon, London, 1999. ISBN 0 85969 827 0.

Travellers health, 3rd edition. R. Dawood. Oxford University Press, Oxford, 1997. ISBN 019 262247 1.

War and public health. P. Perrin. International Committee of the Red Cross, Geneva, 1996. ISBN 2 88145 0776.

Where there is no doctor – a village health care handbook. D. Werner. Macmillan, London, 1993. ISBN 0 333-51651-6.

Where there is no doctor – a village health care handbook for Africa, revised edition. D. Werner. Macmillan, London, 1993. ISBN 0 333-51652-4.

Where women have no doctor – a health guide for women. A. August Brown et al. Mcmillan, London, 1997. ISBN 0 333 64933 8.

## Guidelines and Schedules

British national formulary. Published jointly by the British Medical Association and the Royal Pharmaceutical Society of Great Britain. Regularly updated. ISBN 0 85369438 0.

Clinical guidelines – diagnostic and treatment manual, 3rd edition. Médicins Sans Frontièrs, Paris, 1993. ISBN 2 218 03480 0.

Essential drugs – practical guidelines. Médicins Sans Frontièrs, 1993. ISBN 2 218 02651 1.

Guide of kits and emergency items – decision maker guide, 4th English edition. Médicins Sans Frontières, 1997. No ISBN number.

Minor surgical procedures in remote areas. Médicins Sans Frontières, 1989. ISBN 2 218 02163 3.

Monthly index of medical specialities (MIMS). Haymarket Medical, London, regularly updated. Tel. +44(0)20 7938 0705.

Nutrition guidelines. Médicins Sans Frontières, 1995. No ISBN number.

The medic's guide to work and electives around the world. M. Wilson. Arnold, London, 2000. ISBN 0 340 76098 2 (pb).

## Pamphlets and Booklets

Health advice for travellers. Leaflet T6, 1998. Department of Health, UK, PO Box 410, Wetherby, LS29 7LM.

Health information for overseas travel. Yellow Book, 1995. Department of Health, UK. PO Box 410, Wetherby, LS29 7LM. Available from HMSO, London.

Immunisations against infectious diseases. Green Book, 1996. Department of Health, UK. PO Box 410, Wetherby, LS29 7LM. Available from HMSO, London.

International travel and health, 1996. World Health Organisation. Available from HMSO, London.

# 24. Checklists, Suppliers and Specialist Advice

Jim Ryan, Peter Mahoney and A. J. Thomas

## Checklists

Although pre-packed kits are available (see list of companies below), many will want to personalise their medicines and equipment depending on location, local logistics, risks and length of tour. It is assumed that the organisation deploying you will provide medicines for the population at risk. Therefore, the following recommendations are for personal use.

### Medicines

Pack all medicines with care, label them, and if possible keep them in the containers used for initial dispensing. Check time of expiry.

Detailed lists of commonly needed medicines, including their dosage schedules, can be found in many of the manuals and guides listed in the previous chapter, and also on specialist web sites listed later.

As a rule, your pack should include the items listed below.

> **NB:** non-medically qualified personnel should seek pharmaceutical and medical advice in choosing items for packing, storage and use.

Analgesic tablets or capsules
Antacids
Antibiotics – take expert advice on choice and routes of administration
Antidiarrhoeal tablets and electrolyte replacement salts
Antiemetics (for nausea and travel sickness)
Antifungal creams and powders
Antihistamine creams
Anti-inflammatory tablets and rub-in creams
Antimalarials appropriate to risk
Anti-mountain sickness if at risk
Antiseptic ointments, creams, liquid sachets or sprays
Antiworm medicines – take advice on choice
Bite and itch lotions, creams and repellents

Cold sore medicines – take advice
Drops for sinusitis
Eye drops and ointments
Insect repellents – DEET liquid, spray or gel
Laxatives
Sleeping medicines – take advice
Suntan lotions/creams and sunscreen creams
Vaginal infection medicines – take advice.
Water purification tablets or solutions

## First Aid and Life Support

If making up your own packs, consider the following items.

### First Aid Pack

Contents lists and documentation for customs and security checks
Cotton wool
Crepe bandages – various widths and lengths
Medi-swabs
Non-adherent wound surface dressings
Safety pins
Scissors
Sterile gloves
Steristrips for wound closure – various sizes
Tapes – micropore and zinc oxide
Triangular bandage
Tweezers (tissue forceps) – toothed and non-toothed
Wound cleansing antiseptic solutions, creams and powders
Wound dressing pads and gauze
Wound plasters and band-aids

### Life Support Pack

Airway maintenance devices – oro- and naso-pharyngeal – adult and child sizes
Cannulae for needle decompression – tension pneumothorax
Chest drains (trained personnel only)
Interosseous needles for children under 6 years
Intravenous (IV) administration sets
IV solutions – electrolyte or colloid
Large-bore vascular cannulae (Nos. 12, 14, 16 for adults, Nos. 18, 21, 23 for children)
Large wound pads for haemorrhage control
Needles and syringes – various sizes
Selection of basic limb splints (if space allows)

## Disease Prevention

### *AIDS Prevention*

If you are going to an HIV- or Hepatitis B-prevalent area, specialist packs containing sterile needles, IV administration sets and IV fluids can be purchased. Take advice before travel and discuss the contents with a medical kit supplier and a medical expert.

### *Dental Health*

You should also consider taking an emergency dental kit containing emergency dressings for lost fillings (oil of cloves for example), temporary filling material, analgesics and antibiotics. Some kits contain material for temporary replacement of crowns, bridges and caps.

## Medical and Related Equipment Suppliers

*Although many organisations deploying expatriate volunteers will supply medicines and equipment for the volunteer's personal use, many people will want to travel with a personalised emergency pack. The organisations listed below are useful points of contact for those wishing to purchase proprietary packs or build their own.*

British Airways Travel Clinics. Multiple outlets in the UK and South Africa. Tel. +01276 685040 to find the nearest.

ECHO International Health Services Ltd., 2 Ullswater Crescent, Coulsdon, Surrey CR3 2HR, UK. Tel. +020 8660 2220.

InterHealth, 157 Waterloo Rd, London SE1 8US, UK. Tel. +020 7902 900.

Medical Advisory Service for Travellers (MASTA). London School of Hygiene and Tropical Medicine, Keppel Street, London WC1E 7HT, UK. Tel. +020 7631 4408.

Mission Supplies Ltd., Dawson House, 128-130 Carshalton Rd, Sutton, Surrey SM1 4TE, UK. Tel. +020 8643 0205.

Nomad Travellers Stores. Numerous outlets. Tel. +020 7833 411.

Oasis, High Street, Stoke Ferry, King's Lynn, Norfolk, UK. Tel. +0403 257299.

Safety and First Aid (SAFA), 59 Hill Street, Liverpool L8 5SB, UK. Tel. +0151 708 0397.

SP Services, Unit D4, Horton Park Estate, Hortonwood 7, Telford, Shropshire TF1 4GX, UK. Tel. +01952 288999. Catalogue on request.

# Centres and Organisations Offering Specialist Advice

NB: *Many organisations regularly change their phone numbers or codes.*

Many of these organisations have web sites. These are listed in a later section.

## United Kingdom

British Airways Travel Clinics, 177 Tottenham Court Road, London W1P 0LX, UK. Tel. +020 7637 9899. Multiple outlets. Call 01276 685040 to locate the nearest.

British Foreign Office, Travel Advice Unit, Consular Division, Foreign and Commonwealth Office, 1 Palace Street, London SW1E 5HE, UK. Tel. +020 7238 4503/4504.

Department of Health, Public Enquires Office, Richmond House, 79 Whitehall, London SW1A 2NS, UK. Tel. +020 7210 4850, or PO Box 410, Wetherby LS23 7LN, UK.

Hospital for Tropical Diseases, Mortimer Market Centre, Capper Street, London WC1E 6AU, UK. Tel. +020 7388 9600. Health line 0839 337733 (calls 50 p per minute).

Medical Advisory Service for Travellers, London School of Hygiene and Tropical Medicine, Keppel Street, London WC1E 7HT, UK. Tel. +020 7631 4408.

## United States of America

Center for Disease Control, Travellers Health Section, 101 Marietta Street, Atlanta, GA 30323, USA. New toll-free number: 877-FYI-TRIP.

Travel Clinics Worldwide. The International Association for Medical Assistance to Travellers, 417 Center Street, Lewiston, NY 14092, USA. Tel. +716 754 4883.

## International

World Health Organisation, 1211 Geneva, Switzerland.

# 25. Using the Internet to Access the World Wide Web (www)

Jim Ryan and Peter Mahoney

## Introduction

The web is a growing resource for the humanitarian volunteer and is underutilised. Most aid organisations have web sites – the problem is how to find them and use them to answer questions.

Access to the internet and the web is more and more a routine for the younger generation of health professionals in their daily study and work. In the future, volunteers will expect this facility to be available on deployment, with laptop and hand-held computers linked to mobile phones. Access can also be obtained via internet cafes, which can now be found even in the most resource-constrained environment.

This section attempts to provide a framework for using the web. The sites available vary from those which attempt to list all the aid organisations and provide links to them, to sites provided by individual organisations. Other sites cover such aspects as security, personal preparation, health for travellers and terrorism. The list is almost endless.

### Guide to Humanitarian and Related Sites

The following structure is widely used.
- Directory and gateway sites (points of entry to the topic).
- International and intergovernmental organisations.
- Government/national organisations.
- Non-government organisations.
  - Specialist sites.
  - Preparation and travellers' health.
  - Security.
  - Country information and maps.
  - Training courses.
  - Providers and employers.
  - Essential medicines.
  - Medical and rescue equipment.
  - Vaccinations.

## Directory and Gateway Sites

### The dmoz open directory project

One of the most extensive web directories. It lists 474 humanitarian organisations, broken down and listed by activity. Headings include child welfare, disaster relief, hunger, medical relief and water supply. Organisations are also listed by region. Thumbnail sketches of the major players are provided, and the site also give links to the organisations listed.

http://dmoz.org/Society/Organizations/Humanitarian/

### European Forum on International Cooperation – Humanitarian Aid Gateway

This is an extensive website with links to key resources and organisations. It also issues press releases and bulletins on crisis areas.

http://www.euforic.org/framed/hum_en.html/

### Development Resource Centre

This New Zealand-based site has a link to a site listing development and aid organisations. It includes country agencies, regional agencies, non-governmental organisations (NGOs), development banks and international organisations, and provides links to the organisations listed.

http://www.drc.org.nz/links/devaidorg.html

### Ecumenical Links

This is a site maintained by the World Council of Churches as a service to the ecumenical and humanitarian community. The site is concerned with organisations involved in advocacy aid, relief and development. It provides the most extensive listing of humanitarian and related organisations world-wide. Headings include human rights, peace and conflict resolution, economy and development, humanitarian aid and disaster relief, refugees and migrants, and international/intergovernmental organisations. The site provides links to each other site listed.

http://www.wcc-coe.org/wcc/links/aidorgs.html/

### European Community Humanitarian Office (ECHO)

The EU is the largest humanitarian aid donor in the world, and the EU's humanitarian office coordinates humanitarian aid to populations in need throughout the world. ECHO's website gives useful information on a variety aid programmes and details of collaboration and inter-agency cooperation.

http://europa.eu.int/en/comm/echo/

## Bubl Link

A UK information service for the higher education community. It has humanitarian relief pages containing an A–Z list of articles and monographs on aspects of humanitarian care. It also provides links to many national and international humanitarian organisations.

http://bubl.ac.uk/link/H/humanitarianrelief.html

## Institute of Development Studies

This institute, based in Sussex, is concerned with research and teaching, and the dissemination of information on building and sustaining capacity in less well-developed countries. It has a link page listing agencies involved in multilateral co-operation in the field of development. It lists banks and national and international agencies and provides links to each.

http://ids.ac.uk/eldis/aid/rdb_lorg.html

## Reuters Foundation

Reuters provides a site called AlertNet. This provides global news and other services to the humanitarian relief agencies and personnel, and to the public. It also has a very useful on-line service listing international aid suppliers, and a database of training and job opportunities.

http://www.foundation.reuters.com/aid/main/alertnet.html/

## Community Aid Abroad

This organisation, part of the Oxfam International network, has a website listing its water and sanitation projects, but it also has very useful links to the sites of a variety of other organisations.

Http://www.caa.org.au/world/emergencies/

## Inter-Church Committee for Refugees

This is a coalition of Canadian Churches concerned with the care of refugees. Their site has links to numerous national and international refugee organisations who are the main players concerned with migrants and refugees.

http://www.web.net/~iccr/

### European Council on Refugees and Exiles (ECRE)

ECRE is a coalition of 67 agencies involved in refugee care. Its extensive web site gives an excellent overview of problems associated with refugees and displaced peoples. It also provides numerous links to related websites.

http://www.ecre.org/main.html/

### Voluntary Organisations in Cooperation in Emergency (VOICE)

VOICE is a network of European NGOs which are active across the whole field of humanitarian assistance. VOICE runs seminars and meetings aimed at fostering further cooperation. The site summaries the work of these meetings, provides regular updates from conflict and catastrophe areas, and gives links to other humanitarian resources on the web.

http://www.oneworld.org/voice/

## International and Intergovernmental Sites

### European Parliament

The European Parliament publishes a series of fact sheets on the web. Sheet 6.4.4 concerns humanitarian aid, and is of interest to prospective humanitarian volunteers. It also deals with the legal basis of humanitarian aid.

http://europarl.eu.int/DG4/factsheets/en/6_4_4.html/

### International Committee of the Red Cross

The Red Cross works exclusively with the victims of war and violence. This is a highly recommended web site.

http://www.icrc.org/

### International Federation of Red Cross and Red Crescent Societies

This is the world's largest humanitarian organisation. The web site is extensive and very useful. The federation comprises 176 Red Cross and Red Crescent Societies.

http://www.ifrc.org

### International Labour Organization

This organisation was founded in 1919 to promote social justice, and human and labour rights. The web site is very extensive. We suggest using site map to navigate.

http://www.ilo.org

### Organization for Security and Co-operation in Europe (OSCE)

OSCE is a European security organization with an international remit. Its purposes are early warning, conflict prevention, crisis management and rehabilitation after conflict.

http://www.osce.org

### United Nations Children's Fund (UNICEF)

UNICEF is concerned with all aspects of child health and development.

http://www,unicef.org

### United Nations Economic and Social Development Council

This UN department is concerned with the environment, human rights, human settlement and a raft of other issues surrounding humanitarian assistance. Begin with the site map.

http://www.un.org/esa

### United Nations High Commissioner for Human Rights

The office of this UN department (OHCHR) is concerned with the promotion and protection of human rights for all.

http://www.unhchr.ch

### United Nations High Commissioner for Refugees (UNHCR)

UNHCR was established to care for the world's refugees. An extensive and easy-to-use website outlines its aims and objectives and a great deal more. Highly recommended.

http://www.unhcr.ch/

### World Bank Group

The group's mission is to fight world poverty. It works closely with many NGOs, particularly in the field of development. A useful website with many pertinent links.

http://www.wbg.org

### World Health Organisation (WHO)

WHO's site is one of the most useful. We recommend you to begin by linking to the site map, which will provide directions to pages dealing with diseases, prevention programmes, weekly epidemiological updates and a great deal more.

http://www.who.int

## World Trade Organisation (WTO)

The only international organisation dealing with global rules of trade. It interfaces with NGOs in developing countries and in regions afflicted by war and disaster.

http://www.wto.org

## Worldwide Ministries

The worldwide ministries division of the Presbyterian Church with far-reaching programmes in the fields of human rights, hunger, refugees and development.

http://pcusa.org

## Governmental and National Organisations

Department of Health (UK) – http://www.doh.gov.uk

Department for International Development (UK) – http://www.dfid.gov.uk

Foreign and Commonwealth Office (UK) – http://www.fco.gov/

State Department (USA) – http://www.state.gov/

US Agency for International Development (USA) – http://www.info.usaid.gov/

## Non-Government Organisations (NGOs)

The editors recommend visits to the following NGO web sites, although the list is far from inclusive. Readers are invited to suggest useful additions.

Amnesty International – http://www.amnesty.org

Care International – http://www.careinternational.org

Catholic Agency for Overseas Development (Cafod) – http://www.cafod.org.uk

Doctors of the World – http://www.doctorsoftheworld.org

Doctors without Borders – http://www.dwb.org

International Islamic Relief Organisation – http://www.Arab.net/IIRO/

Leonard Cheshire – http://www.leonard-cheshire.org

Médicins Sans Frontièrs – http://msf.org

Mercy Corps International – http://www.mercycorps.org

MERLIN – http://merlin.org.uk/index.html/

Oxfam International – http://www.oxfam.org

Oxfam UK – http://www.oxfam.org.uk

Red R – http://www.redr.org/

Save the Children – http://www.savethechildren.org

## Specialist Sites

### Preparation and Travel Health

Try any or all of the following sites/

http://www.british-airways.com/travelqa/ – The British Airways travel clinics site. Gives addresses and points of contact in South Africa and the UK.

http://www.cdc.govt/travel/ – The US Government's Centre for Disease Control. Has a search engine and an A–Z of health topics.

http://www.fco.uk/travel/ – The British Government's Foreign and Commonwealth Office. Useful travel information other than medical. Covers security, legal and consular matters. Lists countries not to visit or work in!

http://www.doh.gov.uk/traveladvice/imsum.htm – The UK Department of Health's site for health advice for travellers.

http://www.tripprep.com – The web site of Travel Health Online. US based, but offers information world-wide. Detailed information on specific illnesses, vaccinations, lists of travel medicine providers and destination information.

http://www.indiana.edu/~health/travel.html – The Indiana University Heath Centre, with pages dealing with travel health and links to related sites.

http://pitt.edu/HOME/GHNet/travel.html – The Global Health Network provides a useful site for travel health advice from a variety of sources.

http://www.masta.org/about/index/html – A UK-based organisation set up within the London School of Hygiene and Tropical Medicine. Covers travellers' health, visa and passport information, and travel insurance

### Security

The following sites are worth browsing.

http://travel.state.govt/travel_warning.html

http://travel.state.gov/asafetripabroad.html

http://geocites.com/Athens/Atlantis/7253/Terrorism.html

http://www.state.gov/www/about_state/business/business_travel.html

http://www.redr.org/resources/links/security.htm

http://www.fieldsecurity.com

## Country Information and Maps

http://www.reliefweb.int/mapc/index.html/

## Training Courses

The following sites organise or recommend a variety of training courses.

http://www.redr.org/resources/links/training.htm

http://www.qeh.ox.ac.uk/rsp/

http://www.apothecaries.org/

## Relief Personnel – Providers and Employers

The Red R website below has web pages listing organisations which provide services and employ personnel in the humanitarian aid environment.

http://www.redr.org/resources/limks/hr.htm

## Essential Medicines

The web sites below give expert advice on medicines and related products for use in the field of humanitarian aid.

http://www.who.int/medicines/edl.html

http://www.masta.org

## Medical Equipment

Sites which give information on a wide variety of medical equipment products, from individual items to complex equipment systems.

http://www.999supplies.com

http://www.equipped.com/drperskit.html

http://www.echohealth.org.uk

http://www.dynamed.co.uk

http://www.plysu.com

## *Vaccinations*

The following web sites offer advice on vaccination needs during deployments.

http://www.cdc.govt/travel/

http://www.org/about/index.html

**EDITORS' NOTE** – Readers are invited to submit useful new addresses.

# SECTION 6

## And Finally

The editors and authors recommend the code of behaviour that follows and completes this handbook.

# Code of Behaviour

Humanitarian volunteers are not tourists. They arrive, often uninvited, in a country or region devastated by war or disaster. The atmosphere in a war or disaster setting is unique. Displaced people are vulnerable and dependent on volunteers who may have little knowledge of their religious beliefs, culture and way of life. They may never have encountered foreigners. There is enormous potential for misunderstanding, suspicion and, on occasion, downright hostility. Ideally, expatriate volunteers should be fully briefed on these aspects, but urgency and crisis may mean deployment at short notice without adequate political or cultural briefing. Volunteers must approach displaced people with great sensitivity if they are to avoid gaffes. As an example, a group of soldiers deployed in a humanitarian setting and working with refugees were seen to wear T-shirts with the logo: "Travel the world, see interesting places and people – kill them!". Although meant in jest, the potential for offence is obvious. The following items of advice have been gleaned from a variety of sources and individuals and may help to keep you out of trouble.

- Do your work in a spirit of humility and understanding – keep a low profile.
- Take time to listen and understand the cultural mores of the people you are helping.
- You are not a tourist. Be sensitive when using your camera – always ask permission.
- Avoid displays of wealth and ostentation – do not give gifts of money.
- Do not make promises that cannot be kept.
- Do not collect war souvenirs and keep away from unexploded ordnance (mines and bomblets).
- Avoid drugs and be temperate in your use of alcohol.
- Treat local staff with kindness and respect – listen when they offer advice.
- Avoid political debates and keep away from political meetings and gatherings.
- If provoked, be polite, patient and courteous.

# Conclusion

Medical care in hostile environments encompasses a huge canvas. It is impossible for one individual to have expertise across the varying environments outlined in this handbook. Rapid access to information is increasingly sexpected by informed volunteers. We hope this work will help.

# Index